Preface

This book tries to illustrate the practice as well as the principles involved in applying linguistics to the analysis of language disability. In writing it, I have assumed an audience of professional speech and hearing clinicians who have had little or no formal training in linguistics. Each Chapter therefore begins with a résumé of the main theoretical and descriptive principles needed in order to carry out a clinical linguistic analysis. The relevance of language acquisition studies is a major theme within this résumé. The remainder of each Chapter then applies this information to the study of language disability, as encountered in samples taken from individual patients. I have deliberately devoted a great deal of space to data extracts, and their accompanying analysis. As clinical linguistics is such a new area of study, it seemed best not to spend too much time debating the philosophy of the enquiry, but to get on and show what happens in practice. There is not enough experience yet accumulated for me to be able to say that this book is "what clinical linguistics do"—but it does reflect quite well what *this* clinical linguist does, and (perhaps more accurately) the questions he asks.

The balance of the book is due to my trying to meet current needs. Because semantics is a completely new area to most clinicians, I have devoted most space to expounding that topic and illustrating its applications (Chapter 5). Non-segmental phonology is also relatively unfamiliar ground to many, so that became the next largest chapter (Chapter 3). Grammar would have been as large as semantics (Chapter 4), if I and my colleagues had not published so much on that topic already (see references). And as segmental phonology has also been well treated in previous publications (Ingram 1976, and see Grunwell 1977 and forthcoming), I have kept that chapter fairly short (Chapter 2). Because the relationship between child language acquisition and language disability has been thoroughly addressed in a major work in recent years (Bloom & Lahey 1978), I have kept the acquisitional sections of each chapter fairly brief, and concentrated more than might otherwise be expected on the analysis of adult patients. The newest areas of potential clinical application, sociolinguistics and psycholinguistics (apart from language acquisition), are too unformed to warrant separate chapters; they are reviewed (more briefly than their potential importance warrants) in Chapter 6. Phonetics, on the other hand, as the oldest field of clinical application, I have assumed to be a sufficiently familiar frame of reference to readers of this book that it will not need separate exposition (though a reliance on phonetic concepts and techniques permeates Chapters 2 and 3). Despite these several constraints, the book has achieved its target length without difficulty, and this in itself has brought home to me the enormity of the field I have attempted to introduce and define. To facilitate understanding of the transcription used in the book, a selection of the data is available in tape-recorded form. Further information may be obtained from the author at the University of Reading, Whiteknights, Reading RG6 2AA, England.

Apart from a few examples taken from the clinical literature, the data in this book is based primarily on the analysis of patients from the clinics of the Berkshire Area Health Authority, in particular those attending the Reading University clinic. I have also used material provided for the various in-service courses on clinical linguistics which my colleagues and I have run in recent years. I am therefore most grateful to the many speech therapists who have allowed me access to their patients, and who made recordings on my behalf. Accumulating the right kind of examples was the most laborious part of the present project, and my task was greatly facilitated by their help. In addition, I am conscious of the way in which many of the clinical notions described in the book have come from the detailed discussion of patients carried on with my departmental colleagues over the past few years.

I am indebted to all of them, and especially to Paul Fletcher, Michael Garman and Renata Whurr, who read drafts of this book, and made many valuable suggestions. Lastly, my wife, Hilary, shared much of the labour of this book's preparation, and, in her role as speech therapist, helped shape many of its ideas. To have such double support is an enviable position for any author to be in; I am deeply conscious of my debt to her, and at the same time equally aware of my inability adequately to express it.

Reading, May 1980   **David Crystal**

Preface to the paperback edition

The growing interest in clinical linguistics, illustrated most notably by the appearance in 1987 of a journal devoted to the subject (see References), has prompted the publication of a paperback edition. The subject has not developed its theoretical premises sufficiently since 1981 to warrant a large-scale revision of the book's approach and organisation, but a great deal of relevant research continues to appear, and I have therefore included a set of additional references after the main bibliography. The tape-recording of the prosodic examples and of some of the extracts is still available: further information may be obtained by writing to P.O. Box 5, Holyhead, Gwynedd LL65 1RG, UK.

Holyhead, October 1986   DC

CLINICAL LINGUISTICS

DAVID CRYSTAL

HONORARY PROFESSORIAL FELLOW, UNIVERSITY COLLEGE OF
NORTH WALES, BANGOR

W

WHURR PUBLISHERS
LONDON JERSEY CITY

© 1981 by Springer-Verlag/Wien

First published in Great Britain 1987 by
Edward Arnold (Publishers) Ltd
41 Bedford Square, London WC1B 3DQ

Reprinted 1989 and 1991 by Whurr Publishers Ltd,
19b Compton Terrace, London N1 2UN

British Library Cataloguing in Publication Data
Crystal, David, *1941–*
   Clinical linguistics.
   1. Man. Language disorders. Linguistic aspects
   I. Title
   616.85′5

ISBN 1-870332-65-2

Printed and bound in Great Britain by Athenaeum Press Ltd, Newcastle
upon Tyne.

Contents

List of Transcriptional Conventions and Symbols Used

P	patient/pupil
T	therapist/teacher
/	tone-unit boundary
\	falling tone
/	rising tone
—	level tone
⌃	rising-falling tone
⌄	falling-rising tone
⌐	level-rising tone
⌐	falling-level tone
'	stressed syllable
"	extra stress
* *	overlapping speech
( )	unclear or untranscribable speech (no. of syllables indicated, if audible)
.	brief pause
-	unit length pause
--	double length pause
---	treble length pause
?	doubt about transcriptional accuracy
▬	drawled segment
.	clipped segment
↑	pitch step-up
[ ]	phonetic transcription, segmental or featural
/ /	phonemic transcription

Contextual information is indicated in brackets to the right of the text.
New sentences begin on a new line; sentence continuations being indented.
Phonemic symbols are given in Table 1, p. 24.
Other phonetic symbols are those of the International Phonetic Association.

The Scope of Clinical Linguistics 1

Clinical linguistics is the application of linguistic science to the study of communication disability, as encountered in clinical situations. Unfortunately, almost every term in this definition requires further discussion, in order to identify the orientation and scope of the subject.

Linguistics—and Phonetics?

The title of the book contains an implication which might be questioned: is clinical linguistics a single, coherent subject of study? Might not separate mention be made of the science of phonetics, and the book retitled accordingly? In my view, there is no need for such a division. Linguistics does not need to specify phonetics separately, any more than it does phonology, grammar, semantics, or any of the other branches of the subject. This view is shared by many academic centres, and all introductions to linguistics will have sections on phonetics. On the other hand, apart from university departments named "linguistics", there have also been departments of "phonetics", and also of "phonetics and linguistics", so plainly the matter is not so simple.

The difficulty resides in the way phonetics has developed academically. Under one tradition, it refers to the general study of the articulation, acoustics and perception of speech. Under another tradition, it refers to the study of the phonetic properties of specific languages. Under the first interpretation, phonetics relates clearly to biology, physics and psychology, from which it derives a great deal of its motivation, and much of its methodology: in this sense, its methods of study (of articulation, acoustic transmission, and audition) are valid for all human sounds, regardless of the language or speaker. Because of this concern with general, explanatory processes, the subject is in fact often referred to as "general phonetics", the phonetician's aim being to discover universal principles governing the nature and use of speech sounds, seen as *sounds*. This interpretation, then, contrasts with the second view of phonetics, which closely relates to the study of phonology (see Chapter 2), and which is plainly a branch of linguistics in its motivation and method—an "indispensable foundation", as some would say[1]. Of course, most phoneticians seem to operate happily in both frames of reference, and the topic is no longer as controversial within linguistics as it once was.

When it comes to the analysis of clinical data, however, there are strong reasons why a systematic distinction between linguistic and phonetic frames of reference needs to be drawn. One reason is that there is a major tradition within speech pathology which reflects (apparently) this distinction, namely the classification of disorders into those of *speech* and those of *language*[2]. The speech/language division is not a happy one, as there are too many aspects of language disability which it either ignores or misrepresents (see p. 196), but it does have certain strengths, and it is precisely these which can be illuminated by the use of the distinction between phonetics and linguistics, viewed as qualitatively distinct disciplines of investigation. There is also a second line of reasoning, relevant to this question. For a variety of historical reasons, phonetics has been a routine part of a speech pathologist's training for decades; linguistics, by contrast, is of recent origin. Skills in ear-training and phonetic transcription, and associated descriptive and analytical abilities, can thus be taken for granted in a way that linguistic knowledge cannot—and this affects in a direct way the types of assessment and remediation it proves possible to do, or (at a research level) the kinds of theoretical questions it proves possible to ask. There is a clear contrast at present between most speech pathologists' skills in phonetic analysis and transcription and their corresponding skills in phonological, grammatical, semantic, sociolinguistic or psycholinguistic analysis; and as a consequence, we are much more likely to encounter applications of phonetic techniques in clinical practice than applications of linguistic techniques. Disorders of a purely phonetic disposition are however far outnumbered by those where systematic organisational problems are involved, as definable in phonological, grammatical, etc. terms; and the awareness by clinicians that there is here a domain requiring a wide range of qualitatively different techniques is now widespread. It would therefore seem sensible, in the present book, to take account of the two levels of awareness which have resulted from the way clinical training has developed, and to concentrate on the areas of current progress, rather than reviewing familiar ground. While phonetic techniques and principles will be an essential part of my descriptive framework at several places, therefore, they will be seen as a means to the end of elucidating linguistic structure, and not as an end in themselves[3].

---

[1] The term is from Henry Sweet (cf. Henderson, 1971). For other discussions of the nature of phonetics and its relation to linguistics, see Robins (1971: 76 ff.).

[2] "Apparently" is needed, for the definition of these terms in relation to the data of disability is not without controversy: for a personal view, see p. 196.

[3] A knowledge of basic phonetic descriptive terminology and transcription is assumed in the present book. The above emphasis is not however intended to underestimate the considerable amount of theoretical and empirical innovation in contemporary phonetics. In fact, a book on "clinical phonetics" is very much needed, and might well be as large as this one. Amongst other things, it would include coverage of recent advances in instrumentation (*e.g.* in electropalatography, electromyography); the

Science

What are the implications of the term "science" encountered in the definition on p. 1? Four aims of the scientific approach to language, often cited in introductory works on the subject, are comprehensiveness, objectivity, systematicness and precision[4]. The contrast is usually drawn with the essentially non-scientific approach of traditional language studies—by which is meant the whole history of ideas about language from Plato and Aristotle down to the nineteenth century study of language history (comparative philology). A clinician who encounters this tradition (as represented, for example, by the teaching grammars and manuals commonly used in schools in the early part of the present century) will not find it difficult to see its limitations, if he attempts to introduce it into his clinical practice; and the need for an alternative will quickly suggest itself. The lack of the above attributes is perhaps the most noticeable feature. Traditional grammars and pronunciation manuals, for instance, were in no way comprehensive. The former tended to concentrate on the written language, and moreover on only the "best" styles of writing, often being highly critical of the grammatical features of colloquial speech. Within a grammar, many basic processes of construction were ignored (such as sentence connectivity, the range of word order variations, and most transformational relationships—see Chapter 4). Under the heading of pronunciation, most of the features we would these days refer to as "non-segmental" or "prosodic" would receive no mention (see Chapter 3). Nor were the language features that *were* included dealt with in a particularly objective manner, at least by modern standards. There was a strong tendency to give impressionistic statements about usage, and an overriding concern with notions of correctness. There was an anxiety to preserve the imagined standards of excellence of the linguistic past, and to safeguard the linguistic future by eliminating the imagined slovenliness of the linguistic present. Most clinicians will have encountered this attitude, usually referred to as a *prescriptive* approach to language, and illustrated by such recommendations about usage as to say *I shall* rather than *I will*, or to never split infinitives[5]. The unsystematicness of method and the imprecision of terminology, which also characterized so much of the traditional approach to language, are further serious limitations of its usefulness—but it will be best to illustrate these in relation to particular problems of linguistic analysis below.

Enough should have been said, however, to indicate the irrelevance of this tradition to the clinician. In the vast majority of cases, his concern is precisely with those aspects of linguistic behaviour with which the traditional approach was unable or unwilling to deal. He is not concerned with a static conception of written

---

theory and practice of transcription (especially as applied to deviant speech); the study of phonation types; the study of articulation, and especially coarticulation, through the use of dynamic descriptive techniques; and the development of more sophisticated models of speech perception and production. For recent introductions, see O'Connor (1973), Fry (1977), Ladefoged (1975) and Catford (1977). See also Laver (1970), Lass (1976), Dalton and Hardcastle (1978: Ch. 2), Hardcastle and Roach (1981).

[4] See Robins (1971: Ch. 1), Crystal (1971: Ch. 3), Lyons (1968: Ch. 1).

[5] For a critical review, see Gleason (1965: Part I). This pedagogical trend should be distinguished from the philosophical tradition, well reviewed in Robins (1967), and propounded in support of a particular thesis by Chomsky (1966).

language, but with the dynamic characteristics of connected speech, whether his own or his patient's. He is not concerned with impressionistic or subjective recommendations about conformity with real or imaginary standards of social correctness, but with the systematic, objective and precise description of all aspects of a patient's disability, in relation to the linguistic abilities of his peers. When the clinician's interest is in identifying levels of complexity in language structure or use, or in the nature of language interaction between people, or in language acquisition, there will be little for him to gain from that tradition. In short, the need for some kind of alternative is as pressing in clinical studies as it was in foreign language teaching, mother-tongue education, and other fields which reacted so strongly against this tradition in the middle years of this century.

Linguistics claims to provide an alternative, based upon and constrained by the premises and methods of scientific investigation. But in the early years, this alternative took on a distinctly negative flavour. In its effort to change complacent and purist attitudes to language, fierce criticisms were made of the earlier paradigm of enquiry[6]. In the various fields of applied language studies, such as the teaching of grammar in primary schools, or in foreign language teaching, the weaknesses of the traditional view of language were widely publicised. The criticisms were generally valid, and were often appreciated as such, but what was unfortunate is that they all too often failed to be accompanied by suggestions for constructive alternatives. The situation was early remedied in foreign language teaching, but in the case of the other field referred to, mother-tongue teachers did and still do complain that linguists have as yet produced little to put in the place of the older models.

The situation is somewhat more hopeful in clinical language studies, partly because the clinician's aims are rather more specific and restricted than the mother-tongue teacher's, and thus more achievable in the present state of knowledge. But the contact between linguistics and traditional clinical language studies is still in its infancy, and there are still many areas where criticisms have been made and constructive alternatives are lacking. In such circumstances, collaboration tends to be less in evidence than confrontation. The fact that criticisms of traditional ways of thinking may be correct and desirable, however, is no guarantee that their cogency will be appreciated or accepted. On the contrary, unless it is done tactfully and constructively, the result will be antagonism. For example, it requires little phonetic insight to be able to criticise the traditional terminology for the auditory classification of voice disorders ("harsh", "hoarse", "rough" etc.), and it is not difficult to take some of the classificatory labels in dyspraxia or aphasia, and show inconsistency or ambiguity in their use. What is important is whether a constructive alternative can be provided; the criticisms themselves are not enough. Often, in fact, speech pathologists themselves have been unhappy with the concepts at issue, so that the rephrasing of these criticisms in the terminology of linguistics needs to be done in a particularly positive manner, if the point is to be appreciated. It is the main aim of this book, accordingly, to provide a set of constructive and realistic alternatives, at least with reference to the main areas of linguistic enquiry.

---

[6] For example, Hall (1960), Fries (1952). For a general discussion, see Quirk (1968).

Clinical Situations

It proves difficult to provide a precise account of what should be subsumed under this heading, used in the definition on p. 1. Minimally, it must include all situations and conditions encountered in medical settings. Depending on the definition of "medical", this will include most or all psychiatric investigation. It would also include an appreciable amount of what goes on in remedial education, especially insofar as clear notions of mental or neurological deficit are involved. But the boundary between a "clinical" and an "educational" linguistics is not clear-cut—and, with the increased emphasis these days on the idea of a continuum of learning difficulties between normal and abnormal[7], the boundary is becoming even less clear. The problems are partly terminological, partly conceptual. Given the context of "clinical", and the focus on "language", are we then proposing to deal with linguistic "disorders", "disability", disfunction", "disturbance", "disadvantage", "deficit", "deprivation"...? Each of these terms (and there are several others) has its associations with particular fields, which covers a range of experience stretching from medicine to sociology. Most of the data on which the present book is based has come from situations which are clinical in a strictly medical sense. On the other hand, most of the principles involved are readily applicable to non-medical, remedial settings, and I have included some examples from these backgrounds. To avoid terminological vacillation, I propose to subsume all kinds and degrees of linguistic difficulty under the heading of *disability*, this being in my view one of the more neutral labels available, and one which is capable of interpretation in medical, psychological, social and educational contexts.

A similar arbitrariness surrounds the use of the term *pathology*, to characterise the data encountered in clinical situations, and the chief investigating subject ("speech pathology", "language pathology", etc.). For several years now, this term has been used in the context of linguistic disability in an extended sense from that current in medicine. The medical definition is "a branch of biological science which deals with the nature of disease, through study of its causes, its process, and its effects, together with the associated alterations of structure and function" (Blakistons). This tradition, with its focus on disease, and the underlying organic abnormality, is a valuable one for speech clinicians, as so many of the conditions they treat are the result of disease. And even for those disabilities which lack any obvious organic basis, the application of the term is not without precedent. The Oxford English Dictionary notes the extension of the term to the study of abnormal mental and moral conditions since the 1840s. The Third Webster International Dictionary, likewise, includes the extended sense, where pathology refers to "any deviation from an assumed normal state" (whether there is tissue deterioration or not). The term is therefore a useful one for present purposes, for it lays stress on the relevance of the medical condition which underlies so many linguistically disabled patients, while not insisting on an immediately evident diagnosis in organic terms (and not denying, either, the possibility of organic explanations at neurochemical or other levels). No claim is made in the present book concerning the aetiology of the data considered to be pathological, and confusion should not therefore arise.

---

[7] As illustrated in the Warnock Report (H.M.S.O. 1978), for example.

Application

This notion is fundamental to the orientation and subject-matter of this book, which might, indeed, be viewed as an exercise in applied linguistics[8]. The contrast involved here, in the first instance, is with general linguistics, seen as a "pure" science. From the general linguist's point of view, clinical linguistic data is, first and foremost, *linguistic* data. It would be perfectly possible for him to take samples of linguistic disability, accordingly, and use them for his own purposes—as a corpus of data which can demonstrate the adequacy or otherwise of his analytic techniques and linguistic theories. In teaching students the techniques of, say, transformational grammar, he might attempt to use aphasic or schizophrenic data, instead of material from a range of esoteric languages. This is not often done, for there are difficulties in using clinical data in this way (establishing what the patient's target utterance is, for example); but at a more theoretical level, it has often been said that clinical data are of considerable potential value to the linguist.

This view is perhaps most clearly elaborated in Whitaker's early writing[9]. He gives three reasons for the linguist's interest in pathological data. Firstly, there is a direct contribution to a putative neuroscience:

"Someday man's understanding of the brain and its behavioral mechanisms will progress far beyond the contemporary awareness of a few biochemical properties of neurons, a rough approximation of electrical events and partially specified functions for some of the neuro-anatomic structures. And when that day arrives, the biochemist, physiologist, anatomist, neurologist and all others concerned with brain function will suddenly be in need of a specification of behavioral units that can be correlated with their information" (1969: 135).

Secondly, there is an associated gain, in that such studies will help to provide an explanation for the qualitative differences between human and animal communication (1969: 8). The third and main justification is to provide empirical evidence for linguistic hypotheses (1969: 69). Whitaker argues that we must avoid creating models of language that bear no relation to neurological reality: "the closer we get to the brain, the more likely we are to be discussing the realities of the structure of language" (1969: 135), and again, "there are a priori grounds for bringing neurological information to bear upon linguistic theory ... Ultimately we have to. Certain structures and functions of the nervous system are the substrate of both our 'knowledge' and our 'use' of language" (1969: 7). Once we adopt such paradigms of enquiry (the "aphasia paradigm", as it is sometimes called), a possible evaluation procedure for linguistic theories suggest itself. The point is made by several authors, including Chomsky[10]:

"it is going to be necessary to discover conditions on theory construction, coming presumably from experimental psychology or from neurology, which will *resolve the alternatives* that can be arrived at by the kind of speculative theory construction linguists can do on the basis of the data available to them" (1967: 100, my ital.).

---

[8] The analogies between this and other areas of applied linguistics are discussed in Crystal (1981).
[9] See Whitaker (1969), (1971).
[10] See also Weigl and Bierwisch (1970: 12), Geschwind (1964: 157), and Katz (1964).

Given this large and respected body of opinion concerning the significance of pathological data in relation to linguistics, it is important for me to emphasize at the outset that the present book is *not* an exercise within this paradigm of enquiry. Clinical linguistic analysis, as presented here, is conceived as a much more limited exercise within the domain of linguistic investigation, as conventionally understood. The aim is to take the theories, methods and findings of linguistics, and to use them as a means of elucidating the nature of pathological conditions, insofar as these are manifested in (spoken or written) language. There is no concern in this book to use pathological data as part of the process of illuminating various linguistic theories. The questions raised by Whitaker *et al* are important, as long-term goals; but in my view there is no way in which these questions can be answered in the forseeable future. It is therefore important not to allow these speculations to distract us from matters which *can* be solved or illuminated in the present state of knowledge, by developing applications of linguistics which are already available.

This book, then, is not about the application of clinical language data to linguistic ends: it is about the application of linguistics to clinical ends. But there is an important consequence of this change of direction: the decision to apply these ideas in the first place, the way in which the ideas come to be applied, and the final evaluation of their efficiency all lie in the hands of the clinician. There is one main reason for this, namely that linguistics is only one of a whole range of disciplines which contribute to the understanding and management of linguistic disability. It may be felt to be the central contributing discipline, as Jakobson (1955) argued with reference to aphasia, but as Lesser points out, "Although aphasia may be a linguistic problem, the aphasic patient is a medical problem" (1978: 20). I shall discuss the role of linguistics in relation to therapeutics and management in a later section (see Chapter 6). In the meantime, it is perhaps proper to stress, in view of the occasional ambiguity about the issue, that I take it as axiomatic that it is the clinician who determines all matters in relation to the patient's well-being. It is his responsibility to evaluate linguistic insights, to decide whether to use them with individual patients in specific settings, to integrate them with other techniques of intervention and management, and generally to decide the question of relevance. It is therefore also axiomatic for the clinical linguist to introduce early on in his studies, whether in research or with individual patients, an enquiry into the nature of the clinician's needs. This is not to deny the linguist the opportunity of using his clinical findings as part of his own attempt to develop alternative explanations of linguistic disability to those encountered routinely in clinical settings. There are, after all, many other avenues of enquiry, stemming from the interrelationships between linguistics, psychology and neurology in particular, and the possibility of new research paradigms in these areas is a real one, as Whitaker's discussion indicates. But for the present, the most urgent and practicable task is to develop an initial connection between the two investigating traditions—the linguistic and the clinical—and here the linguist will require information as to the clinician's priorities.

What, then, are the clinician's priorities? The problem here is that the answer to this question varies with the times. There will never be a single answer to the question of relevance: as perspectives on clinical problems change, so different aspects of the contributing disciplines will become more, or less relevant. The situation is now fairly complicated, due to the progress which has been made in patterns of clinical training. In the United Kingdom, for example, the introduction of a syllabus on linguistics into speech therapy training means that there are now two generations of speech therapists, one of which has had little or no formal training in the subject. The question of what kind of and how much linguistics to teach, and at what level, thus has two very different answers, depending on which generation is in mind. However, given the recency with which these developments have taken place, it is perhaps more sensible to assume relatively little knowledge of the subject, and to define the question of priorities for those clinicians who have had little or no formal training in linguistics, and a phonetics training which (for want of a better word) might be called "traditional".

Clinical Priorities

To analyse this notion, we need only begin with any of the characterizations of professional skills presented in the standard textbooks. For example, there is Nation and Aram:

"As a diagnostician, the speech pathologist is a professional who (i) possesses a fund of knowledge relevant to speech and language disorders, (ii) is skilled in applying this knowledge to solving clinical problems, and (3) has an overriding concern in helping a person, his client, understand and manage his speech or language problems" (1977: 3).

Or we might take the American Speech, Language and Hearing Association's requirements for the certificate of clinical competence: "an in-depth knowledge of normal communicative processes, development and disorders thereof, evaluation procedures to assess the bases of such disorders, and clinical techniques that have been shown to improve or eradicate them". From many such specifications, we can readily conclude that the clinical role of linguistics will be evaluated in terms of its contribution to any or all of the following categories: diagnosis, assessment, screening, therapeutic techniques and patient management. But underlying all of these notions are certain more "primitive" requirements which linguistics must meet, if it is to be judged as clinically relevant.

Firstly, it will be judged by the extent to which it provides the clinician with *insight* into the nature of a disability or its management. "Insight" here must of course mean that the observations which the linguist makes must not have been available through the use of traditional paradigms of enquiry, as encountered in initial training, because of their limited range. But obtaining insight is not easy. To count as an insight, an observation must be perspicuous—for example, it must not be obscured by an alien and impenetrable terminology. It must also be productive—that is, provide a basis for future work with the patient. Observations which demonstrate the *systematic* nature of the data of disability, where previously no pattern could be seen, usually count as insights, in this connection, for they contribute directly to assessment and diagnosis. Likewise, observations which make *predictions* concerning a patient's progress are held to be illuminating, for they contribute directly to remedial strategies (*e.g.* by helping to answer the question "What to teach next?"). In both cases, the perspicuity of the analyses is a central concern, and one which linguistics, on account of its necessary technicality, often has considerable difficulty coming to terms with.

Secondly, the clinical relevance of linguistics can be judged by the extent to which it introduces an element of clinical *confidence* into a diagnostic or therapeutic situation. Confidence derives partly from the availability of insights, of course, but it goes much further than this, as it essentially refers to the ability of the clinician to be consciously in control over his patient, and over the clinical situation in which they both participate. It is a point which applies to any technique of intervention, in any field, but in speech pathology the point has often given rise to concern, especially to students in training. The aim of speech pathology, as a professional venture, is not solely to obtain progress in a patient, but to ensure that the progress obtained is due to the clinician's intervention, using the training which qualified him as a clinician in the first place. It is a commonplace observation that many patients can improve given plenty of sympathy from relatives and a rich language environment. Is the clinician thereby redundant? To provide the required counter-evidence, we must be able to show the way in which the improvement has been facilitated by therapeutic intervention. Sometimes it is indeed possible to say with confidence that the therapy "caused" the progress, especially when a rapid change in linguistic ability is produced after a long period of stability or deterioration, when the patient has been lacking therapy. It is even sometimes possible to arrange for comparative studies between groups of patients, though here the ethical problems are well known. But on the whole, verification of the efficacy of most therapeutic strategies is lacking, in scientifically convincing terms. If linguistic techniques are to be valuable, then, they should be able to introduce a greater measure of control over the nature of the patient-therapist interaction, and thus contribute to the development of professional confidence. The detailed description of the patient's linguistic behaviour, before and after the use of a therapeutic strategy, is one, fairly obvious contribution. The correlation of variations in linguistic response with variations in the therapist's linguistic stimuli would provide another example. It would be premature to say how far these techniques can help in achieving these goals. For one thing, the field is in its infancy; for another, linguistic variables are not the only ones involved. But it should still be possible, even in the present state of knowledge, to show *a relative* gain in control and confidence, compared with current practice. This, at least, is my own experience. It is accordingly just such an increased awareness of the linguistic variables involved in the tasks of assessment and remediation that clinical linguistics aims to provide, and by which it should be judged.

The Problem of Time

Insight and confidence are not, however, notions over which we have absolute control. The amount of insight or confidence a clinician has will vary enormously, in relation to such factors as the nature of his initial training and subsequent experience, the complexity of the disability with which he is dealing, the clinical resources available, the setting in which the remediation takes place, his rapport with patient and relatives, and the unpredictability of events affecting both him and the patients (ranging from illness to strikes). It is therefore never possible to guarantee success in the use of a procedure, or even to generalize about its clinical relevance. But there are certain factors which need to be taken into account if *any* degree of success is to be achieved in applying linguistic ideas. Chief amongst these is the question of personal commitment, partly in terms of intellectual energy, but mainly in terms of the much more mundane matter of *time*. It takes time to build confidence, and gain insight; and the linguistic analyses in attaining these ends are always and inevitably time-consuming to use. The reason is simple: clinical linguistic analyses are complex and time-consuming because linguistic disability is a complex and extensive phenomenon. It is only natural for clinicians with heavy case-loads to demand analytic procedures which are as short and as simple as possible—but the operative words are *as possible*. There are limits beyond which it would be unwise to go, and where a procedure would cease to be illuminating and become unreliable. And all linguistically-based procedures which have so far been devised have, in the absence of empirical research which might indicate the nature of these limits, erred on the side of caution. The various components of a linguistic approach to disability (see p. 14) therefore currently demand an outlay of time on the part of the clinician which is far above that which would normally be provided on the basis of traditional practice. While it is possible to do certain types of analyses on certain types of patient in an hour or so, anything at all complex will regularly require a commitment of a half-day or a whole day. How can we justify such an expenditure of time? There are two answers. One is that often there is no alternative: especially in the more complex cases, the limitations of the traditional approach have left the clinician in a position where it is unclear what might be done, and where the only chance to develop a principled therapy is after an appropriately detailed analysis has been made. Secondly, the question of time has to be seen in the long-term, and weighed against the criteria of success: in most cases, quantifiable and explicable progress; but in the absence of progress, the confidence that comes from knowing that no-one else could have done better. A day devoted to linguistic analysis early on in a case may seem trivial by comparision with the overall amount of time devoted to the patient in subsequent months.

The implications of these remarks have yet to be thought through by the remedial professions and the bodies which administrate and pay them. On the one hand, there are several clear statements among the various government reports and professional syllabuses that linguistic analysis is an essential feature of training and professional practice; on the other hand, no-one has attempted to take the time factor into account in carrying out job-analyses of clinical practice, with reference to the numbers of patients requiring therapy. The recommendations of the Quirk Report (H.M.S.O. 1972), for example, suggested a doubling of the number of therapists in Britain to cope with available demand; but if all speech therapists were by some magic to begin doing full linguistic analyses of their patients tomorrow, the effect would be an immediate halving (at least) of their case-load. The choice at both individual and administrative levels is clear: if the quality of service to individual patients is to improve, then *either* this has to be at the expense of the quantity of service throughout the community (with some patients not being seen at all, or being seen less often) *or* more therapists are employed to make good the deficiency. It is fortunately not my job to have to make such decisions; but it *is* the responsibility of linguists to point out the implications to those who wish to use their ideas in clinical situations. And as far as the present book is concerned, it needs to be stated plainly that, if the procedures it outlines prove at all appealing, then the problem of time will be the first barrier that has to be overcome.

An important outlay of time is required by the clinician in a further respect—a once-and-for-all outlay as he first comes to grips with the apparatus of linguistics, whether this be through the medium of a textbook or a tame linguist. To succeed, the enterprise has to be a genuinely collaborative one. Linguist and clinician need to learn as much as possible about each other's metalanguage and strategies of study, and spend time together in the discussion of individual cases. There is effort demanded of both sides. The linguist needs to take time and trouble to familiarise himself with the criteria and pressures of the clinical situation, and one day a book may be written about the best way of doing this *(Speech pathology for linguists?)*. The present book however is attempting to deal with the reverse situation, of the clinician who wishes to find out what the linguistic approach is, and what its clinical strengths and limitations are. It will become apparent, in subsequent pages, that a great deal of "thinking time" is involved—not solely in learning the technicalities of the subject, but also in re-thinking certain aspects of the traditional approach to language (*cf.* above). The motivation to do this is threefold: most obviously, there may be a formal motivation, in the sense that these subjects are now part of examination syllabuses which define the modern criteria of professional competence in the field; and there may also be a personal motivation, in the sense that the clinician may have perceived for himself the confusion which surrounds certain aspects of the traditional paradigms of enquiry, and wish to sort it out; but ultimately the best motivation comes from having seen the benefits of using this approach with patients, and wish to do likewise. That is why I spend so much space on case studies, in the course of the book.

Communication and Language

This remaining term from the definition on p. 1 also requires careful handling. Linguistics is the science of language, and not of communication, for which such terms as *semiotics* have been proposed. Communication is a much broader notion than language, as is the associated notion of "communication disability". Communication refers to the transmission of information (a "message") between a source and a receiver using a signalling system; restricting this notion to "human communication", it may be interpreted in terms of the use of any of the modes which humans have available for information transmission—auditory/vocal, visual, tactile, olfactory and gustatory[11]. Of these, the last four (especially the second and third) are of-

---

[11] For an account of this method of enquiry, and of semiotics as the study of "patterned human communication in all its modes", see Sebeok, Hayes and Bateson (1964), Crystal (1969: Ch. 3), Lyons (1977: Ch. 2).

ten grouped under the heading of "non-verbal" communication, especially in psychological studies. The notion of "language proper" is defined with reference to the first mode, namely as a system of spoken communication, or its encodings in written or signed form. The field of linguistics is thus circumscribed with reference to the notions of spoken and written language, in the first instance. Other forms of visual or tactile communication would be included only insofar as it could be shown that they displayed a range of structural and pragmatic properties comparable to those demonstrated by these primary notions[12].

What particular properties might be said to characterize linguistic, as opposed to non-linguistic communication—to distinguish between spoken and written language, on the one hand, and such behaviour as facial expression and bodily gesture on the other? Out of a wide range of criteria which have been proposed[13], two have been viewed as crucial. The first is to point to the major difference in *productivity* between spoken language and gestural, etc. communication. Productivity refers to the creative capacity of language users to produce and understand an indefinitely large number of words and sentences. Words in spoken language are continually being invented and dying out; and fresh combinations of words are continually being produced and understood. By contrast, gestural communication lacks productivity, in this sense: there are a very limited range of gestures that can be made using the body, and a similarly limited range of meanings that can thus be communicated. The second criterion of difference is one of structural organization. Spoken language displays *duality of structure,* which is lacking in non-linguistic modes of communication. Duality of structure refers to the way language is organized in terms of two abstract levels. At one level, language can be seen as a sequence of units which lack meaning, *e.g.* the segments *p, t, k, i.* But when these meaningless units are put together into certain sequences, meaning is attributable to the larger units formed, *e.g. pit, pat.* It is this capacity to produce meaningful units out of meaningless entities which identifies a behaviour as being a language. By contrast, normal gestural communication lacks duality of structure. The minimal units of "body language" (such as a wink) are meaningful in themselves, and this meaning is preserved, usually with little change, in the few cases where gesture sequences are used.

What does this imply for the clinician? It does not of course mean that he need not be bothered with the non-linguistic aspects of communication. On the contrary, as his role is to understand the whole of his patient's communicative ability, these other factors will need to be systematically considered in evaluating such matters as comprehension, or in motivating patients in the earliest period of meaningful expression. But working with the "non-verbal" aspects of behaviour is no substitute for working with language. If a patient is restricted to his natural "body language", there is very little meaning that he can unambiguously communicate. To develop his potential for communication, the clinician has to come to grips with

---

[12] The main field to which this extension has been made is that of deaf signing, where recent studies are gradually bringing to light the structural and pragmatic complexity of the behaviour. See Schlesinger and Namir (1978).

[13] See especially Charles Hockett's "design features" of language: Hockett (1958), Hockett and Altmann (1968); for further discussion, Lyons (1977: Ch. 3), Crystal (1975: Ch. 3).

language sooner or later; and when he does, the qualitative distinctions discussed above will require the patient to cope with a fresh learning situation. Because of the major differences between language and other forms of communication, there is very little that can be carried over from one learning situation to the other. The sounds, structures and meanings of spoken language (and the corresponding forms of writing and signing) present the patient, and of course the clinician, with a much more complex, multi-faceted and long-term problem, and it is this which is the focus of the present book. A book on "clinical semiotics" would be a fascinating, but altogether different enterprise, and one to which psychologists and anthropologists would make major contributions[14].

This emphasis on language as auditory-vocal communication needs to be qualified in two important respects. Firstly, it does not follow, from what has been said, that *all* aspects of auditory-vocal communication should be included under the heading of language. We must exclude the range of physiological reflexes which may have vocal expression, such as coughs and sneezes, and also the notion of *voice quality*—the permanently present "background" feature of our speech, which enables people to recognize us and derive certain conclusions about us, *e.g.* how old we are, what sex we are. Voice quality is the auditory consequence of the anatomical and physiological differences between individuals, and it is against such a background that we learn to speak and to identify the spoken language of others. In a strict sense, therefore, voice quality is not part of language; rather, it is a permanent accompaniment to spoken language[15]. Once we have "tuned in" to voice quality, we discount it; because it does not affect the meaning of what we say, it does not have to be listened to. Instead, we concentrate on listening to the sounds, words and structures which are in the "foreground" of speech. Confusion of background and foreground features thus constitutes an important clinical problem, within the field of voice disorders (see further, Chapter 3).

The second qualification to the notion of language as auditory-vocal communication concerns the way in which other forms of idiosyncrasy manifested in spoken form must also be discounted. Idiosyncrasy is not just a matter of voice quality: every sound we produce, at a certain level of phonetic detail, is idiosyncratic to the speaker—but as these characteristics are usually not audible, and demonstrable only on an acoustic record of the speech, they do not affect the nature of the communicative activity. Similarly, hesitations, pauses, self-corrections and other "mistakes" in our production of spoken language, while they may cause minor irritation on occasion, do not usually interfere in any radical way with the communication of meaning. Only when such features exceed certain norms would we wish to investigate them, and then by definition we would be involved in clinical work. In normal

---

[14] See for example the papers by Ostwald and Mahl and Schulze in Sebeok, Hayes and Bateson (1964); also Shapiro (1979). It follows from the account above that the contribution of linguistics to genuine communication disorders (*i.e.* disturbances in which other modes of communication are also involved) may be quite limited. For example, given the range of characteristics associated with autism, only some will be capable of elucidation using linguistic techniques (see further, p. 204).

[15] There is an analogy, to a certain extent, in handwriting, which may be idiosyncratic—but as formal handwriting styles are often taught, the analogy is by no means exact. For further discussion of voice quality, see Crystal (1969: Ch. 3), Laver (1968), (1980), and Giles and Powesland (1975).

circumstances, however, the study of these features adds little to our understanding of the structure of language[16], and a definition of language would generally exclude them. Linguistics, accordingly, is not concerned, in the first instance, with the personal characteristics of the language-user, but only with those aspects of his auditory-vocal expression which are shared by other members of his community. In order for linguistic communication to take place, there must be a single set of rules, or conventions, which the parties to the communication need to follow; and it is the study of these which constitutes the primary subject-matter of linguistics.

Aims

The clinical and communicational perspectives outlined above indicate several important long-term goals for clinical linguistics. But in order to achieve these goals, several intermediate aims must be recognized. As a first step, it is useful to identify seven specific aims for the subject, which constitute the linguist's interpretation of the clinical demands made upon him. These aims, easy to state, more difficult to achieve, are as follows:

(i) the clarification of areas of confusion arising out of the traditional metalanguage and classification of speech pathology;

(ii) the description of the linguistic behaviour of patients, and of the clinicians and others who interact with them;

(iii) the analysis of these descriptions, with a view to demonstrating the systematic nature of the disabilities involved;

(iv) the classification of patient behaviours, as part of the process of differential diagnosis;

(v) the assessment of these behaviours, by demonstrating their place on scales of increasing approximation to linguistic norms;

(vi) the formulation of hypotheses for the remediation of these behaviours, insofar as the therapy and management of patients requires reference to linguistic variables, and evaluating the outcome of these hypotheses, as treatment proceeds;

(vii) the evaluation of the remedial strategies used in intervention, insofar as linguistic variables are involved.

Ultimately, only success in relation to aims (vi) and (vii) will justify the introduction of linguistic techniques into clinical work. Unless we can demonstrate remedial progress, and moreover ascribe this progress to the use of these techniques, the linguist's claims for his subject will necessarily remain unconvincing. But what must not be forgotten, in this respect, is the dependence of success in the remedial aim on success in the other aims listed. Systematic remediation is obviously dependent upon the foundation laid by insightful assessment; this in turn is dependent on an accurate classification and analysis of patient behaviour, which in

---

[16] Experimental studies of the psychological and neurological processes underlying these "performance" errors can make a contribution to our understanding of what happens in speech production (see, *e.g.* Laver 1970), but this kind of information is in principle different from the characterization of language as an abstract system for the communication of meaning; see further below, p. 18.

turn presupposes a satisfactory initial description of that behaviour. And every-thing is dependent on the clinician's awareness of the existence of a problem that necessitates a description in linguistic terms in the first place.

However, as might be expected, the apparently straightforward way in which these interdependencies can be stated obscures several theoretical and methodol-ogical problems. In particular, the first three aims—clarification of the problem, de-scription and analysis—raise several difficulties, and as a consequence it is not sur-prising to find that most of the efforts of linguists have been devoted to making progress in these areas. In fact, it is only recently that linguistically-inspired contri-butions to diagnosis, assessment and remediation have been forthcoming.The point has sometimes been made by way of criticism, that clinical linguists have not devoted sufficient attention to the daily problems of clinical practice; but the an-swer is plain—that without an adequate descriptive and analytical foundation, remedial procedures are scientifically worthless, being dependent for their success on the fortuitous combination of an individual therapist's charisma and the avail-ability of resource excellence. Without this foundation, there is no way of persuad-ing the lay sceptic of the relevance of professional expertise in remedial language work.

What, then, are the difficulties which must be overcome in order to achieve the basic aims of description and analysis of a patient's language? Insofar as technical issues are raised by this question, the answer will be postponed until later chapters; but there are certain general considerations which apply to all the special areas covered later in this book, and these may be summarized here. Chief among these is the need to achieve a synthesis of several different kinds of information, which to a considerable extent cross-cut the inventory of aims given above. What provides the optimum setting to elicit a sample of language from the patient that is representative of his behaviour? What subject-matter should be introduced into the discussion? How should the sample be recorded? How should it be transcribed? At what level of detail should the descriptive observations be made? Within what kind of theoreti-cal framework? In what kind of experimental or naturalistic setting? The task of description is a deceptively complex one, as it presupposes a whole range of other, interlocking decisions, some practical (such as the availability of recording equip-ment), some theoretical (such as the purposes for which the description is to be made).

This last point is especially important. It is not as if there is an optimal kind or level of description which will automatically satisfy the needs of all clinicians. For example, the question of how much detail to introduce into a phonetic transcrip-tion (*i.e.* how "narrow" should the transcription be?) cannot be answered without knowing something of the analytic and remedial demands which will be placed upon it. For some purposes, a very narrow transcription will be desirable (as in the initial study of articulation disability—see Chapter 2); for others, a broader tran-scription will suffice (in identifying patterns of stuttering, for example). In other cases still, a phonetic transcription will be either unnecessary (as in doing grammati-cal analysis, where for most purposes the data can be represented in traditional orthography) or need to be supplemented by alternative descriptions of the speech data (such as provided by acoustic or articulatory instrumentation, as used, for instance, in the study of dysarthria). One measure of the success of a transcription is the extent to which it supplants the tape from which it derives: if we have made a transcription at the right level for our purposes, it should be unnecessary to have to refer back to the tape in carrying out our analyses later. Another criterion is the extent to which every symbol introduced into the transcription turns out to have a role to play in the later analysis. Getting the level right at the outset is, however, often very difficult in clinical work, a great deal depending on whether a reasonably accurate preliminary diagnosis can be made.

The same problem arises in deciding on the depth of detail at which to make a grammatical description of patients' language. The difficulty is not so marked when describing a sample from an individual patient, as once an orthographic transcription has been made of the tape, it is a relatively easy matter to look again through the pages of transcription to check on the use of a grammatical category or structure previously thought not to be significant. The problem becomes acute when we are comparing samples, either of the same patient at different times, or of different patients. With aphasic patients, for example, because we do not have, in the present state of knowledge, a clear conception of how many *linguistic* categories of aphasia there are, it is often difficult to decide how detailed to make our description. Is it necessary to describe the only occasionally disturbed syntax of some "fluent" aphasics at the same level of detail as that required for their grossly agrammatic counterparts? If the distinction between "fluent" and "non-fluent" were linguistically clearcut and uncontroversial, there would be no problem; but it is not, and as a consequence we continually run the risk of omitting to describe the frequency and distribution of a grammatical feature in a patient, the seriousness of the omission emerging only when we later attempt a comparison with another patient for whom precisely that feature is an important index of progress. To go back over the earlier data and re-code it for the omitted aspect may be possible in theory, but it is usually impracticable (especially if we have processed the data computationally) and it is always dispiriting. Most of the time, the omission stays an omission, and the subsequent analytic account, to that extent, remains incomplete or misleading.

In the absence of clear guidance from clinical literature or experience as to the level of description required, it pays to be cautious, and to include as much as there is time to process. Analytic procedures (such as those used in assessment) also need to be comprehensive, at least in outline. In devising such procedures, it is always wise to follow the dictum that "anything that *can* go wrong, *will*, sooner or later", whatever area of language we are investigating. It is simply not realistic to exclude on principle a particular linguistic feature, or set of features, on the grounds that it is clinically unimportant. It might be rare, and thus not worth giving it prominence in our procedure; but it is not by that criterion unimportant. When it finally is observed as a characteristic of a patient's linguistic difficulty, it may turn out to be very important—for him. And our analytic procedure must be able to cope with it, if a fair description of the patient is to be obtained[17].

---

[17] See further Crystal 1979 a: 11 ff.; also Crystal, Fletcher and Garman 1976: 14 ff., where the limitations of selective commentary are discussed. The value of the clinical case presentation remains, but it needs to be carried out within an explicit theoretical framework, so that the inevitable comparisons can be made.

It is for this reason that the clinician needs to be aware of more than just the descriptive facts of the language in which he happens to be working. These descriptive facts—of the normal adult language, and of the stages of development in its acquisition by children—are absolutely essential, but they are not the whole story, because patients do not stay within these norms, and thus the clinician needs to be in a position to anticipate the nature of departures from the norms, and to evaluate them. The relevant perspective, in other words, derives partly from what we know about the *universal* characteristics of human language. Faced with a highly deviant patient, it is desirable to establish whether what he is doing is at all constrained by factors which are conceivably those that could be used in one of the world's languages (though not necessarily English), or whether he.is operating in a manner which is outside or marginal to this frame of reference (but characteristic, say, of animal communication). Often, in the present state of knowledge, it is not possible to be sure; but it is in principle always useful to aim for a comparative perspective in clinical studies, not only because particular clinical issues might be clarified[18], but also because it gives a sense of the idiosyncratic logic which a patient might be using in his attempts to impose order and interpretation on the linguistic world around him. The view of linguistics which we must bring to bear on clinical situations, in other words, is not a language-specific one (*e.g.* "English linguistics") but a general one, in order to achieve the aims listed at the beginning of this section.

General Principles

Looking back over the history of linguistics in the present century, it is possible to identify two main emphases, both of which are of considerable clinical relevance. On the one hand, there is a concern to develop reliable procedures for the collection, transcription, description and analysis of quantities of linguistic data *(corpora)* from a wide range of languages. On the other hand, there is a concern to develop plausible models and theories capable of accounting for these data, and (at a higher level of abstraction) criteria which will enable the linguist to evaluate the efficiency of his analyses. These three levels of achievement have been summarized by Chomsky in terms of levels of *adequacy.* A grammar (in the sense of a theory of the whole of language—see p. 97) is said to be "observationally adequate" if it can account for the whole of a particular sample of data; it is said to be "descriptively adequate" if it goes beyond the limitations of particular samples, and accounts for the intuitions that native speakers have about their language; and it is said to be "explanatorily adequate" if in addition to this, a principled basis is established for deciding on the relative merits of alternative grammars[19]. The same levels of achievement might be postulated in handling clinical data—though the stage that clinical analysis has reached to date, due to its preoccupation with individual case

---

[18] For example, comparing French and English aphasics could help to indicate which of their difficulties are purely linguistic and which due to deeper cognitive deficits that cut across linguistic boundaries. For more on universals, see Lyons (1968: Ch. 8), Huddleston (1976: Ch. 13).

[19] See Chomsky (1964), and for an introductory account Huddleston (1976: Ch. 1).

studies, is nowhere near the level of sophistication that can be achieved, hardly any studies even approaching observational adequacy.

Several basic theoretical distinctions need to be drawn, in order to develop adequate frameworks for clinical linguistic analysis.

1. Language System/Language Act

We have already seen (p. 13) how linguistic analysis focuses on the systematic aspects of language, and plays down the idiosyncratic. A somewhat more generalized conception of this difference is basic to all linguistic enquiry, emerging most clearly in de Saussure's distinction between *langue* and *parole,* and Chomsky's distinction between *competence* and *performance*[20]. Competence refers to a person's knowledge of his language, the system of rules which he has mastered so that he is able to produce and understand an indefinite number of sentences, and to recognize grammatical mistakes and ambiguities. It is an idealized conception of language, which is seen as being in opposition to the notion of performance, the specific utterances found in an act of speaking, which will contain features irrelevant to the abstract rule system arising out of the various psychological and social pressures acting upon the speaker (*e.g.* memory lapses). According to Chomsky, linguistics before generative grammar had been preoccupied with the study of performance as represented in corpora, instead of with the underlying competence involved. The aim of generative grammar, as a consequence, was to focus directly on this competence, and thus to replace observationally adequate statements with descriptively adequate ones.

As a general conception, this distinction has been widely used; but increasing criticism has come from linguists who feel that the boundary between the two notions is not as clear-cut as their definitions would lead us to believe. There are problems, often, in deciding whether a particular speech feature is a matter of competence or performance, and these problems loom large in clinical language studies, where direct access to the intuitions of the patient is often difficult or impossible. But the aim to think predictively about the clinical performance of patients is certainly important: the aim is not simply to describe exhaustively the properties of a sample of the patient's output, but to use this sample to extract regularities which are predictive of the patient's future behaviour. The analysis of a language sample enables us to make hypotheses about the patient's limitations, which subsequent interaction confirms or disconfirms. Clinicians invariably have intuitions about the system which is present in their patients' behaviour, and can make observations about the representativeness and consistency of data samples. The clinical linguist too must make an assumption about the system in a patient: unless he assumes that system is present, he is in no position to proceed. Having made the assumption, his job is then to explicate it.

---

[20] See de Saussure (1916: Ch. 3), Chomsky (1965: Ch. 1). There are certain differences between langue and competence which do not affect the present discussion. For a critique of Chomsky's conception of competence, see Matthews (1979). For a useful discussion of the notion of idealization, see Lyons (1972). Several specific criticisms have been directed at the particular model of competence originally proposed by Chomsky, especially the conception of a syntactic deep structure; as this notion is no longer felt to be central by most generative linguists, it will not be further discussed here.

2. Synchronic vs. Diachronic

This distinction refers to the two main temporal dimensions of linguistic investigation introduced by de Saussure (1916). In synchronic linguistics, languages are studied at a theoretical point in time: we describe a "state" of the language, disregarding whatever changes might be taking place (*e.g.* the language of the 18th century, or of "the present day"). In diachronic linguistics, languages are studied from the point of view of their historical development. For example, the changes which have taken place between Old and Modern English can be classified and described in terms of grammar, vocabulary, pronunciation, etc. The importance of carrying out adequate synchronic description before proceeding with a diachronic enquiry has been repeatedly stressed: if we are comparing the changes between two states of a language, we need to know first of all what the two states are. This point bears directly on procedures in clinical linguistics, where diachronic information is critical at two points (though we are now talking about language change in the individual, and not in society as a whole). Firstly, information about the normal development and decay of language in a person provides an essential perspective for remedial work. As pointed out elsewhere [21], it provides the only practicable means of bridging the gap between techniques of assessment and those of remediation, and provides a realistic alternative to oversimplified models of developmental "complexity". This is why an acquisitional framework is considered so important in later Chapters. Secondly, rate and quality of language change is the essence of clinical concern; but to study change as an end in itself, without seeing it within a proper synchronic perspective, can be distorting. It is only natural for a clinician to notice progress, especially if this has been a recent focus of remedial activity. What is less noticeable is the accompanying areas of lack of progress, or, at times, those areas which are being hindered *on account of* the progress being made elsewhere (*cf.* p. 114). Only a synchronic analysis can provide the frame of reference within which such weaknesses can be isolated.

3. Language Structure vs. Language Use

The interdependence of these notions is regularly stressed in linguistic analysis, and in this respect the view contrasts with that common in mother-tongue teaching, where structure and use are seen as in opposition to each other[22]. Under the heading of language structure is included the formal organization of spoken or written language, and the meanings conveyed by this organization. Three main branches *(components,* or *levels)* of linguistic organization are recognized by most theories:
(i) *grammar,* comprising the sub-fields of syntax and morphology (see Chapter 4);
(ii) *semantics,* the study of the meanings conveyed by the syntactic and morphological features (see Chapter 5);
(iii) *phonology,* the study of the way sounds are organized by a language to enable the transmission of grammatical (and thus semantic) structure to proceed (see Chapters 2 and 3)[23].

---

[21] See Crystal, Fletcher, and Garman (1976: 25 ff.), Crystal (1979a: 3), Rees (1971).

[22] See the discussion in Crystal (1976: Ch. 3).

[23] The equivalent notion for the study of the written language is *graphology.*

In addition, the physical properties of sound, and the articulatory and auditory factors involved in its production and perception by human beings, constitutes the field of *phonetics*.

The importance traditionally given to these three levels of structural organization is sufficient justification for the attention paid to them in this book, where they constitute its main organizing principle. It will undoubtedly be on the basis of these distinctions that a more satisfactory, behavioural account of linguistic disability will emerge as an alternative to that traditionally provided by the medical model of enquiry[24]. But without a systematic study of the way these structural features are *used* in communication, such an account would be sterile. "Language in use" is a heading under which is subsumed a wide range of factors to do with the social and psychological determinants of linguistic behaviour—what the native speaker needs to know, and how he needs to develop, in order to communicate effectively in socially distinct settings. Included would be such environmental matters as the relationship between speaker and hearer, and the pressures which stem from the time and place of speaking[25]. There are now two major fields within linguistics which study language in use.

(i) *Sociolinguistics,* which studies all aspects of the relationship between language and society, such as the linguistic identity of social groups, social attitudes to language, standard and non-standard forms of language, the patterns and needs of national language use, social varieties and levels of language, the social basis of multilingualism, and so on[26].

(ii) *Psycholinguistics,* which studies the correlation between linguistic behaviour in the individual, and the psychological processes thought to underlie that behaviour. From the linguistic (as opposed to the psychological) point of view, the subject is basically seen as the study of the mental processes underlying the planning, production, perception and comprehension of speech, with its most well-developed branch being the study of language acquisition in children[27].

The clinical relevance of psycholinguistics is obvious, given the close relationship between psychological and linguistic disability in a very large proportion of the patients encountered in speech clinics. The role of sociolinguistics is perhaps less immediately obvious, in the context of the clinic, but there are several points of contact in the handling of individual patients (*e.g.* in relation to immigrants, dialect-users) and it is only through a sociolinguistic perspective that a proper approach to clinical interaction will develop. Both psycholinguistics and sociolinguistics need to be involved, if we hope to explain what the patient does when undergoing remedia-

---

[24] For an account of the medical vs. the behavioural approaches, see Crystal (1980: Ch. 2). For the notion of structural level, and the structuralist view of language as a system of interdependent categories, see Lyons (1968: Ch. 2), Lepschy (1970), Robins (1971: Ch. 1), Halliday, McIntosh and Strevens (1964).

[25] The notion of "communicative competence" summarises one approach to the study of such variables—the term being a reaction against the restriction of linguistic theory to the analysis of structure in purely formal terms (as in the Chomskian notion of competence above). See Lyons (1977: Ch. 14), Gumperz and Hymes (1972).

[26] See Trudgill (1974), Gumperz and Hymes (1972).

[27] For an introductory account, see Clark and Clark (1977), Glucksberg and Danks (1975); see also Flores D'Arcais and Levelt (1970).

tion: we need to study the nature of the interaction between clinician and patient in its own terms, as well as what the clinician and the patient each bring to the interaction in terms of their individual backgrounds and expectations. The study of linguistic structure needs to be integrated within a social and a psychological frame of reference in order to provide the foundation for the long-term goal—a theory and praxis of linguistic management. This theme is resumed in Chapter 6.

4. Syntagmatic vs. Paradigmatic

Far more attention has been paid to the way linguistic structure should be modelled than to language in use, and consequently later chapters will deal predominantly with the application of structural insights and criteria. Perhaps the most useful of these is the view of linguistic structure in terms of two intersecting dimensions. The syntagmatic dimension deals with the sequential characteristics of speech (or writing), seen as a string of units, usually in linear order. The relationships between the constituents in a string are referred to as "syntagmatic relations". The paradigmatic dimension refers to the set of relationships which a linguistic unit has with other units in a specific context—the "paradigmatic relations" of the unit. The two types of relations, taken together, constitute a statement of a linguistic unit's identity within the language system. For example, the function of /p/ in English phonology can be summarized by identifying its syntagmatic relationships (*e.g.* its ability to occur initially, medially and finally in a word: *pit, apt, rip*) and the paradigmatic relationships it contracts with other elements (*e.g. pit, bit, sit*). The intersection is most obviously represented thus:

$$p \leftrightarrow i \leftrightarrow \quad \text{(syntagmatic)}$$
$$\updownarrow$$
$$s$$
$$\text{(paradigmatic)} \quad \updownarrow$$
$$h$$
$$\vdots$$

The same principle applies to the study of all levels of linguistic structure, and the procedures involved in establishing these relationships (especially the principle of *substitution* illustrated above) are also universally used[28].

Linguistic Profiles

Keeping in mind both the long- and the short-term aims for our subject, and working within a framework derived from general linguistic considerations, we may now proceed to investigate the different levels of the organization of language in greater detail. At all points, our aim will be to develop a theoretical and descriptive frame of

---

[28] See Lyons (1968: 70 ff.), Robins (1971: 44 ff.). For further illustration, see pp. 146 ff. below. Cf. also Jakobson (1964), who used this basic idea to construct a typology of categories of aphasic impairment.

reference based upon recent research into these levels. As child language acquisition provides an essential perspective for investigating linguistic disability, we shall then proceed to a review of the main trends and findings in that field, for each of the levels. Lastly, we shall attempt to synthesize the descriptive, theoretical and acquisitional findings into a procedure for the analysis of patients' language. Throughout, we shall be concerned to make a selection from the available information that is clinically relevant, in the sense that the linguistic observations made would be agreed as contributing to the tasks of assessment, diagnosis or remediation. As research into clinical linguistics is in its infancy, it will often be possible only to construct outline sketches of areas of disability—linguistic *profiles*.

A profile, as its name suggests, is no more than a first approximation to an accurate description; but it does at least imply that the salient, identifying features of a problem area have been isolated. To be useful, a profile of linguistic behaviour needs to be discriminating—to indicate the main differences between normal and abnormal, and to identify different categories of abnormality. The most useful profiles are those which are based on an acquisitional dimension, because they can then be used simultaneously for assessment and remediation: by showing where a patient *is* on a profile chart, we can see immediately where he ought to be, and perhaps see paths which would enable us to get him there. Wherever possible, then, we shall think of clinical linguistics as an exercise in profile-building. There is also a corollary: at no point will we think in terms of *scores*. The number of clinically relevant variables, as we proceed through our examination of the different linguistic levels, will be seen to be extremely large, and at present it seems impracticable, and certainly unilluminating, to try to collapse all of these variables into a single "value", as would be represented by a score. While quantitative indices of disability have their merits, the present book is very firmly an exercise in qualitative description, with the occasional statistical excursus very much a means to an end[29].

---

[29] To facilitate exposition in the following pages, two abbreviations will often be used: T refers to therapist or remedial teacher; P refers to patient or pupil.

2 Segmental Phonology

Theoretical Background

Phonology is the study of the sound systems of languages. Out of the very wide range of sounds that the human vocal apparatus can produce, and which are studied by phonetics, only a relatively small number are used distinctively in any one language. The sounds are organized into a system of contrasts, which signal differences of meaning within the language. The aim of phonology is to establish on what basis this contrastivity operates, to describe the patterns of distinctive sound used in a language, and to make as general statements as possible about the nature of sound systems in the languages of the world. Putting this another way, phonology is concerned with the range and function of sounds in specific languages (and is often therefore referred to as "functional phonetics"); it is also concerned with the rules which can be written to show the types of phonetic relationships that relate and contrast words and other linguistic units[1].

Within phonology, two branches of study are usually recognized. *Segmental* phonology studies the way speech can be analyzed into discrete units, or segments, that constitute the basis of the sound system; and this, along with the analysis of the various phonetic features and processes which relate and differentiate these segments, is the subject-matter of this chapter. *Non-segmental*, or *supra-segmental* phonology studies those features which extend over more than one segment, such as intonation and rhythm; and these are the subject-matter of Chapter 3. This, at least, is the traditional mode of division within the subject. Some phonological theories cut across this division in various ways, and have important implications for clinical analysis. But for the most part, clinical applications of phonology fall neatly into one or other of these divisions, and we shall therefore continue with the distinction here.

---

[1] For introductions to phonology, see O'Connor (1973), Robins (1971: Ch. 4), Fudge (1973), Hyman (1975). "Functional phonetics" is discussed in Martinet (1949) and Haas (1968).

If sound systems are the immediate object of study, the basic question would therefore seem to be: what are the fundamental units that are in systematic use? Very early on in the history of linguistics, it was recognized that the obvious answer to this question ("sounds") was insufficient and misleading. There were too many distinguishable sounds used by the speakers of a language for a single system to be clearly demonstrated. Different speakers used different sounds, because of the different configurations of their vocal tracts; and even within the same speaker there could be considerable differences between his articulations from one time to another. It proved essential to conceive of the notion of "sound system" at a more abstract level than the physical conception of a set of acoustically distinct units would suggest. The notion had to allow, at least, for the principle that sets of physically identifiable sounds were *variants* of single, underlying units; and it was on this principle that the phonemic theory of phonology came to be established[2].

According to traditional phonological theory, then, a phoneme is the minimal unit in the sound system of a language. Its main purpose is to allow linguists to group together sets of phonetically similar sounds, or *phones*, as variants of the same underlying unit. The phones were said to be "members of" or "realizations of" the phonemes, and the variants were referred to as *allophones* of the phonemes. Each language could be shown to operate with a relatively small number of phonemes—some languages having as few as 15 phonemes, others as many as 50. The variety of British English usually described in textbooks on English pronunciation ("received pronunciation") has, according to one influential analysis, 44 phonemes[3]. These are listed in Table 1, along with a list of the phonemic symbols used for transcriptional purposes later in this book.

Table 1. *The vowel and consonant phonemes of British English (R.P.)*

ɪ	hid	ɜː	bird	t	*t*oo	ʒ	measure
e	head	eɪ	paid	d	*d*o	h	*h*ot
æ	had	aɪ	hide	k	*c*ap	m	*m*um
ɒ	hod	ɔɪ	coin	g	*g*ap	n	*n*o
ʊ	hood	əʊ	load	f	*f*an	ŋ	si*ng*
ʌ	bud	ɑʊ	loud	v	*v*an	l	*l*ay
ə	sof*a*	ɪə	beard	θ	*th*in	r	*r*ay
iː	bead	ɛə	bared	ð	*th*is	w	*w*in
uː	food	ʊə	poor	s	*s*oon	j	*y*et
ɑː	bard	p	*p*at	z	*z*oo		
ɔː	board	b	*b*at	ʃ	*sh*oe		

A fundamental issue in early phonology was on what basis sounds could be considered to be members of the same phoneme. The main criteria were that the sounds should be phonetically similar, and not occur in the same environment in a word—or if they do, that the substitution of one sound for the other should not cause a change in meaning (*i.e.* the sounds are in "free variation"). The principle of not occurring in the same environment was referred to as "complementary distribu-

---

[2] For the main conceptions of the phoneme, see Trubetskoy (1939), Jones (1950), Bloomfield (1933).

[3] See Gimson (1980). For the notion of "received pronunciation", or R.P., see that book (p. 89 ff.), and also Trudgill (1974).

tion". So, for example, in the R. P. pronunciation of *dad* in normal speech, the sounds at the beginning and at the end of this word could be said to be members of the same phoneme. They are different sounds (the initial sound being fully voiced, and the final sound having a much reduced degree of voicing), but they still have a great deal in common, and can thus be said to be phonetically similar. Each sound is restricted to the environment in which it occurs (in normal speech): the fully voiced sound is not normally heard at the end of the word, when the word is spoken in isolation, and the devoiced sound is not normally heard at the beginning of the word; so the sounds are in complementary distribution. Moreover, if a context arose where a speaker *did* replace one of these sounds by the other, there would be no confusion of meaning: the word *dad* would still be heard as such (albeit with an "odd" pronunciation), and not confused with *cad, dab, dat* or other such sequences. These principles, and especially the principle of distribution, are crucial guidelines in the analysis of phonological disability, as we shall see.

There are however several ways in which we can take the apparently simple notion "members of the same phoneme". To take an analogy, we can talk of a group of people as being members of the same family on grounds of their physical similarities (facial features, genetic code) or of their functional similarities (where they live, their mutual status). Early on in the history of phonology, different views of the phoneme developed: one view saw the phoneme as a "family" of related sounds; the other main view saw it as a "bundle" of abstract oppositions between sounds; and there were various intermediate positions. It is the second approach mentioned that has exercised most subsequent influence[4], and which holds most promise for clinical application. The sounds which cause differences in meaning are viewed as being made up of sets of *features*. A feature is an element of a sound which can be used in a language to help make contrasts in meaning: in English, for example, voicing, nasality, bilabial place of articulation, and so on are all features which are used to help distinguish consonant contrasts. The phoneme /p/, for instance, can be seen as the result of the combination of such features as bilabiality, voicelessness, and plosiveness, in particular. Other phonemes will differ from /p/ in respect of at least one of these features.

Depending on your theoretical viewpoint, the set of *distinctive features* a language uses may be seen as a supplementary specification of the phonemes of the language, or as a complete replacement of the notion of phoneme. In so-called "distinctive feature" theories of phonology[5], the phoneme is in fact eliminated as a relevant unit of explanation, and symbols such as *p, b,* etc. are seen simply as convenient abbreviations for particular sets of features. It is the features which are the minimal units of phonological analysis, not the phonemes. The main reason for this is the argument that by substituting features for phonemes in this way, generalizations can be made about the relationships between sounds in a language, which would otherwise be missed. Moreover, because features are phonetic in character, it should be

---

[4] The original statement was made by members of the Prague School of linguistics, especially by Trubetskoy (1939). Later developments included the approach of Jakobson and Halle (1956), which was a formative influence on generative phonology.

[5] See Hyman (1975), Schane (1973), and for the main theoretical statement, Chomsky and Halle (1968).

possible to make inter-language comparisons (both of a historical and dialectal kind), and ultimately statements about phonological universals, more readily than by using a phonemic model of phonology.

Distinctive feature analysts claim that there are several advantages over the traditional phonetic alphabet approach to phonological description, which analyses utterances as a sequence of segments. For example, it was originally suggested that a relatively small set of abstract feature oppositions (a dozen or so) would account for all the phonological contrasts made in languages: it would not then be necessary to recognize so much phonetic classificatory detail, as exists on, say, the I.P.A. chart, where the phonological status of the segments recognized is not indicated. (In fact, it has turned out that rather more features are required, as new languages come to be analyzed.) Another advantage, it is suggested, is that consonants and vowels can be characterized using the *same* set of phonetic features—unlike traditional descriptions, where the classificatory terminology for vowels (high, low, etc.) is quite different from that used for consonants (labial, palatal, etc.). By using a system of this kind, some quite specific predictions can be made about the sound systems of languages. For example, using the Jakobson and Halle system (1956) enables us to distinguish phonologically two degrees of front/back contrast in the consonant system and three degrees of vowel height. But what follows from this is a universal claim, that no languages permit more than these numbers of contrasts in their phonological systems. These are empirical claims, of course, and in recent years much effort has been spent on investigating these claims and modifying the nature of the feature inventory required.

Two major statements concerning the distinctive feature approach have been made: Jakobson and Halle (1956) and Chomsky and Halle (1968). The former approach set up features in pairs, defined primarily in acoustic terms (as could be detected on a spectrogram), but with some reference to articulatory criteria. Examples of their features are listed in Table 2. The emphasis in this approach is firmly on the nature of the oppositions between the underlying features involved, rather than on the description of the range of phonetic realizations each feature represents. In the Chomsky and Halle approach, more attention is paid to the phonetic realizations of the underlying features recognized, and a different system of feature classification is set up. Some of the earlier features are retained (*e.g.* voice, consonantal, tense, continuant, nasal, strident), but many are modified, and new features added, some of which overlap with the earlier approach (see also Table 2). The application of these features to languages is not without controversy, and in recent years further suggestions have been forthcoming as to the need for additional features (such as labiality). But several attempts have been made to use distinctive feature frameworks (or "matrices", because of the tabular presentation of the data, as in Table 2) in contexts of assessment and remediation.

A quite different approach to phonological analysis from either the phonemic or the distinctive feature theories discussed above is *prosodic phonology*[6]. This approach also to some extent cuts across the distinction between segmental and

---

[6] See Firth (1948), Palmer (1970), Robins (1971: Ch. 4), Waterson (1971).

Table 2. *Distinctive features and their use in English*

Jakobson and Halle (1956)

vocalic (vs. non-vocalic)	free passage of air through vocal tract; most radical constriction in oral cavity not exceeding [i] and [u]; vocal cords positioned to allow spontaneous voicing; sharply defined formant structure
consonantal (vs. non-consonantal)	major obstruction in middle of vocal tract; low acoustic energy
compact (vs. diffuse) (Chomsky and Halle low vs. high)	stricture relatively far forward in the mouth; relatively high concentration of acoustic energy in a narrow, central part of the sound spectrum
grave (vs. acute)	peripheral articulation in vocal tract; concentration of acoustic energy in the lower frequencies
nasal (vs. oral)	released through the nasal cavity
discontinous (vs. continuant)	complete closure of the vocal tract
strident (vs. mellow) (Chomsky and Halle non-strident)	relatively complex stricture; relatively high frequency and intensity
flat (vs. plain)	relatively narrow mouth opening with accompanying velarization; weakening of the high frequency components of the sound spectrum
sharp (vs. plain)	tongue raised towards hard palate; relatively wide area behind the stricture; greater intensity of some of the higher frequencies of the sound spectrum
voiced (vs. voiceless)	vocal cords in a position which will enable them to vibrate in an air-flow

Chomsky and Halle (1968): new contrasts

delayed release (vs. instantaneous release)	gradual release sufficient to produce a sound with acoustic turbulence of a fricative
anterior (vs. non-anterior)	stricture in front of the palato-alveolar area
coronal (vs. non-coronal)	blade of the tongue raised from its neutral position
distributed (vs. non-distributed)	stricture which extends for a considerable distance along the direction of air-flow
syllabic (−vocalic) (vs. non-syllabic)	segment containing a syllabic nucleus
sonorant (vs. obstruent/ non-sonorant)	relatively free air-flow; weak cord position such that spontaneous voicing is possible

Distinctive feature matrix for English consonants (after Chomsky and Halle)

	p	b	f	v	m	t	d	θ	ð	n	s	z	ʧ	ʤ	ʃ	ʒ	k	g	ŋ	h	r	l
vocalic	−	−	−	−	−	−	−	−	−	−	−	−	−	−	−	−	−	−	−	−	−	−
consonantal	+	+	+	+	+	+	+	+	+	+	+	+	+	+	+	+	+	+	+	−	+	+
high	−	−	−	−	−	−	−	−	−	−	−	−	+	+	+	+	+	+	+	−	−	−
back	−	−	−	−	−	−	−	−	−	−	−	−	−	−	−	−	+	+	+	−	−	−
low	−	−	−	−	−	−	−	−	−	−	−	−	−	−	−	−	−	−	−	+	−	−
anterior	+	+	+	+	+	+	+	+	+	+	+	+	−	−	−	−	−	−	−	−	−	+
coronal	−	−	−	−	−	+	+	+	+	+	+	+	+	+	+	+	−	−	−	−	+	+
round																	−	−				
voice	−	+	−	+	+	−	+	−	+	+	−	+	−	+	−	+	−	+	+	−	+	+
continuant	−	−	+	+	−	−	−	+	+	−	+	+	−	−	+	+	−	−	−	+	+	+
nasal	−	−	−	−	+	−	−	−	−	+	−	−	−	−	−	−	−	−	+	−	−	−
strident	−	−	+	+	−	−	−	−	−	−	+	+	+	+	+	+	−	−	−	−	−	−

non-segmental phonology, made at the outset of this chapter. "Prosodies", in this approach, refer to phonological features extending over stretches of utterance, such as the sentence, or the syllable. The term covers far more than does the notion of "non-segmental": it includes not only such phenomena as pitch, stress and juncture patterns, but also such articulatory effects as lip rounding and nasalization, when these are used to account for restrictions on sequences of phones, or to relate phonology to grammatical structure. Examples of "vowel harmony" or "consonant harmony" are illustrative: a word or phrase displaying consonant harmony would have all or most of the consonants it contained sharing certain properties, *e.g.* all articulated with lip-rounding, or all voiced. Such processes may be of considerable importance in phonological acquisition (see below), and are certainly widespread in the characterization of phonological disability.

The other main category in prosodic phonology is the "phonematic unit". This notion comprises those linear features of utterance which cannot be handled in terms of prosodies—consonants and vowels. Despite the resemblance of the term to "phoneme", the two notions are conceptually quite different, as no attempt is made with this unit to analyse speech totally into a single system of phonological oppositions, valid for all places in structure (as is the case with the phoneme), and some features which would be included in a phonemic analysis would not be included in an analysis into phonematic features (*e.g.* lip-rounding). The principle which permits different phonological systems to be set up at different places in grammatical, lexical or phonological structure is known as *polysystemicism*. This view is based on the observation that the contrasts which occur at the beginning of a word may not be the same as those which occur in the middle or at the end. Rather than attempt to conflate them all into a single system, therefore, separate systems are set up. In a language like English, where most of the phonemes which occur initially may also occur finally (apart from the well-known exceptions, such as /ŋ/ and /h/), this method of analysis is not so illuminating as in other languages where the differences are marked. But in the context of disability, where there are often gross differences between initial and final consonants in a syllable or word, the method has much to commend it.

Whether we talk in terms of phonemes, phonematic units, features or prosodies, all of the above approaches have one thing in common: they are "static" descriptions of the phonological system. They do not allow for the possibility that phonology should also have a dynamic dimension, in which statements about the *processes* affecting these units would be made. In a process model of phonology, certain units or structures are postulated as "basic" and the range of data found in the language shown to be derivable from these basic entities through the application of a set of processes, or rules. The aim is to make statements about the language that are much more general (and, it is claimed, psychologically meaningful) than those produced by the static approach. The differences in emphasis can be seen in the following example. The word *bib*, as normally pronounced, contains different articulations of *b*, one fully voiced (initial) and one devoiced (final). The phonemic model would handle this by saying that the phoneme /b/ has two allophones, [b] in initial position, and [b̥] in final position. But at no point would a statement be made in which these two allophones were related to each other. In a process approach, however, one of these articulations would be set up as basic, and the other derived from it. There are two possibilities:

[b̥] $\longrightarrow$ [b]   in initial position
[b] $\longrightarrow$ [b̥]   in final position

Because the voiced articulation seems the more general one (*i.e.* the devoiced [b̥] can often be heard fully voiced—if a vowel follows, for example—whereas the initial [b] is *not* usually devoiced), it is the second possibility which would usually be given, in a process statement about this relationship. Process statements of this kind

X $\longrightarrow$ Y   usually stating the context in which the process occurs

are known as *phonological rules.*

It should be noted that all static statements can be reformulated as phonological rules. We could introduce the notion of phoneme, and handle the above example by saying that the phoneme /b/ "becomes" [b] initially and [b̥] finally, or:

/b/ $\longrightarrow$ $\begin{cases} [b]/\# \underline{\quad} \\ [b̥]/ \underline{\quad}\# \end{cases}$

(where the symbol "{" means "either/or"; "/" means "in the context of"; and "#" means "boundary of the word", its position relative to _____ indicating whether initial or final position is involved). Exactly the same formalism could be used to handle statements about the relationship of sounds to each other using distinctive features. For example, instead of saying that P says *blue* as [bu:], we could summarize the essential characteristics of the relationship in feature process terms, as follows:

[+sonorant] $\longrightarrow$ ∅ / [+consonantal] _____

In other words, sounds containing a sonorant feature (*i.e.* [r], [l], [w], [j]) are deleted ("become zero", for which the symbol is ∅) after a sound containing a consonantal feature (*i.e.* after a consonant).

Process ideas in phonology have been around a long time, and are integral to many routine notions in clinical analysis. Terms such as "substitution", "omission", "distortion" and "transposition" are process terms, though the way in which these notions are usually applied is an extremely limited one (see below, p. 44). The full potential of a process approach is best illustrated in the phonological component of a generative grammar, where the aim is to make maximally general and economical statements about languages in particular, and language in general (the idea of phonological "universals"). The field is a controversial one, partly because of problems in motivating the distinction between what is basic in a phonological system and what is derived, and partly because of difficulties in achieving the aims of generality and economy, given the many types of "exceptions" which a language presents. But its main principles, and much of its method, have been a formative influence on phonological studies in language acquisition.

A particularly fruitful use of process thinking has been in the notion of *rule-ordering.* In order to explain the phonological shape of a word or phrase, it is often necessary to postulate more than one process as being applicable. Sometimes the processes which apply seem independent of each other, but sometimes there is a clear interdependence, with one process being applicable only if a previous process has operated. In such instances, the rules we would set up to capture this effect would have to be ordered. An example of unordered rule application would be if P, instead of saying [bɪb], said [b̥ɪbʰ]. Here he has devoiced his initial /b/ and overaspirated his final /b/. In rule terminology we might propose the (abnormal) application of a devoicing rule initially and an aspiration rule finally, to handle this word:

(i) [b-] ⟶ [b̥-]   (devoicing)
(ii)[-b] ⟶ [-bʰ]   (aspiration)

But there are no ordering constraints here: it would not matter if we applied (ii) before (i); the same result would obtain. The opposite situation may be seen in a patient whom we know (let us assume, for the sake of illustration) regularly aspirates his final voiced plosives, as above, and also perseverates on initial plosives (*e.g.* cat becoming /kak/—what we shall refer to below as "consonant harmony"). This patient produces the word [babʰ] for *bat*. How is this to be analyzed? We might of course simply put it down to an odd substitution: /t/→[bʰ]. But this would not be a very satisfying analysis: a rule set up to handle just one word is not as helpful to assessment and remediation as demonstrating the operation of a rule that applies to large numbers of words (and, maybe, to the language as a whole). Is [babʰ] an exception, then? That it is not can be shown using the notion of rule-ordering. We may postulate that at an early stage in our representation of this patient's phonology, *bat* is represented as [bat]. Due to his perseveration rule, his output realization of this form becomes [bab]. But once he finds himself with a voiced plosive in final position, his aspiration rule then applies, and he finally comes out with [babʰ]. This sequence may be summarized in the following way (the rules are ordered, this time):

(i) [-t] ⟶ [-b]   (perseveration)
(ii)[-b] ⟶ [-bʰ]   (aspiration)

It should be noted that to apply these rules in reverse order would be to predict forms for this patient that do not occur: if the aspiration rule applied first, then *bat* would stay [bat], as there is no voiced plosive at the end of it; the perseveration rule would then apply, and we would have [bab]. But [bab] does not turn up as the output form for *bat* in this patient. Smith (1973) and Ingram (1974a, b) provide many other examples of this kind of reasoning, in their child studies, with often several intermediate stages between input and output forms being postulated.

    Lastly, by way of theoretical background, we need to recognize the importance of certain higher-order phonological notions in carrying out any of the analyses that have been outlined above. When we investigate the relationships of phonological units to each other, we need to postulate some kind of larger unit as a frame of reference. To talk of a phoneme, say, being replaced by another phoneme, or being followed by another phoneme, only really makes sense if we know *where* the substitution or sequence takes place. This frame of reference is provided by either the notion of *syllable* or that of *word,* one or other of which is presupposed in the descriptive statements made above. When something happens "initially", "medially" or "finally", we must mean "in a syllable" or "in a word"[7]. When we talk of the way a vowel or consonant behaves when it is stressed or unstressed, we presuppose a syllable or word sequence. The notion of consonant "cluster" can be interpreted only with reference to syllable or word. Opinion is divided as to which of the two is the most useful, in devising phonological models of language acquisition, or descriptive frameworks for clinical use. In many ways, the syllable is a more basic and universally applicable notion, and has received a great deal of attention by theorists involved in constructing models of speech production. On the other hand, the notion of a phonological word[8] is important in explaining several processes (such as consonant harmony or vowel harmony) which are not restricted to single syllables. It is also receiving increasing attention in studies of the early period of phonological development in children[9]. A comprehensive clinical investigation will doubtless have to utilize both.

It is indeed this eclectic attitude which needs to be held in all clinical phonological studies. Because of our training, one or other of the above approaches will be preferred, as an initial tool of enquiry; but it is important not to allow ourselves to be blinkered by our background. No single approach is capable of presenting all the facts of phonological behaviour in a maximally efficient manner. If insights are not to be obscured, analysts must be in a position to move from one frame of reference to another, when required. And a phonological profile of a patient should not shirk from incorporating notions from different theoretical models. "Eclectic" does not mean that these notions are in some miraculous way transmuted into a new phonological theory: it means simply that all the possible ways in to an analysis are systematically considered. At the very least, then, in analysing a sample of clinical data, we will need to have available:

(1) *An inventory of phones:* as phonetically accurate a statement as is possible about what P is doing with his articulators.

(2) *An inventory of features:* a statement concerning the phonetic features used, which will cut across the phone inventory above. The features of place of articulation,

---

[7] But it should be noted that initial, medial and final will have different meanings, depending on which notion is used: cf.

c u p f u l		c u p f u l
syllable model ❘ ❘ ❘ ❘ ❘ ❘	word model ❘	❘ ❘
I M F I M F		I M F

A similar confusion can arise in relation to consonant clusters (see below), which will mean different things depending on which notion is used, *e.g.* /pf/ is a cluster only in the word model above. A much broader conception of cluster may also be found if word boundaries are ignored, *e.g. ties today* (/-zt-/): see, for example, Olmsted (1971).

[8] See, *e.g.* Robins (1971: 188 ff.). For discussion of the place of the syllable in phonological analysis, see Kohler (1966), Anderson (1969), Fudge (1969), Hooper (1972). An important early study is O'Connor and Trim (1953). The point is discussed in relation to language acquisition by Moskowitz (1970); see also Priestley (1977). There are basically two issues that have to be decided: do the same syllable patterns turn up regardless of the syllable's position in the word? To what extent is syllable division arbitrary? We shall be making use of both notions in the analysis later in this chapter (as does Grunwell [1977]).

[9] See Menyuk and Menn (1979), Ingram (1979).

manner of articulation and voicing seem to be universally regarded as the most important, but precise specifications of these notions vary between models (see further, Table 3)[10].

Table 3. *Four ways of indicating the inventory of phones*[a]

Connor and Stork (1972: 45)

	Bilabial	Labio-dental	Dental	Alveolar	Palatal	Velar	Glottal
	I M F	I M F	I M F	I M F	I M F	I M F	I M F
Stop							
Affricate							
Fricative							
Nasal							
Lateral							
Other							

Cruttenden (1972: 32)

		Labial	Dental	Alveolar	Palatal	Velar	Glottal
Plosive	Fortis						
	Lenis						
Fricative	Fortis						
	Lenis						
Nasal							
Lateral							
Approximant							

Grunwell (1975: 35-6)

	I M F		Stop	Nasal	Fricative	Affricate	Lateral	Approximant
Stop								
Nasal		Bilabial						
Fricative		Alveolar						
Affricate		Palatal						
Lateral		Velar						
Approximant								

Beresford and Grady (1968: 30)

	Bilabial	Labio-dental	Alveolar	Velar	Glottal
Stop					
Nasal					
Fricative					
Lateral					
Continuant					

[a] I, M and F refer to "initial", "medial" and "final"

[10] The idea of an "inventory" is not an elementary one: inventories have to be made on the basis of certain theoretical principles, and there are several ways in which phonetic inventories can be made to look very different, with phonological factors influencing decisions. For example, in a list of P's phones, should [ʧ] be regarded as a separate manner category ("affricate") or as a type of palatal plosive (as in Cruttenden, 1972); if the former, should it be placed in the inventory adjacent to plosive (cf. Connor and Stork, 1972) or fricative (Grunwell, 1975)? Is [s] to be classified along with other alveolars, or as a

(3) *A statement of distribution:* both (1) and (2) need to be viewed in terms of their positional variability—initially, medially and finally in syllables and words. A set of criteria have to be established for handling the ambiguous cases which turn up, whichever higher-order unit is used, *e.g.* is *sister sis+ter, si+ster* or *sist+er?* A separate statement may be made to handle the further modifications which take place in connected speech, *e.g.* assimilation and elision, as when *and* becomes [m] in a phrase like *dad and mum.*

(4) *A statement of relationship to the normal adult target.* This may be presented statically or dynamically, or both. A static view will give a list of the targets (phones, phonemes, features, etc.) alongside a statement of their use by P—whether there is identity (*e.g.* [p] turns up as [p]), overlap (of 1 or more features, *e.g.* [p] turns up as [f]), or no overlap (none of the main features shared, *e.g.* [p] turns up as [a])[11]. A dynamic view will attempt to summarize the data in the form of phonological rules, which will operate on phones, feature matrices, or syllables[12]. Various types of rules may be recognized, as in the language acquisition studies reviewed below.

(5) *A statement of relationship to other linguistic levels*—where, that is, factors at these other levels are influencing the phonology. Chief amongst these will be the role of stress, or accent, in view of the well-recognized tendency for phones to behave differently in stressed vs. unstressed syllables. But we should also allow for the influence of grammar (*e.g.* whether /s/ as the exponent of a morpheme, such as plurality, should be handled differently from its use elsewhere) and lexicon (*e.g.* if a phone is used only in an individual lexical item, such as a proper name). We will certainly want to know whether the total words analyzed in a sample should be "number of different words", or just "number of words", regardless of the frequency with which a particular word turns up in the sample. And we may choose to exclude certain words, on the grounds that their behaviour is in some way atypical (*e.g.* grammatical words such as *the*).

(6) *A statement of indeterminacy.* Analysts ought not to be scared of recognizing that a fair proportion of any sample of data will contain data impossible or ambiguous to analyze. It is often difficult to hear whether a feature contrast is being made (such as an element of aspiration), and acoustic analysis (if available) may not always help. We may choose to exclude certain aspects of the data, or to handle them differently, *e.g.* incomplete words, unintelligible stretches of speech. We may be uncertain what the target word is (a common problem in spontaneous conversation with patients). Or, we may know what the target is, but be unclear how P's production relates to it, *e.g.* [emp] is produced for "elephant".

(7) *The role of interaction.* It may be important to know whether phonological units turn up only in certain interaction situations. The main factor for phonology seems to be the role of direct imitation of T's stimulus; but there are other variables, such as delayed imitation, or P's self-repetition.

---

separate "post-alveolar" category? Is [w] labial or velar? And so on. Table 3 gives some possible inventory frameworks.

[11] Cf. Beresford and Grady's (1968) realization tables, *e.g.* slt ~ d ~ k; Cruttenden's (1972) matrix of target and realisation; Ferguson, Peizer and Weeks' (1973) statements in a "model and replica" approach.

[12] Cf. Hyman (1975), Schane (1973), Chomsky and Halle (1968).

Phonological Acquisition

From the above discussion, we can see that the apparently simple question "what is it that is being acquired?" turns out to quite complicated. There will be many different answers, depending on whether we see the child as acquiring phones, phonemes, oppositions, features, prosodies, and so on, and on what range of other factors we introduce into the analysis (*cf.* the grammatical, lexical, etc. factors referred to above). It is not possible to make definitive statements, because not all the variables have been investigated properly (individual children being made to carry a great deal of theoretical weight, in some instances)[13]. All that can be done is reflect the main findings of the recent literature, where certain theoretical paradigms have attracted particular attention.

(i) Transitional phenomena. The transition from phonetic to phonological abilities in the first year of life has been one focus of study. Here, the traditional descriptions of early utterances, whether vocalizations, babbling or speech, in terms of an undifferentiated notion of "phone" or "phoneme" has come to be replaced by models of development in which phonetic and phonological skills are kept distinct, though allowing for a transitional period between the two. The importance of babbling as a precursor for speech is stressed, as systematic, language-influenced trends within it have been observed (*e.g.* Oller, Wieman, Doyle, and Ross 1976). The study of the transitional period has led to several proposals for handling the very diverse kinds of data obtained: "phonetically consistent forms" which seem to lack referential content, "prewords" which do seem to have reference, but which are not based on any obvious adult form, and "protowords", which are early attempts at adult forms, are just three of the constructs that have been recognized for this period "between babble and speech"[14].

(ii) The acquisition of phonemes. It is now plain that the early attempts to list the order in which the various phonemes of a language are learned by a child have not been as illuminating as was expected, and it is instructive to examine why. Here is an example of one such ordering[15].

By 2	p	b	m	n	w	
By 2½	t	d	k	g	ŋ	h
By 3	f	s	l	j		
By 4	ʃ	v	z	r	ʧ	ʤ
By 5	θ	ð				
Later	ʒ					

---

[13] For example the prosodic approach to phonological acquisition seems wholly based on a single child (Waterson 1971). An example of a factor which has been little considered in the context of phonological disability is the notion of "variable rule" (Labov 1972).

[14] See the review in Fletcher and Garman (1979: 4 ff.), and the paper by Menyuk and Menn in that volume. The traditional view is illustrated by Irwin and his colleagues (*e.g.* Irwin and Chen 1943). Much of the linguistic interest in babbling and speech stems from Jakobson (1941), but his discontinuity theory concerning the relationship between the two is no longer convincing, in view of the recent studies. For early (pre-babble) phonetic development in production, see Stark, Rose and McLagen (1975); on early phonetic and phonological perception, see Morse (1974).

[15] It is based on a synthesis of Sander (1961), Templin (1957), Olmsted (1971) and Ingram (1976: Ch. 2); see further below.

What is wrong with such a summary as this? Basically, the diagram simplifies too much, and omits information of importance to development. For example, what would it mean to say that /t/ has been "acquired" by 2½? Does it mean that for every adult word containing /t/, the child also has /t/? Does it mean that all the various allophones of /t/ are being correctly articulated? in all positions in the word? for all words? Does it mean that all children achieve a certain level of mastery by this age? The answer to each of these questions is no. Despite the limited samples analyzed to date, it is evident that there is a great deal of individual variation between children in the rate and the order of acquisition of phones. Moreover, there is a great deal of variation within an individual child, at any given age. Phonemes are not produced with absolute phonetic consistency from one word to the next (often, several repetitions of the same word will produce several phonetically distinct forms); and variations in ability between initial, medial and final positions in a word are marked. There are several empirical difficulties of this kind. And then there are the theoretical problems, of how much learning needs to have taken place before we can say that a particular phoneme has been "acquired". How consistently in how many positions in how many words does a phoneme have to be used before we can talk about acquisition[16]?

Of course, many of these problems may prove to be temporary. Individual differences are always more noticeable in small samples, and it may be that, with many more children being studied, trends and age-based norms may be more in evidence. It is thus premature to reject the phonemic approach out of hand (*cf.* the arguments of Menyuk and Menn, 1979). It would also be possible to apply the phonemic model so that it would take into account information about distribution and free variation. Table 4 illustrates a possible order of acquisition for single segments within syllable structure, based primarily on Olmsted (1971). It is obviously a much more illuminating statement than that given on p. 34, despite its limitations. On the basis of this kind of description, several interesting hypotheses might be formulated, such as:
- acquisition order is basically: labial→velar→alveolar→postalveolar→dental;
- the vowel system is acquired by 3½;
- fricatives in final position are easier than those in initial position;
- contrasts which are particularly important for the early period are voiced vs. voiceless, and oral vs. nasal.

An analysis of the errors the children in this study made would produce such generalizations as the following:
- labial consonants produce few place of articulation errors;
- postalveolar and dental consonants display mainly place and voicing errors;
- diphthongs produce more errors than pure vowels;
- there are few errors in semi-vowels;
- in the early period, voiced consonants substitute for voiceless ones, rather than the reverse.

---

[16] Olmsted (1971), for example, defines acquisition as when at least half of the child's attempts at a phone are successful. This study should also be referred to for its information about developmental trends in the distribution of phones—on the whole (apart from fricatives) initial phones → medial → final.

3*

Other phonological units might be included, such as clusters:
— clusters are acquired first in final position;
— in cluster simplifications, it is usually the second element that is affected, whether the cluster is CC or CCC.

Table 4. *Postulated order of acquisition for single segments in syllable structure*[a]

	Initial	Medial	Final
1	p b 　　d k g 　　m 　　n f h	ɪ ʊ æ ɒ iː 　　　ɔː 　　　ɑː aɪ	p b k 　　n f
2;0	t w̥ w	əʊ	g s ʃ 　　m
2;6	s ·ʃ 　j	ʌ uː eɪ aʊ	t d 　　v 　　z
3;0	l	e ə ɔɪ	θ ʃ
3;6	ʃ θ ð 　z 　dʒ 　v 　r 　ʒ		ŋ ð dʒ l ʒ

[a] Within a stage, the organization of phones is based on phonetic, not on developmental criteria

Many conclusions of this kind might be formulated, some quite specific (*e.g.* /f/ vs. /s/ is the earliest fricative contrast acquired), and they are obviously worth using as guiding hypotheses in remedial work, in the absence of anything more systematic. What seems impossible, in the present state of knowledge, is to construct a single theoretical system capable of accounting for the order of emergence described. Jakobson's (1941) account of phonemic development, for example (the child starts with two consonants and a vowel, and gradually builds up his system by a process of binary splitting), is difficult to subject to test (mainly because it is unclear how much free variation is to be permitted under each "opposition") and is weakened by many recently observed counterexamples[17].

[17] The same comments apply to studies of the development of phonemic perception, as opposed to the production studies, some of whose results are given above. Here too it is possible to establish acquisitional hypotheses concerning the order of phonemes or features. For example, Olmsted used work by Miller and Nicely (1955) to predict children's errors in consonant discrimination. Miller and Nicely had shown that adult perceptual confusions were greatest on place of articulation, less on

(iii) The acquisition of phonological rules. One way in which the phonemic model of development is inadequate is that it does not enable us to see how different strategies used by different children can produce the same phonological result. The suggestion was therefore made that a study of the strategies themselves would be more illuminating, and the main way in which this approach has been tried is by use of the formalism of the phonological rule. These rules summarize processes in which the adult linguistic forms are taken as the input, and the child's forms are taken as the output. The assumption, in other words, is that the child is "doing something" to the adult forms, and this in turn makes certain assumptions about the relationship between perception and production (which will be discussed below)[18].

Three main classes of rule are proposed:

(a) *Substitution processes,* such as

stopping, whereby fricatives are replaced by stops, *e.g. say*→/teɪ/;

fronting, whereby velars and palatals are replaced by alveolars, *e.g. coat*→/dʊt/, *shoe*→/suː/;

gliding, whereby /l/ and /r/ are replaced by /w/ or /j/, *e.g. leg*→/jeg/;

vocalization, whereby syllabic consonants are replaced by vowels, *e.g. apple*→ /apʊ/.

(b) *Assimilatory processes.* Ingram (1974a) makes the important point that substitution rules, such as those above, play only a limited role in accounting for the phonological patterns in children's data. They miss out certain aspects of development altogether, and may be misleading, in that they will not show that the incorrect use of a phoneme may at times be the result of a beneficial general process. He suggests that substitution rules need to be supplemented by "phonotactic" rules, in order to account for the way in which consonants or vowels working in combination within a word may develop certain problems that the units in isolation would not have (see also Vihman, 1978). This is a particularly important change of emphasis for clinical language work, where for so long the notion of substitution has held sway. Examples of these rules are:

consonant harmony, whereby a consonant in one position within a word or syllable becomes more like or identical with one from another position in the same word/syllable. Several types of harmony can be identified: "velar assimilation" (or "deapicalization"), in which apical consonants become velars, *e.g. dog*→/gɒg/; "labial assimilation", in which apicals become labials, *e.g. think*→/fɪŋk/, *table*→ /babuː/;

vowel harmony, whereby a vowel in one position within a word or syllable becomes more like or identical with one from another position in the same word/ syllable, *e.g. rabbit*→/wawa/, *flower*→/faːwa/ (the latter being referred to as "progressive vowel assimilation" by Ingram);

---

sounds involving a fricative component, and least on voicing and nasality, and Olmsted finds a similar predictiveness for the errors in his child sample (supported by Timm [1977] on Russian). Cf. also the progression of stops → voiceless fricatives → voiced fricatives found by Edwards (1974). But there are many exceptions to these trends. See also Menyuk and Menn (1979).

[18] The following is based mainly on Ingram (1974 a, 1974 b, 1979), Smith (1973, 1974); only the main processes are illustrated. I shall use phonemic notation for the examples, for convenience: see Smith's studies for examples in feature notation.

voicing, whereby a consonant becomes voiced before a vowel, and devoiced in syllable-final position, *e.g. pig*→/bɪk/, which illustrates both processes happening in the same word.

The analysis of words in terms of harmony rules is a major principle of Waterson (1971). In some children, it seems, the earliest period of word production may display harmony rules that are almost total, *i.e.* in a word, the consonants must be identical, and the vowels identical; the progressive weakening of these harmony rules then follows.

(c) *Syllable structure processes,* generally seen as processes of simplification of the adult form, such as

cluster reduction, whereby elements in an adult consonant cluster are omitted or blended, so that a singleton consonant is produced. Examples of omission are /s/ followed by a consonant, *e.g. sky*→/kaɪ/, and /l, r, w, j/ preceded by a consonant, *e.g. quick*→/kɪk/. In cases of blends, features from each segment combine, *e.g. smile*→/maɪl/;

final consonant deletion, whereby the last consonant in a CVC syllable is omitted, leaving the so-called "open syllable", *e.g. bike*→/baɪ/;

unstressed syllable deletion, e.g. banana→/naːna/;

reduplication, common in the earliest period of word production, in which a syllable (usually CV in form) is repeated and a disyllabic word thus produced, *e.g. water*→/wawa/, *ball*→/bʌbʌ/; see Schwartz, Leonard, Wilcox, and Folger, 1980.

Several other individual processes have been suggested in the literature, some of fairly general applicability, some that seem to be idiosyncratic (*e.g.* Priestley, 1977). In addition, there have been several proposals arguing for a hierarchical organization of these processes, *e.g.* Smith (1973, 1974), where harmony and cluster reduction are seen as primary.

(iv) The relationship between production and perception. Obviously both perceptual and production abilities are prerequisite for normal phonological learning; but what is the relationship between the two? The various answers which have been given to this question constitute a further theme in the research literature. The primary issue is the extent to which the child's skills in production presuppose a prior perceptual ability, and if so, the nature and extent of this ability. There are three main positions.

(a) The child is credited with an efficient ability to perceive adult contrasts from the outset, perhaps all adult contrasts[19]. The fact that all sounds do not emerge at once is to be explained by the child's problems in speech production, which is a much slower ability to develop. The main evidence for this view is the fact that the child seems to understand a great deal of adult speech, though he is unable to produce it, and that he is intolerant of adults who fail to make required phonological distinctions (the "fis" phenomenon: see Priestley, 1980, for a review). In Stampe's proposals concerning "natural phonology", it is also assumed that the child represents words internally exactly in their adult form. In addition, he is ascribed a set of innate processes, hierarchically ordered, which he uses to simplify the adult forms when he wishes to produce them. In the earliest period, for instance, these processes

---

[19] See Smith (1973), Kornfeld (1971). The "natural phonology" approach is in Stampe (1969).

will combine to mean that his attempt at *tractor* will come out as, say, /taːtaː/. As the child matures, some of these processes are lost (for example, he learns *not* to reduplicate), some come to be restricted to certain contexts (*e.g.* devoicing applies only to final consonants), and so on.

(b) In the second view, the child is credited with not nearly so efficient a perceptual ability as in the first; he is still seen as trying to learn adult contrasts, but this is a gradual and patterned progress, over several years[20]. The evidence here is in several studies which have shown that the "across-the-board" pattern of phonological learning expected as an outcome of the first position does not materialize in practice. In an across-the board view, once a phoneme has been used correctly in one context, it will then automatically carry over to other lexical items where the phoneme would be expected in the adult language. Rather, a slow process of "lexical diffusion" is apparent, with the child sometimes producing the phoneme correctly (in some words, in some tasks, *e.g.* imitation) and sometimes not—the "coexistence of success and error", as Olmsted put it (*cf.* 1971: 244). Cruttenden (1979: 21), for example, outlines four stages for the development of the *sell* vs. *shell* opposition: (i) both are produced as [s]; (ii) there is free variation between [s] and [ʃ]; (iii) *sell* is produced consistently as [sɛl] but *shell* has either [s] or [ʃ]; (iv) correct production, for this pair of words, at least. It is not possible to explain such developments solely on the basis of a growing efficiency in speech production; there must be some kind of developing proficiency in perceptual discrimination as well.

(c) This view also accepts that perception acts as an important constraint on production, but does not model perception, at the outset, in terms of adult categories; rather, the child's early output is held to be based on the particular way he perceives, which is not the same as the adult way[21]. Specifically, in this model, it is proposed that the child perceives whole words—"auditory images formed by word gestalts" (Menyuk and Menn, 1979: 69). From these words, he extracts certain phonetic features which he then applies to the word as a whole, *e.g.* "make everything nasal", "make the consonants plosive", using the kinds of primitive harmony rule referred to above (p. 37). The approach is an attractive one, but to be convincing it needs a great deal of empirical support, and an indication of how the transfer from child-based to adult-based perceptual categories takes place.

Two important general points can be extracted from the above literature, both of which have immediate clinical implications. Firstly, we must avoid a direct relationship between production and perception, as far as phonology is concerned. To have good auditory discrimination ability does not necessarily mean that there will be swift learning of a phonological contrast. Conversely, efficient motor production of sounds does not necessarily mean that there is good phonological perception. Secondly, there is no easy parallelism between production and perception learning. There is a general trend for production to follow the same developmental path as perception, but there are many categories of exception. The danger, as ever, is of our underestimating childhood ability, not only on the perception side (as was argued

---

[20] See Shvachkin (1973), Garnica (1973), Edwards (1974). The lexical diffusion view below is in Ferguson and Farwell (1975), Hsieh (1972).

[21] See Waterson (1971), who cites a parallel in Piaget's (1926) notion of verbal syncretism; also Menyuk and Menn (1979).

by Smith *et al.*) but also on the production side (as argued, for instance, by Macken and Barton, 1980). It seems that children can utilize phonetic distinctions in ways that adults are unable to hear, and which can only be demonstrated instrumentally. This kind of evidence, which is only now beginning to emerge, has major implications for future discussion of this topic[22].

(v) Factors influencing acquisition order. From the amount of variability observed in the studies on individual children, it is evident that there must be a great many interacting influences on phonological acquisition. The main factors which have been suggested are as follows.

(a) Frequency of use of a phone or phoneme in the adult language—or, at least, that sub-set of sentences used by parents. The general view here is to minimize the role of frequency: while not denying it some influence in individual cases, there seems little correlation between the order of emergence of sounds and what is known about the frequency of their use in the language as a whole. In colloquial R. P., for example, the relevant statistics are as follows (from Fry, 1947):

	%		%		%
/ə/	10.74	/n/	7.58	/ʤ/	0.60
/ɪ/	8.33	/t/	6.42	/ʧ/	0.41
/e/	2.97	/d/	5.14	/θ/	0.37
/aɪ/	1.83	/s/	4.81	/ʒ/	0.10
/ʌ/	1.75	/l/	3.66		
/eɪ/	1.71	/ð/	3.56		
/i:/	1.65	/r/	3.51		
/əʊ/	1.51	/m/	3.22		
/æ/	1.45	/k/	3.09		
/ɒ/	1.37	/w/	2.81		
/ɔ:/	1.24	/z/	2.46		
/u:/	1.13	/v/	2.00		
/ʊ/	0.86	/b/	1.97		
/ɑ:/	0.79	/f/	1.79		
/aʊ/	0.61	/p/	1.78		
/ɜ:/	0.52	/h/	1.46		
/ɛə/	0.34	/ŋ/	1.15		
/ɪə/	0.21	/g/	1.05		
/ɔɪ/	0.14	/ʃ/	0.96		
/ʊə/	0.06	/j/	0.88		

Certain of the more frequent phonemes turn up early in child speech (*viz.* /n/, /d/, /ɪ/, /aɪ/) and certain of the least frequent ones turn up late (*viz.* /ʒ/, /θ/, /ʧ/, /ʤ/, /ɔɪ/); but for counter-examples we need only look at /t/, /s/, /l/, /j/, /g/, /ʃ/, /ə/, /e/ and /ʌ/.

(b) The *functional load* of a phoneme or feature in the language—that is, the number

---

[22] See further, on the interdependence of production and perception, Eilers (1975), Eilers and Oller (1976). The Macken and Barton research (on the learning of word-initial plosives, as measured by voice-onset-time) generally provides support for the lexical diffusion model of acquisition, though aspects of their findings suggest a rapidity of acquisition which might support the across-the-board model.

of words which are actually distinguished using the phoneme/feature. For example, the distinction between /p/ and /b/ in English is important, in the sense that there are very many words which are kept apart solely by this contrast (*pin/bin, pat/bat,* etc.): this contrast is thus said to have a high functional load. On the other hand, there are very few cases of words in the language which are distinguished by, say, /ʃ/ vs. /ʒ/: this contrast would thus be said to have a low functional load. It would be possible to work out a scale of functional loading for all the contrasts in a language, on the basis of a sample of data, although the precise quantification of the notion is difficult (*cf.* Lyons, 1968: 81 ff.). Such a scale would very likely bear some correlation with the order of emergence of phonological contrasts, but (as the tense form of this sentence implies) the relevant counting in the relevant samples of parental language has not been done.

(c) Articulatory complexity is an obvious variable, but one which it has proved extremely difficult to define. One of the consequences of the dynamic approach to the study of articulatory phonetics (see p. 3) has been to extend the notion of articulatory complexity to include neurological, as well as physiological and anatomical constraints; the dimension of temporal organization has also to be considered (for a summary, see Dalton and Hardcastle, 1977: Chs. 2, 3). Thus, while this factor might readily be referred to to explain the late development of those phonemes whose articulation requires fine motor control (such as certain fricatives), it is not so easy to apply the notion to plosives or vowels. Instrumental studies of the development of children's control over individual parameters are needed, along with more detailed models of speech production than are so far available[23]. The application of this factor in the analysis of individual cases should therefore proceed with caution.

(d) Physiological maturity, referring to the maturational developments in the size and shape of the vocal tract, and in the neurological system supplying it, is a further factor whose significance is only beginning to be understood. The point however seems relevant not only for the period of maximal development (the first year of life), but also later, *e.g.* attempts have been made to explain the relatively late appearance of certain high frequency sounds on the basis of the degree of myelination of the auditory nerve and the cortical areas to which it connects[24].

(e) Auditory complexity, in the sense of some overall measure of discriminability, sonority, resonance, etc., is another relevant factor, but one which is also difficult to quantify. Some of the grosser sound contrasts can be explained by reference to this notion (as Jakobson aimed to do), but it proves difficult to carry the idea through the phonological system as a whole[25].

(f) Phonological complexity, as defined by one or other of the models discussed above,

---

[23] However, several studies of one important variable, voice-onset-time, have taken place: for production, see Gilbert and Purves (1977), Menyuk and Klatt (1975), Gilbert (1977), Macken and Barton (1980); for perception, see Eilers, Wilson and Moore (1979). It should also be pointed out that a child may have excellent motor control, and still have phonological problems, *e.g.* he may have a well-formed articulation in some words, but be unable to use it contrastively. Note also distributions such as *puddle* → [pʌɡəl], but *puzzle* → [pʌdəl], which illustrates the priority of phonological over phonetic issues.

[24] See Salus and Salus (1974). For a relevant general account of physical maturation in the infant, see Lenneberg (1967), Bosma (1975).

[25] See Jakobson (1941), Jespersen (1926), Ladefoged (1975: 219–220).

will be relevant. For example, the number of allophones a phoneme has may affect the rate at which it is learned; /f/, for example, is a phoneme with little allophonic variability, and is also the first fricative to be acquired in English (or so it would seem). On the other hand, there is a fair amount of allophonic variability in relation to /k/ and /g/, and these emerge early. Alternatively, we might define phonological complexity in terms of distinctive features, and compute orders of emergence on that basis. But there are several theoretical problems which make it difficult to work safely with this notion[26].

(g) *Lexical factors* have now been shown to be extremely important in accounting for the patterns of development noted in young children. In the output of a child, we may simultaneously observe several historical "stages" of phonological matura- tion: some lexical items will appear stereotyped or "frozen" in an immature form; others will appear advanced; and between there will be a range of phonological ability that is so divergent, it is argued, that only an analysis in terms of individual items is sensible. Ferguson and Farwell (1975), for example, stress the importance of lexically-orientated learning in the early stages of development of a child's phono- logical system, strictly phonological processes emerging only later[27]. It is unclear how far the notion needs to be extended into later development: certainly there are many examples of frozen forms to be observed, *e.g.* a child may have learned initial /j/ for most words, but still makes an immature substitution on the word *yellow* (usually /leləʊ/).

(h) *Grammatical factors* may account for the erratic performance of certain sounds, *e.g.* having to learn that, on top of its purely phonological status, sounds such as /s/ and /z/ have also a morphological status.

(i) *Social factors* may be shown to be important—for instance, whether certain social situations facilitate acquisition or hinder it. The way some older children adopt the immature pronunciations of their younger siblings illustrates the relevance of this point. The role of accent variation in the language around the child would be another issue. Also, the domesticity of the subject-matter may be important: a child might perform better (both in terms of perception and production) if he were asked to focus on words with which he has some familiarity or which he has some motiva- tion to use[28].

(j) *Individual differences* are often cited casually as an escape-route by the analyst, but in the case of phonological acquisition there does seem to be plenty of justification for the notion. Authors repeatedly cite it: Ferguson and Farwell (1975: 438) talk of the "idiosyncratic paths which particular children follow in learning to produce their languages", and the point is echoed by several others[29].

---

[26] See the discussion of phonological complexity in Hyman (1975: Ch. 4).

[27] See also Shibamoto and Olmsted (1978), though they conclude that the Ferguson and Farwell lexical principle must be restricted to the first phone in a word: once this is chosen, they argue, phono- logical processes take over and govern the developing structure of the rest of the word.

[28] Cf. the study by D. Barton (referred to in Menyuk and Menn [1979: 51]), who found in a dis- criminiation study that responses were better in the case of familiar words as opposed to nonsense words.

[29] For example, Shibamoto and Olmsted (1978: 454) talk about individual "strategies", Ingram (1979) of "phonological preferences" for particular articulatory patterns; and then there is Priestley's detailed study (1977). See also the discussion in Menyuk and Menn (1979: 52).

(k) Task effects are another well-known variable in explaining anomalies in a set of data, and here too the phonology literature provides plenty of examples of its relevance. Whether children perform better in their spontaneous imitations of adult speech, in induced imitations (the "say what I say" context) and in other circumstances has been considered an important factor, in both normal and clinical settings. On the whole, analysts deal with imitations separately, on the grounds that imitated forms tend to introduce phonological features not otherwise found in a sample of spontaneous speech, which thus obscure the presence of genuine patterns and may lead to overestimates of production ability[30]. A similar point might be made concerning perception experiments: the child's ability to identify contrasts in isolated words may be far in excess of his ability to discriminate them in connected speech.

What might we conclude from this review of the factors involved on phonological acquisition? Given the range of factors, it is perhaps remarkable that the child data is as consistent and predictable as it is—even more remarkable when we bear in mind the speed at which the process of learning is taking place. There may not be a universal order of acquisition, but there is certainly a great deal of correspondence across children. Individual children's behaviour, moreover, is far from random. We are, I think, justified in the view that phonological acquisition is systematic, even though we are at present unable to state precisely what the properties of the system are, and how the child tackles the task of learning it. It is perhaps too extreme to see the task as resembling foreign language learning (*cf.* Haas, 1963), given the nature of the adult linguistic environment in which the child comes to learn. On the other hand, the "internalized adult system" view would seem to be an untenable opposite extreme. Several intermediate positions are possible. We may see the child as operating with a reduced version of the adult system, or with a system which is largely his own[31]. Whichever view we adopt, one thing is clear: the behaviour involved is to a large extent systematic, but its complexity often obscures its systemicness. The need for meticulous analysis and careful statement of the rules governing the behaviour is paramount, and is in my view the main conclusion to be given practical application in the study of phonological disability.

Phonological Disability

Much of the motivation to develop accounts of disorders of pronunciation has come from an increasing awareness of the limitations of the traditional process of articulation testing, and the associated notion of articulation disorder. Characteristically, definitions refer to P's abnormal substitutions, omissions and distortions of

---

[30] See, *e.g.* Shibamoto and Olmsted (1978: 419–420). On the other hand, Leonard, Schwartz, Folger and Wilcox (1978) adopt a more optimistic attitude, and support the inclusion of imitation data in corpora of spontaneous speech—though they do advocate caution. A similar division of opinion is found in the literature on articulation testing: see, for example, the review in Johnson and Somers (1978), who conclude that there is a need to keep the two modes apart.

[31] See Cruttenden (1972), Priestley (1977), and the general discussion in Ingram (1976) and Grunwell (1977).

speech sounds[32], with the tests providing a quantitative (and sometimes a qualitative) index of error on the basis of P's responses to a predetermined set of lexical stimuli. Both empirical and theoretical criticisms of this tradition have been made in recent years. Empirically, the limitations of the sample of articulation elicited have been stressed: a small number of (usually drawable) lexical items, produced in isolation (as opposed to connected speech), with little or no opportunity for free variation to be observed (if P were to use the item repeatedly), and involving only a sub-set of the phonological contexts in which sounds are used. Theoretically, there are problems of definition over the main descriptive categories (e.g. the distinction between substitution and distortion) and limitations in the amount of information that test procedures can determine: error patterns which extend across several words might be noticed only fortuitously, and phonetic patterns which bear a complex relationship to their targets might be mis- or un-analyzed[33]. The pragmatic value of articulation tests on this basis evidently is sufficiently great to keep them in routine clinical use, but it is becoming increasingly plain that the information they provide is only a fraction of what we need to know in order to understand the nature and extent of an abnormal pronunciation system. Traditional studies of articulation thus need to be supplemented by more sophisticated phonetic and phonological analyses, and it is under the heading of phonology that most attention has recently been focussed.

The distinction between the abstract phonological system (however defined) and the phonetic realization of that system is central to the enquiry. There are three main ways in which the relationship between these two levels of language organization can be abnormal:

(i) the phonological system is normal, but its phonetic realization is abnormal (e.g. immature or deviant pronunciations of phonemes, but without the range and pattern of phonemic use being affected);

(ii) the phonological system is abnormal, but its phonetic realization is normal (e.g. the range of phonemes used may be considerably delayed, but their pronunciation is within normal limits);

(iii) both the phonological system and its phonetic realization are abnormal, delay or deviance affecting both aspects of the analysis.

The notion of "phonological disability" could be applied to all three of these abnormal relationships, but it is more useful to restrict it to categories (ii) and (iii) only—that is, to cases where there has been a failure to learn or retain the underlying system. Category (i) problems would then be referred to as "phonetic disability". It is this emphasis which underlies Grunwell's (1977) definition of phonological disability as "the use of abnormal patterns in the spoken medium of language" (p. 115)—*language* being the operative word.

This conception is easy to characterize, but more difficult to define precisely. The phonological system available to the patient is inadequate to cope with the

---

[32] For example, the 1959 terminology leaflet of the College of Speech Therapists, Powers (1957: 713), etc. Other categories (e.g. transposition) are sometimes added to this list, but these are generally reducible to types of substitution.

[33] See further Higgs (1970), Beresford and Grady (1968), Grunwell (1975), (1977: Ch. 2), Lund and Duchan (1978).

normal demands made upon it, by children or adults, in that P is unable to produce (and possibly to discriminate) the expected range of sound contrasts required for the expression of meaning. But how exactly should the notion of "phonological system" be defined? In the context of disability, both the phonemic and the feature approaches have been applied to the analysis of individual cases, and their respective strengths and weaknesses evaluated[34]. Their common aim is to demonstrate systemicness in clinical data, and to provide a way of evaluating its deviant character, relative to our expectations about child/adult linguistic norms. Each of these approaches has its own insights to offer the clinician, and there is much to be gained by considering all of them before arriving at a decision concerning assessment, diagnosis or remediation.

1. Correspondence to the Adult Target

The first kind of abstraction that can be made is a statement of the kind and degree of correspondence which exists between the patient's pronunciation and that which would be expected from a normal adult from his speech community. Grunwell (1977) observes three main patterns in her child data, but these can be extended to adult samples also:

(a) Zero correspondence: a phonological unit (syllable, phone, feature, etc.) in the adult language is not used at all by P; or, P uses a phonological unit not to be found in the adult language. The former is common enough, as it subsumes the familiar notion of phoneme omission; the latter has been less observed, but is common in certain syndromes, *e.g.* the abnormal use of glottalization or nasalization as feature contrasts in cleft palate speech. For example, place of laryngeal stricture was observed as a relevant variable in the speech of one cleft palate child of 3. His voicing contrast was regularly realized as a distinction between glottal and pharyngeal places of articulation, *viz.: voiced consonant*→[ʔ], voiceless consonant→[ħ]. Examples were:

two	[t̪ħūː]	*do*	[t̪ʔūː]
Sue	[ṣħūː]	*zoo*	[ṣʔūː]
cot	[g̊ħo̅ħ]	*got*	[g̊ʔo̅ħ]

etc.
(̥ indicates a vague attempt at the co-occurring articulation).

(b) Gross inclusion: a range of phonological units differentiated by the adult language is subsumed under a single form by P, *e.g.* all vowels might be produced with a single, central quality. A consequence of this reduction will be a marked increase in the number of homophones: *bad, bed, bid, bud,* etc. will all be /bʌd/, in this example.

(c) Extreme variability: a single adult contrast may be given a range of realizations from one phonological context to another, and P may operate with this wider range either consistently or inconsistently. This distinction can be illustrated as follows:

[34] For phonemic analysis, see Haas (1963), Hartley (1966), Beresford and Grady (1968), Beresford (1971, 1972), Connor and Stork (1972), Panagos (1974). For feature analyses, see Compton (1970), McReynolds and Huston (1971), Pollack and Rees (1972), Oller (1973), Smith (1973). For a general review, see Grunwell (1977: Ch. 2), Walsh (1974). The threefold division below is the main organizational principle of Grunwell.

adult /t/   P₁ (consistent)   initially ⟶ [tʰ]
                                      medially ⟶ Ø
                                      finally   ⟶ [ʔ]

                 P₂ (inconsistent)   initially ⟶ [tʰ], [t] or [ʔ]
                                      medially ⟶ [ʔ] or Ø
                                      finally   ⟶ [ʔ] or Ø

2. Correspondence to Normal Child Development

The second kind of abstraction that can be made concerns the kind and degree of relationship between the patient's pronunciation and that expected in normal child development. While this perspective is obviously most beneficial in relation to cases of phonological disability in children, it can also be used as a convenient frame of reference for work with adults. The model most often invoked for investigating this relationship is the process model described above (p. 28). Several types of correspondence have been noted:

(a) *Unknown processes:* processes completely outside the normal course of development, as so far observed. An example is "lateral insertion", observed in one of the subjects studied in Grunwell (1977: see S5), *e.g.* [pli] for *beach.* Smith (1975) refers to processes of "segmentalization" and "perseveration" which apply to the speech of the 11-year-old dysphasic boy analyzed. Perseveration is of course common in adult disorders.

(b) *Uncommon processes:* processes not completely outside the normal course of development, but certainly not commonly observed. An example, again from Grunwell (1977: see S2), is the process of labiodental substitution used by one of her subjects (*e.g.* draw→[fɔ]). Lisping and other examples are discussed by Ingram (1976: 116).

(c) *Persistence of early processes:* a process that we would normally expect to have disappeared by a given age stays in use. A common example is cluster reduction, which should be well on its way out in the fourth year of life, but which is frequent in the speech of much older children displaying phonological disability. Some analysts distinguish cases of "pure delay" from those where there is an imbalance of processes from various stages of development: examples of such "chronological mismatches" are given by Ingram (1976: 117 ff.). The abnormally early use of a late process, and the under-use of late processes also need to be considered in relation to this view.

3. The Patient's Own System

The third kind of abstraction from the patient's data concerns the extent to which it is possible to see a consistent pattern of relationship, regardless of the nature of the adult language around him or of the processes of development he might normally be expected to use. His phonological productions may be constrained by certain general factors, which may conform to the properties of phonological systems in general (*e.g.* always having more consonants than vowels) or may seem quite "alien"[35]. Alternatively, his phonological output may be random, *i.e.* totally unintelligible and unsusceptible to any kind of decoding—but this is (a) most unusual, and (b) not a conclusion we would draw until every available analytic procedure had been tried. Some of the factors which are felt to be of importance in this respect are as follows:

(a) Polysystemic variability: the range of contrasts which P uses at one place in structure is different from that used in another, the entire range being much greater than would be expected in normal language use. Patients often have radically different consonant ranges in initial, medial and final positions within words, for example, with each range being used in a systematic way, but not readily explicable with reference to normal developmental processes.

(b) Phonemic overlapping: the range of allophones from different phonemes may overlap in ways which go well beyond the tolerance limits of the normal language, but which are nonetheless systematic. For example, the loss of voicing as a contrastive feature would cause immediate confusion, because of the way certain phones would expound both /t/ and /d/, /p/ and /b/, etc., but not all contrasts would be equally affected (the nasals, for example) and the speech would still have system. A similar situation would arise if an abnormally wide range of phones was used by a patient, some perhaps from outside the normal articulatory possibilities in his language, with a situation of overlap developing as a result—a bilabial trill, for example, sometimes being used for /p/ and sometimes for /b/.

(c) Asymmetry: given the tendency for normal phonological systems to display symmetry (or "pattern congruity", as Chao [1943] expressed it), a markedly asymmetrical appearance in an analysis would suggest its disordered character. Nonetheless there may be perfectly systematic reasons for the asymmetry, *e.g.* the overuse of a particular phonological contrast, or overreliance on a particular feature or phone. It should be noted, too, that *complete* symmetry is abnormal: phonological systems typically display "gaps in the pattern" (*e.g.* there is no voiced glottal fricative phoneme in English, though a voiced/voiceless distinction operates elsewhere with the fricatives). This, along with a certain amount of normal instability, is an important factor in motivating phonological change[36].

By combining the results of analyzing clinical data using these three approaches, very full profiles can be obtained of a patient's phonological disability. For example, in the "prototypical" cases discussed by Grunwell, Ingram and others, the following characteristics stand out:

— a restricted range and frequency of segments, with consequently fewer potential contrasts and many homophones;
— a restricted range and frequency of segmental combinations;
— a restricted range of features, especially affecting place of articulation (often, one place of articulation is predominant);

---

[35] On the general properties of phonological systems, see Greenberg (1966), Grunwell (1977: Ch. 3).

[36] See Hockett (1958: Ch. 11), Hyman (1975: Ch. 1). The lack of this normal instability in much clinical data is noteworthy, the phonological system showing signs of developmental arrest, and thus presenting little potential for change. See Grunwell (1977: Ch. 7).

- an extremely limited range of fricatives;
- an extremely limited range of non-nasal sonorants;
- the likelihood of voiced/voiceless (aspirated/unaspirated, or fortis/lenis) confusion;
- syllable structure tends towards a canonical CVCV form, open syllables being the norm (apart from the use of final nasals);
- consonant clusters are generally absent;
- use of the glottal stop as a substitute form is pervasive;
- the vowel system is relatively well-developed, apart from a tendency to centralize;
- a relatively wide range of sounds from outside the normal articulatory possibilities of the language.

These characteristics, it should be noted, obtain in "pure" cases of phonological disability, *i.e.* where the data has not been "contaminated" by problems of articulation arising out of abnormalities of an anatomical, physiological or clearly neurological kind. There may of course be phonological problems alongside these other abnormalities, though their existence has often tended to be overlooked.

The current approach to phonological disability is both a help and a hindrance, as far as the classical delay/deviance distinction is concerned. It is a help, in that a much more systematic and comprehensive approach to the notion of phonological deviance has been proposed. It has been a hindrance, in that it is no longer possible to talk in a simple manner about cases of phonological delay. But of course, this might be a very good thing! Certainly, it seems from the above that there may *never* be cases of delay, pure and simple: there always seems to be some sign of deviance. The notion of delay, also, is problematic in the absence of a consensus of opinion as to the order of emergence of phonological units and processes. It is not unusable, for it is still helpful to look for gross resemblances between a patient and a young child, at different stages; but detailed phonological assessment and remediation work must proceed on rather different lines. More illumination is obtained from a detailed synchronic analysis of the observed deviance, in terms of (a) the amount of variability in the data, (b) the degree of symmetry in the use of contrasts, (c) the amount of overlapping, (d) the regularity of phonetic realizations, and (e) the range of lexical units differentiated. The aim is to establish those places in P's phonology where there seems to be maximum stability and absence of growth, and those where the system is undergoing change. Whether the change is in the right direction (*i.e.* directed towards the appropriate child or adult norm) may then be investigated, through the use of further samples at later periods.

An Example

The various stages involved in the theoretical account given above can be illustrated from the case of Alex, a boy of 4;4, referred as a problem of "language delay". A sample of spontaneous speech was obtained from an unstructured play session (with toy animals, doll's house, etc.) lasting 30 minutes. Of the 149 sentences obtained, 44 proved unintelligible, in whole or in part. From the remaining sentences, the first 100 different words were given a fairly broad phonetic transcription, as follows[37]:

big	bɪg̊	*lemon	ˈvəʊfm̩	sister	ˈtʰɪçtə
	b̥ɪʔ	*tomatoes	ˈsʃezʒuː	mum	mʌm
yeah	jɛə	remember	əˈmembə	mum's	mʌmẓ
in	ɪn	sleeping	ˈteɪtɪn	room	duːm
car	gɑː	what	wɒʔ		(r)uːm
farm	fɑːn	this	dɪː	fat	fæʔ
pig	pʰɪg̊	washing	ˈfɒfɪn		fæp
down	daʊn	*ball	ˈbɒbɔːl	know	nəʊ
	daʊˈnə	tractor	ˈfæʔtə	mummy	ˈmʌmiː
cow	faʊ	pram	fæm	animal	ˈæmɪməl
	saʊ	painting	ˈfw̥eɪtɪn	more	mɔː
farmer	ˈfɑːmə		ˈkʲeɪtɪn	come	kəm
	ˈfɑːbə		ˈfr̥eɪtɪn	plaster	ˈfw̥ɑːtə
*chicken	ˈbəkʃən		ˈfweɪtɪn	*running	ˈbʊʌnːtɪn
no	nəʊ		ˈbreɪtɪn		ˈvʌnɪn
	næʊ	walking	ˈfwɔːkɪn	*sitting	ˈdɪpʰdɪn
fence	vetʰ	shoes˒	fuː	girl	gɜːl
fire	faɪ(ə)	up	ʌʔ	sit	sɵɪtʰ
engine	ˈɪndʒɪn	trip	ʃɪp	wash	θw̥ɒtʃ
he	iː	blood	fl̥ʌd	arm	ɑːm
not	nɒʔ		b(ə)lʌd	hand	ænd̥
	nɒtˀ	hay	ʔeɪ	bed	bed̥
be	bɪ	go	dəʊ	a	ə
out	aʊʔ		gəʊ	do	duː
	aʊ(t)	sleep	s(l̩)iːpʰ	dinner	ˈdɪnæ
and	ən(d)	dogs	dɒgẓ	kitchen	ˈtɪtʃɪn
dog	dɒg̊	lay	leɪ	bedroom	ˈbedrəm
*horsie	ˈtʰɒpsiː	on	ɒn	upstairs	ʌpˈtɛə
eat	iːtʰ	there	dɛə	chair	d̥ʒɛə
some	sm̩		nɛə		tʃɛə
bit	bɪʔ	loo	luː	soft	sɒf
crowded	ˈkr̥aʊdiː	my	maɪ	where	wɛə
stay	fw̥eɪ	one	wʌn	funny	ˈ(f)ʌnɪ
scarecrow	ˈfɛəfəʊ	two	tʰuː	noise	nɒɪ
	ˈtçɛətçəʊ	door	dɔː(ə)	lounge	laʊnː
man	mæn	daddy	ˈdæʔtɪ	into	ˈɪntə
lap	læpʰ		ˈdædɪ	hot	ɒʔ
rip	ʋɪpʰ	beans	biːn	plaster	ˈbwʌːʔdə
yellow	ˈ(j)eləʊ	toast	tʰəʊ(h)	Max	mætʰ
sausage	ˈvɒʋiːd	baby	ˈbeɪbeɪ	nothing	ˈnʌfɪŋ
					ˈnʌtˢɪŋ

---

[37] Items repeated during the sample are given in sequence; items with an unclear segmentation relative to the target are marked *.

Table 5. *Inventory of phones in Alex's sample*[a, b]

Initial C				V			Final C			
Target phone			Substitute	Target phone		Substitute	Target phone			Substitute
p	1	0	fw̦ (2), kʮ, fɽ, br	ɪ	30	eɪ, iː (2), ə, ɪː	p	2	0	pʰ (3), ʔ, t
b	9	0	b̦	e	5		b	0	0	
t	3	0		æ	11		t	1	0	tʔ, tʰ (2), p, ʔ(5)+
d	9	0		ʊ	0		d	6	1	ʔt
k	1	0	g, f, s, t	ʌ	12		k	1	0	
g	2	0	d	ɒ	11		g	3	0	ʔ
ʃ	2	0	ʤ	ə	12		ʃ	0	0	
ʤ	1	0		iː	5		ʤ	0	0	d
f	7	0	v	ɑː	6		f	0	0	
v	0	0		ɔː	3		v	0	0	
θ	0	0	f+, tˢ	uː	6		θ	0	0	
ð	0	0	d (2)+, n	ɜː	1		ð	0	0	
s	2	0	tʰ, ʊ (2), sθ	eɪ	9		s	0	1	
z	0	0		aɪ	1		z	0	3	
ʃ	0	0	f	ɔɪ	1		ʃ	0	0	ʃ, f
ʒ	0	0		əʊ	8		ʒ	0	0	
h	0	3+	ʔ+	aʊ	8		—	—		
m	9	0		ɪə	0		m	11	0	n, ɓ
n	9	0	m	ɛə	9		n	11	0	nə
—	—			ʊə	0		ŋ	2	0	n (7)+
l	5	0		eɪə	0		l	2	0	
r	2	1	d, ʊ (2)	aɪə	1		m	1	0	
w	3	0	f, fw̦, θw̦	ɔɪə	0					
j	2	0		əʊə	0					
				aʊə	0					

Initial CC				Medial CC			Final CC			
pl	0	0	fw̦, bw	st	0	ʔd, çt, t	ks	0	0	tʰ
pr	0	0	f	kt	0	ʔt	st	0	0	(h)
tr	0	0	f, ʃ	nt	0	t (4)	ft	0	0	f
kr	1	0	f, tç				gz	1	0	
st	0	0	fw̦, t				mz	1	0	
sk	0	0	f, tç				nd	2	0	
bl	0	0	fl̩				nʤ	0	0	n:
sl	0	0	s(l̩), t				ns	0	0	tʰ
							nz	0	0	n

[a] ( ) unclear phones, + items probably normal for Alex's dialect.

[b] All CVCV disyllables were divided CV/CV, unless there was a clear morphological boundary after C. Medial clusters were left undivided.

A distributional summary of the phones in these items is given in Table 5. The data were transferred onto a phonological profile chart, on which the following kinds of information are represented[38]:
(i) realization of target phones as correct (within normal adult limits), omission and substitution;

[38] This profile chart is explained in detail in Crystal (1982). Several details are omitted in the present discussion.

(ii) distribution of phones in syllable structure, consonants being classified as single-tons, two-element clusters, and three-element clusters;
(iii) phones are organized as phonetic classes: for consonants—plosives, affricates, fricatives, nasals and continuants; for vowels—short vowels, long vowels, diph-thongs and triphthongs;
(iv) distribution of phones in stressed vs. unstressed syllables;
(v) assimilation or elision features affecting word sequences in connected speech;
(vi) feature analysis in terms of place of articulation, manner of articulation and voicing;
(vii) prosodic (*i.e.* consonant/vowel harmony) processes;
(viii) syllable structure processes;
(ix) abnormal functional load;
(x) free variation in repeated lexical items.
The complete profile is gradually built up by a series of separate scans through the data, information relevant to the first four scans being presented in Tables 6 and 7.
(a) The total number of phones in the sample is 366, about which little can be said, apart from noting the relatively high proportion of consonants to vowels: C 167, V 149, CC 50[39].

Table 6. *Inventory of phones*

(a) Consonants

	C—			—C		
	✓	x	Ø	✓	x	Ø
Plosives	25	11	0	13	11	1
Affricates	3	1	0	0	1	0
Fricatives	9	8	0	0	2	4
Nasals	18	1	0	24	3	0
Continuants	12	6	1	3	0	0
Totals	67[a]	27	1	40[a]	17	5

(b) Vowels

	✓	x	Ø
Short	81	9	0
Long	20	2	0
Diphthong	36	0	0
Triphthong	1	0	0
Totals	138	11	0

(c) Clusters

			Omissions				
	✓	x	C₁	C₂	Both	Blend	?
Initial	1	4	1	0	0	8	1
Medial	0	3	5	0	0	0	0
Final	4	2	0	2	0	0	2
Totals	5	9	6	2	0	8	3

[a] Plus a further 4 dialect forms initially, and 12 finally.

[39] Throughout, C = consonant, V = vowel, and CC = 2-element consonant cluster. The figure of 50 is reached by including the indeterminate cases, and (debatably) counting [n:] for /-ndʒ/ as a single phone.

4*

Table 7. *Feature analysis of singleton consonant errors*

	Voicing					Place				Manner			
	Maintained			Lost		Maintained		Lost		Maintained		Lost	
	C–	–C	?	C–	–C	C–	–C	C–	–C	C–	–C	C–	–C
Plosives	7	8	7	3	1	3	2ª	8	9	4	11	7	0
Affricates	0	1	0	1	0	1	0	0	1	1	0	0	1
Fricatives	8	2	1	3	0	3	0	9	2	4	1	8	1
Nasals	1	10	0	0	0	0	1	1	2ª	1	3	0	0
Continuants	3	0	0	3	0	4	0	2	0	2	0	4	0
Totals	19	21	8	10	1	11	3	20	14	12	15	19	2

ª Cases of dialectal [-ʔ] for /-t/ and [-n] for /-ŋ/ have been excluded.

(b) The proportion of correct phones : incorrect phones : omitted phones is 250 : 75 : 14, possible dialect forms being included as correct[40]. These totals again tell us little, apart from suggesting that the disability is not particularly severe.
(c) The proportion of correct to incorrect phones within the main categories is more illuminating:
vowels almost totally correct (though the "almost" is worth noting, given the traditional neglect of this area);
consonants: 107 correct; 50 incorrect (either omissions, or falling outside of the normal adult allophonic range);
clusters: 5 correct; 28 incorrect or indeterminate.
This indicates the reason for the misleading impression given by *(b)*: the large number of correct vowels obscures the fact that nearly one out of two consonants is in error, and clusters are in error in nearly 90% of cases.
(d) Distributional information introduces a further clarifying element:
for consonants, initial position is correct in 71 cases, incorrect in 28 cases (*i.e.* 40% error); final position is correct in 40 cases, incorrect in 22 cases (*i.e.* 55% error);
for vowels, 10 of the 11 errors are evenly distributed between medial and final positions in the syllable;
for clusters, half of the errors are in initial position.
(e) The next step is to relate distributional information to phone type, this usually being a very important stage in our understanding of the disability:
vowels: almost all the errors relate to the use of short vowels;
consonants: there is a gradient of error between the various phonetic categories, viz. nasals (11.5% error), continuants (31%), plosives (38%), affricates (40%)[41], and fricatives (61%). However, these proportions differ greatly between initial and final positions:

---

[40] The omissions total includes cases of one C omitted in clusters. There were no cases of clusters being omitted completely, though this may be due to ambiguity in the target, *e.g.* if P used [kɑ:] with reference to a picture of two cats, it would not be entirely clear whether the target were *cat* or *cats*.
[41] This is hardly a real figure, in view of the small numbers. It will not be further considered in (f) and (g) below.

— there are twice as many nasal errors in final position (5% vs. 11%);

— continuant errors occur entirely in initial position (not very surprisingly, as only /-l/ is a possible final unit, in this dialect);

— plosive errors are much more frequent in final position (nearly half [48%], as opposed to less than a third [31%]);

— there are no correct fricatives in final position; in initial position, nearly half (47%) are in error.

(f) A feature analysis of consonant errors is next made (for present purposes, only voicing, place of articulation and manner of articulation are analyzed): see Table 8.

Table 8. *Feature analysis of consonant clusters*

(a) Voicing

		Maintained			Lost		
		C_1	C_2	Blend	C_1	C_2	Blend
C_1	C_2-	3	3	8	2	2	0
$-C_1$	C_2	5	2	0	1	0	0
$-C_1$	C_2-ª	1	7	0	0	1	0
Totals		9	12	8	3	3	0

(b) Place

		Maintained			Lost		
		C_1	C_2	Blend	C_1	C_2	Blend
C_1	C_2-	2	3	0	3	3	8
$-C_1$	C_2	4	0	0	2	2	0
$-C_1$	C_2-	0	8	0	3	0	0
Totals		6	11	0	8	5	8

(c) Manner

		Maintained			Lost		
		C_1	C_2	Blend	C_1	C_2	Blend
C_1	C_2-	5	3	1	2	1	7[b]
$-C_1$	C_2	5	1	1[b]	1	0	0
$-C_1$	C_2-	2	8	0	1	0	0
Totals		12	12	2	4	1	7

ª [?] was unanalyzed.
b Using the first element in the target cluster as comparator.

This provides the following trends:

voicing: maintained in 68% of cases—more, if the 8 cases of [?] are interpreted as voiced. Almost all errors are in initial position.

place: lost in 71% of cases, the loss being more noticeable in initial position;

manner: lost in 44% of cases, which are almost entirely due to errors in initial position.

Of the different phonetic categories:

plosives are mainly affected by loss of place in both initial and final positions, and by loss of manner in initial positions only (there are no errors at all in final position);

fricatives are mainly affected by loss of place and manner in initial position;

nasals display some minor problems of place in final position;

continuants have problems involving all three feature classes.

A follow-up analysis of the features lost in clusters showed a similar trend for voicing (maintained in 83% of cases) and place (lost in 58% of cases), but produced a better result for manner (maintained in 68% of cases).

(g) Certain trends can be clearly identified under the heading of processes:

voicing: voiceless phones are much more vulnerable: two-thirds of the errors affect voiceless targets in singleton consonants; and there was only one correct articulation out of 19 voiceless clusters (compared with 8 out of 13 for voiced clusters). Devoicing of final consonants and in consonant clusters was within normal limits.

place: several types of articulatory substitutions could be identified:

bilabialization (*e.g.* /-t/→[-p]) 2

dentalization (*e.g.* /w-/→[θw-]) 1

labiodentalization (*e.g.* /k-/→[f-]) 18 (11 in C, 7 in CC); as half of these instances involve a movement from bilabial position, the phenomenon cannot easily be subsumed under the heading of "fronting".

alveolarization (*e.g.* /k-/→[t-]) 12 (9 in C, 3 in CC); this is "fronting"—the one apparent exception (/-p/→[-t]) being explicable (see below).

postalveolarization (*e.g.* /k-/→[s-]) 6 (2 in C, 4 in CC); this is usually "fronting", but there are two exceptions—/-s-/→[-ç-] in *sister*, and /tr-/→[ʃ-] in *trip*.

velarization (*e.g.* /p-/→[k-]) 1

glottalization (*e.g.* /-t/→[-ʔ]) 5 (2 in C, 3 in CC).

The focus on labiodental and alveolar areas is notable, and the former particularly so, in view of its rarity in normal development.

manner: stopping (*e.g.* /s-/→[t-]) 6 (4 in C, 2 in CC)

frication (*e.g.* /k-/→[f-]) 16 (8 in C, 8 in CC)

affrication (*e.g.* /-ʃ/→[-ʧ]) 9 (7 in C, 2 in CC)

nasalization (*e.g.* /ð-/→[n-]) 1 (in C)

gliding (*e.g.* /l-/→[w-]) 4 (2 in C, 2 in CC)

glottalization[42] (*e.g.* /-t/→[-tʔ]) 2 (in C)

overaspiration (*e.g.* /t-/→[tʰ]—more than would be expected for the normal realization of this phoneme) 9

weak articulation (indeterminate quality, indicated by the use of brackets in the transcription) 10

front vowel lengthening (as in *crowded, sausage* and *this*, though this may be no more than a consequence of other processes affecting final consonants).

---

[42] To be distinguished from place glottalisation above, where the *whole* of a segment is replaced by a glottal. In the present category, the two cases of medial clusters involving a glottal stop have not been analysed as glottalised.

plosive insertion (as in *horsie, running* and *sitting*).

fricative insertion (as in *sit* [sθɪtʰ]).

The last three processes are certainly uncommon in normal development, and may not occur.

(h) Harmony processes are apparent in the data, and account for some of the anomalies encountered above. There is labial assimilation in *washing* ['fɒfɪn], *animal* ['æmɪməl], *scarecrow* ['fɛəfəu], and one of the unanalyzed items, *lemon* [vəufm̩]. There is alveolar assimilation in *scarecrow* ['tɕɛətɕəu], *sleeping* ['teɪtɪn] (this explaining the apparent counter-example to fronting referred to above), and possibly in *sister* and *kitchen* as well: ['tʰɪçtə], ['tɪʃɪn]. At times, the effect is one of perseveration: for example, at one point in the session, when P is naming objects in a book, he seems to fix on [f] and is unable to stop this interfering with his normal phonological processes: see the sequence from *washing* to *shoes* in the transcription above.

(i) Syllable structure processes are not well illustrated from this sample. There is cluster reduction in *lounge* [laun:] (or so it might be argued); final consonant deletion in *noise* [nɔɪ] and possibly in *shoes* [fu:] (depending on what the target word is thought to be); there is unstressed syllable deletion in *tomatoes* (about the only thing we can say with certainty about this item!); reduplication seems to appear in *baby* ['beɪbeɪ] and certainly in *ball* [bɒ'bɔ:l]; the latter item also displays syllable addition, as does *down* [dau'nə] and possibly *blood* [b(ə)lʌd]; there are two cases of syllabic [m̩]. Stress patterning is always correct: there are 42 polysyllabic words in the sample, 39 with a strong-weak pattern. Stress in this patient does not seem to be affecting the analysis in any way.

(j) While it is not possible to estimate functional load in any precise manner, it is nonetheless evident that certain phones are being used in a way which is bound to lead to considerable overlapping and homophony. Particularly serious are:

[f]   which on occasion realizes /f-, k-, θ-, ʃ-, w-, -ʃ, pr-, tr-, kr-, sk-, -ft/
[fw]   /p-, w-, pl-, st-/
[t]   /t-, k-, s-, ?θ-, -p, -t, st-, sl-, -st, -nt-, -ks, -ns/

(k) P's repetitions of words display a great deal of free variation, far in excess of what would be expected in normal children:

/b-/ is on occasion realized as [b-] and as [b̥-].
/-t/   [-t], [-ʔ], [-p] and [-t²].
/-d/   [-ʔt] and as [-d].
/g-/   [d-] and as [g-].
/k-/   [f-] and as [s-].
/ð-/   [d-] and as [n-].
/θ-/   [f-] and as [tˢ-].
/ʧ-/   [ʤ-] and as [ʧ-].
/-m/   [-m] and as [-ɓ].
/r-/   [bʊ-] and as [ʊ-].
/sk-/ and /kr-/   [f-] and as [tɕ-].
/bl-/   [fl-] and as [b(ə)l-].

There is no particular relationship with stressed/unstressed syllables. What *is* noticeable, however, is that all of this variability involves a plosive component somewhere or other, suggesting an instability somewhat more severe than that already identified above.

These comments have excluded the very interesting *painting* sequence, as it was not entirely spontaneous: on the first occasion, T did not understand P and asked for a repetition twice. The variability does however indicate P's problem, as he tries to avoid his [f] perseveration: first of all the labiality is located in C_2, but at the expense of place and manner ([fw̥]); then, in attempting to improve manner, he loses place a little ([kv̥]), and this reinforces the [f] tendency ([fɾ]); a second attempt ([fw̥]) goes in the other direction, with place and manner maintained, but for the first time a loss of the voicing contrast ([br]). This "pendulum" effect is a fairly common observation in clinical phonological analysis.

Alex, on this account, emerges as a much more severe case of phonological disability than the initial quantification of error suggested. It is doubtful whether traditional tests could even begin to capture the complexity of his behaviour. He displays several areas of normal development (*e.g.* devoicing, cluster simplification), but also several highly abnormal processes (*e.g.* labiodentalization). He is extremely variable in certain circumstances, and his system is quite asymmetrical. Just taking the analysis this far illustrates very well the need to consider the whole range of phonological factors described earlier in this section. And there is still plenty of scope, with these data, for further kinds of phonological enquiry, which might show "deeper" levels of structural organization in his speech.

New Directions

An analysis of the kind presented above carries several important implications for clinical practice. Its "multidimensional" character allows for a sophisticated typology of disability to be established (though that is not the purpose of this chapter)[43]. It also provides several hypotheses about the nature of the deviance in P's system, and thus suggests possible paths for remedial work. Suggestions concerning the directions in which remediation might proceed have been made by Ingram (1976: 148 ff.), and also by Grunwell (1977: Ch. 7.3). In the present state of knowledge, the point that must be stressed is the need to see the problem as an individual one: the patient must be seen in his own terms, and an individual treatment programme developed, using the guidelines from phonological theory and phonological acquisition reviewed above. With so many variables involved, it is most unlikely that the treatment programme devised for one patient will automatically carry over to another. We may take Ingram's advice in general terms (*e.g.* to eliminate processes

---

[43] For more on typology, see Ingram (1976: Ch. 5) and Grunwell (1977). Cf. also Lund and Duchan's (1978) "multifaceted" approach. One of the problems of typological statements to date is that they are very restricted, through the use of only one descriptive framework. The author thus sees only what his descriptive framework lets him see, and classifications and generalisations are made accordingly. It is a permanent danger, of course, but it is as well to be aware of it.

that seem to promote instability, to reduce homonymy), but this immediately needs to be interpreted with reference to a meticulous analysis of a data sample[44]. A lot here depends on the way concomitant investigations of the patient yield hypotheses which might help to explain the nature of the deviance. If Alex had been deaf, for example, it might suggest why he was focussing so much on labial articulations. Further investigation of his auditory processing skills might bring to light particular kinds of mismatch between his perception and production ability. By providing a precise specification of the abnormality of a pronunciation system, phonological analysis can make a major contribution, not only to our understanding of linguistic disability *per se,* but also to the interaction between linguistic and non-linguistic factors underlying patients' behaviour.

---

[44] Note that the data sample used above fell midway between spontaneous conversation and predetermined production (as in an articulation test): P was free to talk about whatever he wanted in the play situation, but the range of possibilities in his universe of discourse was very much constrained by T.

3 Non-Segmental Phonology

Theoretical Background

The study of non-segmental contrastivity in language, viewed as a coherent field of study within phonology, has a much shorter academic history than has segmental phonological analysis, and consequently has so far received only limited clinical application. The field is not unfamiliar, as is clear when reference is made to such notions as "prosody", "intonation", "stress", "rhythm" and "tone of voice", all of which would be subsumed under this heading. What is novel is the integration of all of these effects within a single framework, and the systematic analysis of the relationship between these effects and other levels of linguistic analysis, especially grammar and semantics[1]. The importance and complexity of this field of study has clearly emerged in the process, and its neglect in the routine investigation of speech and hearing disability is more noticeable and regrettable as a result.

"Non-segmental" (or "suprasegmental") phonology, as its name suggests, is usually defined in a negative way—what is left *after* we have studied the segmental sounds in a language, *i.e.* the vowels, consonants, and their combinations as syllables and syllable-sequences. More positively, we can define non-segmental phonology as dealing with any linguistically contrastive sound effect which cannot be described by reference to a single (phonemic) segment, but which either (i) continues over a stretch of utterance (minimally, a syllable) or (ii) requires reference to segments in different parts of the utterance. Examples of the former are utterances spoken louder, higher or slower than usual, where the contrast affects the meaning. Examples of the latter include whispered speech (only the voiced sounds being affected) and labialized speech (*e.g.* in using extra lip-rounding on certain sounds when talking to babies and animals). While technically only a selection of sounds is

---

[1] For a historical review of the field, see Crystal (1969: Ch. 2). This book, along with its sequel (1975), provides the detailed account of the theoretical frame of reference used in this chapter. The sections below dealing with language acquisition are based on two further papers, (1978, 1979b).

affected by such contrasts as whisper and labialization, the overall impression is of a single phonological and semantic effect. The two types of effects are thus grouped together for most purposes.

An essential phrase in the above definition is "linguistically contrastive": we are dealing only with sound contrasts which systematically realize a set of meaning differences, for speakers of the language. There are of course many non-segmental variations in a person's voice which do not do this—tones of voice and levels of speech which relate only to the speaker's physiological state or personal preferences—and these a phonological study would aim to exclude (just as it would in analyzing the segmental phonemic system). In the clearest cases, there is no problem. A phonologist would not be particularly interested in the high pitch or huskiness which permanently characterized a speaker, and which thus set him apart from other speakers of the language. On the other hand, he is certainly interested in the way in which speakers of the language use the distinction between falling and rising pitch, or between whispered and non-whispered speech, to make contrasts in meaning. A particular focus of theoretical attention in recent years has been on the indeterminate cases—those non-segmental effects whose linguistic status is difficult to establish, but which are not wholly idiosyncratic either. Such cases constitute an important problem area in clinical investigation (see p. 76). The main focus of this chapter, however, will be on those cases of non-segmental contrastivity whose linguistic status is in no doubt, and where problems of expression and comprehension cause major difficulties in a patient's intelligibility.

We can summarize this issue by constructing a model of non-segmental vocal effect in which a clear distinction is made between phonetic and phonological description. General phonetics, first of all, provides us with a classification of features of sound into *attributes* of sound sensation, three of which are traditionally taken as central:

pitch, perceived in terms of "high" vs. "low";
loudness, perceived in terms of "loud" vs. "soft";
duration, perceived in terms of "long" vs. "short".

More complex effects, based on combinations of pitch, loudness and durational characteristics, are usually summarized under the heading of *rhythm*, perceived in terms of "rhythmic" vs. "arhythmic" speech. The importance of *silence* in helping to identify salient features of utterance must also be recognized. All other phonetic effects in speech can be grouped under the heading of *timbre* which, because of its multi-dimensional properties, is not capable of perceptual analysis in terms of a single scale. It subsumes the whole range of laryngeal, pharyngeal, nasal and oral non-segmental effects other than those described above, *e.g.* whisper, huskiness, nasal resonance. The distinction between effects of *phonation* and those of *resonance* is one traditional way of making a subclassification under this heading[2].

To avoid confusion, the terminology of phonological analysis should be different from that used in the phonetic description of these effects. The linguistic use of

---

[2] As in speech pathology, *e.g.* Travis (1957: Ch. 22), Greene (1964). For the phonetic theory underlying the distinction, see Catford (1977). It should be noted that the notion of phonation is also applicable to pitch and loudness features, and is thus less useful for present purposes, where a distinction between these and timbre effects is being maintained.

pitch, accordingly, will be referred to as *intonation* (this being a fairly standard definition for this term). The linguistic use of loudness will be referred to as *stress* (though some texts refer to *accent* here). The linguistic use of duration (other than that encountered in segmental phonology, *e.g.* vowel or consonant length) will be referred to as *tempo*. The linguistic use of rhythm will be referred to as *rhythmicality*. The linguistic use of silence will be referred to as *pause*. Each of these notions is viewed as a system of contrasts (the "intonation system", the "stress system", etc.). The usual term to characterize this whole area within non-segmental phonology is *prosody* (the "prosodic systems" of language), though both narrower and broader definitions of this term will be encountered. The linguistic use of the remaining characteristics of speech will be referred to as *paralanguage* (the "paralinguistic systems" of language). Research has made little headway in sub-classifying the range of effects operating within this heading. One distinction which will be useful is to group laryngeal and pharyngeal effects together, in their linguistic use, as *voice qualifiers* (*e.g.* the use of whisper, huskiness, creaky voice, and so on, when used in a controlled way by the speaker for semantic effect). The remaining nasal/oral effects, in their linguistic use, are usually identified using the process affix *-ization* (*e.g.* labialization, nasalization, velarization).

These distinctions between phonetic and phonological modes of description can be summarized in the form of a table (Table 9), to which has been appended the relevant clinical nomenclature to be used later in this chapter. It is particularly important to note the difference between the phonetic notion of *dysprosody*, taken from the literature on voice disorders, and the phonological notion of *prosodic disability*, introduced to handle the range of clinical problems presented below.

Table 9. *Phonetic and phonological analysis of non-segmental vocal effects*

	DISORDERS OF	
	phonetic attributes	phonological systems
DYSPROSODY	pitch	intonation
	loudness	stress
	duration	tempo
	rhythm	rhythmicality
	silence	pause
DYS-PHONIA / **timbre** — laryngeal effects		voice qualifiers
pharyngeal effects		
RESO-NANCE — nasal/oral effects		*-izations*
	VOICE	NON-SEGMENTAL PHONOLOGY

Right-hand vertical labels: **PROSODIC DISABILITY** (intonation, stress, tempo, rhythmicality, pause); **PARALINGUISTIC DISABILITY** (voice qualifiers, *-izations*).

Misconceptions

The intuitive significance we attach to non-segmental phonological effect, reflected in such catch-phrases as "It's not what he said, but the way that he said it", is a major motivation for its formal study. We have only to consider its role in the expression of our attitudes, or in the organization of our grammatical expression (where it has been called the "punctuation of speech"), to see how fundamental and pervasive a phenomenon it is. Perhaps because of the difficulty involved in subjecting it to analysis, several misconceptions about its character have developed, which it is important to expose, if a clinically useful analytic procedure is to emerge.

The first fallacy is the view that units of non-segmental form represent in a one-to-one manner units of syntactic or semantic function. A common example of this way of thinking is the claim that in English intonation the change from a falling to a rising tone corresponds to a grammatical or speech-act distinction between statement and question. It may even be believed that the rising tone "expresses" the meaning of question. However, there is no isomorphism between such variables. Several adult studies have shown that rising intonations signal a great deal more than questions, and questions are expounded by a great deal more than rising intonations[3]. Interpretations depend on several factors, of which the lexical, grammatical, non-verbal (especially kinesic), and situational contexts are the most relevant. We also have to be extremely careful about the use of such terms as "question". If the term is already being used in a formal syntactic sense (covering the use of question-words and subject-verb inversion in English, for example), then it would be misleading to use it for the semantic effect produced by an intonational change. To say that *he's còming/→he's cóming/* is a change from "statement" to "question" may seem plausible at first, but when we consider the identical intonational substitution on the sentence-pair *what's he dòing/what's he dóing,* the usage becomes confusing. We could hardly say that the "question" has become a "question". Rather, we need to talk in terms of the addition of "questioning", "puzzled", "surprised", etc. elements of attitudinal meaning. The problem is not a grammatical one; it is one of identifying and delimiting the emotional nuances involved. An identical problem would affect any analysis involving speech-act terminology (*cf.* p. 201).

Another reason why a one-to-one analysis of non-segmental form and meaning is unjustified stems from the way in which certain features have been selected for study, at the expense of other areas of non-segmental phonology. Intonation and stress are the main features involved, and while the focus on these systems can be justified, in view of their importance in communication, they should not be studied to the exclusion of the other formal systems. Ultimately, we have to adopt an integrated view, seeing intonation as but one exponent of meaning, along with the other prosodic and paralinguistic features of language. From a formal point of view, the distinction between intonation and these other features is clear; but from a semantic point of view, it is often irrelevant, a given "meaning" (such as sarcasm, or parenthesis) being signalled by a range of prosodic and paralinguistic features, pitch being just one. Over the first two years of life, and often in adult clinical contexts,

---

[3] For example, Fries (1964), Crystal (1969: Ch. 1). For speech-act, see p. 201.

non-intonational features (such as variations in loudness, duration, rhythmicality) are of considerable importance in the expression of meaning. This is so not only for attitudes, but also for grammatical patterning, where any adequate phonological discovery procedure for sentences at around 18 months (see below) has to refer to far more than sequences of pitch contour and pause. Two lexical items could be linked in several ways, *e.g.* both being pronounced with extra pitch height, loudness, longer duration, marked rhythm, or with some shared paralinguistic feature—all of which would make the use of pitch contour and pause less significant. Only these last two features are ever given systematic attention in the literature on early syntax in assessment and remediation, however.

Of all the non-segmental systems referred to above, it is intonation which has attracted most attention. This is as it should be, for, as we shall see, the intonation system has a much more complex formal organization, and a much subtler potential for conveying semantic distinctions, than any other system. A major misconception thus concerns the tendency to oversimplify the phenomenon, by viewing intonation as if it were a single, homogeneous phenomenon, formally and functionally, as is implied by such phrases as "the intonation shows . . .", "intonation is an early development" and "intonation disorder" (see further below). The oversimplification can be seen both with reference to the formal analysis of intonation and with reference to its functional role.

Intonational Form

Although terminology varies, almost all theories of intonation recognize certain core characteristics of the intonation systems of English.

(i) Firstly, a basic distinction is made between pitch *direction* and pitch *range*. A pitch may fall, rise, stay level, or perform some combination of these things in a given phonological unit (*e.g.* falling-rising on a syllable), and these directional *tones* provide one system of intonational contrastivity. But any of these tones may be varied in terms of pitch range, which is seen as a separate system of contrasts. A tone may be uttered at an average pitch level for a speaker, higher/lower than his norm (to various degrees), or widened/narrowed to various degree (the ultimate degree of narrowing being, of course, monotone).

(ii) The intonation contrasts perceived in connected speech are not all of the same kind, and some carry more linguistic information about the organization and interpretation of the utterance than others. The primary organizational distinction is the analysis of speech into *tone-units* (also known as *tone-groups* or *pitch contours*). A tone-unit is a finite set of pitch movements, formally identifiable as a coherent configuration, or contour, and used systematically with reference to other levels of language (especially syntax). Tone-units provide the most general level of organization that can be imposed upon non-segmental data, equivalent in status to the notion of "sentence" in grammatical analysis. For example, the normal tone-unit segmentation of the utterances

when he comes/tell him I'm out/

John came at three/Mary came at four/and Mark came at five/
is as indicated by the slant lines. In general, the assignment of the tone-unit
boundary seems motivated by syntactic reasons, *e.g.* to mark the boundary between
clauses (see further, Crystal, 1975: Ch. 1). We might accordingly expect such a fundamental notion to be an early characteristic of prosodic development, and tone
unit disturbances to be an important characteristic of prosodic disability (see
below).

(iii) Given the analysis of utterances into tone-units, the next decision is to identify
the prosodic feature which seems to carry the next most important kind of linguistic
contrastivity, namely *tonicity*—the placement of maximum prominence on a given
syllable (or, occasionally, on more than one syllable). This is primarily a matter of
pitch movement, but extra loudness is involved, and duration and silence may be
used to heighten the contrast between what precedes and follows. The prominent,
or *tonic* syllable may be seen capitalized in the utterances

it was a *very* nice party/ vs.
it was a very *nice* party/ vs.
it *was* a very nice party/.

This was the focus of most of the discussion on intonation in the context of generative grammar, where the aim was to demonstrate that tonicity had a syntactic function[4]. The alternative view (maintained below) is that the factors governing tonic
placement are primarily semantic (*e.g.* the signalling of new information in context),
although it is possible to find cases where tonic placement is obligatory or dis-
allowed for syntactic reasons, *e.g.*

*it was a nice party/
*he's going/ isn't *he*/.

(iv) Given an analysis of an utterance into tone-units and tonic syllables, the next
most noticeable prosodic characteristic is the specific direction-range of the tonic
syllable, *e.g.* whether the tone of the syllable is high-falling-wide, low-rising-narrow,
etc. These features seem to signal primarily attitudinal information, although certain tonal contrasts can expound grammatical contrasts, *e.g.* utterance end vs.
continuation, as in

would you like béer/ or whískey/ or tèa/

compared with

would you like béer/ or whískey/ or téa/.

In written English, the former would be concluded with a period, the latter probably with a dash or dots (. . .). Another example is the "asking" vs. "telling" distinction
in tag-questions, as in

you're còming/ áren't you/
you're còming/ àren't you/.

---

[4] See, for example, Bresnan (1971) and Bolinger's (1972) reply; the debate is reviewed in Crystal
(1975: Ch. 1).

Different systems of intonation analysis recognize different numbers and types of these "nuclear" tones (*i.e.* they constitute the "nucleus" of the tone-unit). The system used in the present book (*cf.* Crystal 1969: 210 ff.) makes a threefold division of nuclear tones into *simple, complex* and *compound* types. Simple tones are the three possibilities of unidirectional pitch movement: *falling, rising* and *level.* Complex tones are those nuclei where there is change in the direction of the pitch movement within a syllable, the main categories in English being the *falling-rising* and the *rising-falling* tones. Compound tones are combinations of certain of the above tones used on different syllables within a tone-unit, but acting as if they were a single tone, *e.g. fall-plus-rise, rise-plus-fall.* Examples of each of these categories, along with one possible interpretation in terms of attitude, are:

he's a fòol/ (neutral; matter-of-fact statement)
he's a fóol/ (with a high start to the rise; questioning or surprised)
he's a fōol/ (routine, bored)
he's a fǒol/ (warning, caution)
he's a fôol/ (definite)
hè's a fóol/ (extra emphasis on *he,* along with above meaning)
hé's a fòol/ (extra emphasis on *he,* along with above meaning)

The frequency of occurrence of these tones in adult conversational data (according to Crystal, 1969) should be noted:

\ 51.2%   / 20.8%   \/ 8.5%   \+/ 7.7%   /\ 5.2%   − 4.9%   /+\ 1.7%

An important point is that one out of every two tones is simple falling. A further classification into *high* vs. *low* pitch range is also possible for each tone (*e.g.* low falling vs. high falling, low rising vs. high rising).

(v) Other pitch features of the tone-unit may then be decided, the most important being the height of the first prominent syllable, the change-points within the overall contour, and the height of any unstressed syllables.

Intonational Function

In contrast to the traditional view, in which intonation is seen as the means of expressing attitude and emotion, and little else, it is possible to distinguish at least five roles for this system in English.

(i) The *grammatical* role is primary. Here, intonation, along with certain other non-segmental contrasts (such as rhythm and pause), is being used to mark the demarcation and integration of grammatical structures, such as sentence and clause. More specifically, intonation may be used to signal a contrast, the terms of which would be conventionally recognized as morphological or syntactic in the rest of a grammar, *e.g.* singular/plural, present/past, or positive/negative. These contrasts are common in tone languages, but they may also be found in English, where tone-units, tonic syllables and tones can perform a grammatical role of this kind, as in the distinction between restrictive and non-restrictive relative clauses:

my bróther/ who's abróad/ wrote me a lètter/(*i.e.* I have one brother)
my brother who's abróad/ wrote me a lètter/(*i.e.* I have more than one brother).

In a secondary sense, intonation may also be used to reinforce a grammatical distinction already overt in word order or morphology, as in the obligatory tone pattern on parallel coordinations, such as

I liked the *green* dress/ and she liked the *red* one/.

(ii) The *semantic* role of intonation subsumes both the organization of meaning in a discourse, and the reflection of the speaker's presuppositions about subject-matter or context. Under the first heading, the highlighting of certain parts of an utterance is often carried out by intonational means (and analyzed in terms of such distinctions as "given" vs. "new" information, or the "focus" on marked patterns of word order)[5]. This includes the use of intonation to emphasize the relatively unfamiliar item in a sequence, as Bolinger (1972) argues in his critique of the generative account of tonicity (with reference to such contrasts as *clothes to wash* vs. *clothes to burn).* Under the second heading is included the interactional use of intonation, as when the focus on a specific lexical item presupposes a specific context immediately preceding, *e.g.*

there were *three* books on the table/

implying a context in which the number of books was in doubt (*cf.* Chomsky, 1970).
(iii) The *attitudinal* function of intonation is usually distinguished from (ii) above, on similar grounds to the classical distinction between denotation and connotation. Personal attitudes and emotions are signalled concerning the subject matter or context of an utterance, *e.g.* anger, puzzlement, surprise. It is unclear how far such emotions use prosodic features specific to a language, and how far they rely on universal characteristics of emotional expression (*cf.* Bolinger, 1964). Their linguistic status is thus often somewhat indeterminate.
(iv) The *psychological* function of intonation is evident from the several experiments which have shown that certain prosodic variables (especially tonicity) have an important role to play in controlling performance, *e.g.* in recall, paraphrase, comprehension and imitation. Varying the prosodic input does influence response patterns, as has been shown both for normal children and adults, and in the context of disability[6]. For example, there is a strong tendency for lexical items containing tonic syllables to be more readily recalled than those which do not.
(v) The *social* function of intonation signals information about the sociolinguistic characteristics of the speaker, such as his sex, class, professional status, and so on (see Crystal, 1975: Ch. 5). The importance of this function in facilitating social interaction in dialogue is being increasingly recognized, *e.g.* when the intonation of a stimulus sentence prompts someone to respond, or implies that no further comment is needed. Several studies have now been made which show the significance of prosody in the variety of language adults use in talking to children, and varying

---

[5] See Quirk, *et al.* (1972: Ch. 14), Halliday (1967–1968).
[6] For children, see du Preez (1974); adults, Cutler (1976), Leonard (1973); disability, Goodglass, Fodor, and Schulhoff (1967), Stark, Poppen, and May (1967).

forms of intonation in relation to differing social roles have been described in young children[7].

In short, there are evident grounds for a more sophisticated awareness of both the form and function of non-segmental patterns when commencing the analysis of early child speech or speech disability in children and adults. In particular, being aware of the main issues of theoretical debate in the literature on normal adult intonation (such as the relevance of "emic" models of analysis, or the relationship between intonation and syntax) would provide a perspective that might forestall the premature construction of theories of acquisition or language breakdown, where non-segmental phonology is often made to take a weight it cannot legitimately bear (see below). The limitations of empirical research should also be borne in mind. In fact, as almost the whole of this research has focussed on intonation, it is difficult to make other than anecdotal observations about the clinical relevance of other non-segmental systems. The attention paid to intonation in the rest of this chapter, therefore, is solely a consequence of the bias of the research to date, and does not imply that other systems are uninvolved in the assessment and remediation of language disability.

The Acquisition of Intonation

Given the limited empirical study which has taken place (almost entirely within the first two years of life), talk in terms of clear stages of development in this area may well be premature. On the other hand, the evidence which is available does agree so far on several points, hence the following progression. Five stages can be distinguished, of which the last two are particularly important.

Stage I. There have been many studies of the prelinguistic antecedents of prosodic features, usually under the heading of "infant vocalization". On the whole, these studies recognize a period of biologically determined vocalizations[8], and a period of differentiated vocalizations which permit general attitudinal interpretation only (*e.g.* "pleasure", "recognition"). Systematic variation in these vocalizations can be ascribed to such factors as the baby's sex or environment. There seems to be little difference in their physical characteristics and attitudinal function across languages. This stage, from birth until around 6 months, is reviewed in detail in Crystal (1975: Ch. 8).

Stage II. The first sign of anything linguistic emerging is the awareness of prosodic contrasts in adult utterances directed to the child. This has long been known to be present in children from around 2 to 3 months, as the reports in Lewis (1951) testify. But this literature is rather anecdotal, and experimental studies are lacking which

---

[7] For example, Sachs and Devin (1976) report the use of higher pitch and wider intonation patterns when 3—5 year-old children talk to a baby or doll, or role-play a baby. For the characteristics of intonation in adult speech to children, see Blount and Padgug (1977), Garnica (1977), Ferguson (1977).

[8] For example, the "basic cry" pattern, underlying hunger, pain, etc. states, described in Wolff (1969: 82). For a recent phonetic description, see Stark, Rose and McLagen (1975).

attempt to separate prosody from other semiotic features of the stimuli, and to identify the roles individual prosodic features might play within the adult utterance, *e.g.* whether pitch or loudness are discriminated first. Kaplan (1970), for example, demonstrated that a contrast between falling and rising tones could be discriminated from around 4 months, but it is difficult to be sure of the relative roles pitch and loudness had to play.

Stage III. The increasingly varied vocalizations of children around 6 months have begun to be studied in detail, using a combination of acoustic, articulatory and auditory criteria, and it is possible to isolate a wide range of non-segmental parameters in terms of which the patterns of crying, babbling, etc., can be classified. Stark, Rose and McLagen (1975), for example, cite breath direction, pitch, loudness, and several kinds of glottal and supraglottal constriction; within pitch, they distinguish contrasts of range, direction and continuity.

Gradually, these non-segmental features come to resemble prosodic patterns of the mother tongue—from as early as 6 months, according to most scholars (see the review in Crystal 1975: 136). Initially, the resemblance is only hinted at, by the occasional use of a language-specific prosodic characteristic within a relatively long stretch of non-linguistic vocalization. Such instances are very striking when they occur on a tape, as they stand out as something much more familiar, discrete and transcribable than the general background of utterance. Increasingly, at this time, babbling patterns become shorter and phonetically more stable: accordingly, when a babbled utterance of only one or two syllables is used in conjunction with a language-specific prosodic feature, the result is going to be very much like an attempt at a meaningful utterance. Such combinations are quickly focused on by parents, who will comment on what they think the baby is "saying", often providing lexical glosses. It is, however, very difficult to be precise about the nature of the development at this stage. To say that a language-specific feature has been detected is to say very little: recognition of language-specificity involves both phonetic notions (*e.g.* the "community voice quality" or characteristic "twang" of a language) and phonological notions (*e.g.* the selection of contrasts which produce an identifiable accent), and it is by no means clear how to distinguish these in the child's vocalization at this stage. The boundary area between the phonetic use of pitch, loudness, etc., during the first 6 months of life, and the phonological use of pitch that has emerged by around a year, is totally uncharted territory (*cf.* Olney and Scholnick, 1976).

Stage IV. However the transition to phonology takes place, it is evident that learned patterns of prosodic behaviour are characteristic of the output of the child during the second half of the first year. These patterns can be studied both formally and functionally. From the formal viewpoint, the increasingly determinate and systematic character of these patterns is readily statable: a configuration of features is involved, using primarily pitch, rhythm and pause. This configuration has been variously labelled a prosodic "envelope", "matrix" or "frame"[9]. Lenneberg (1967: p. 279) describes the process thus:

"The first feature of natural language to be discernible in a child's babbling is contour of intonation. Short sound sequences are produced that may have neither any

---

[9] See Bruner (1975: 10), Dore (1975). Weir (1962) also talks about the splitting up of utterances into "sentence-like chunks", at this stage.

determinable meaning nor definable phoneme structure, but they can be proffered with recognizable intonation such as occurs in questions, exclamations or affirmations. The linguistic development of utterance does not seem to begin with a composition of individual, independently movable items *but as a whole tonal pattern*. With further development, this whole becomes differentiated into component parts . . " (my emphasis).

The important point is that these primitive units have both a segmental and a prosodic dimension, but it is the latter which is the more stable, and the more readily elicited. In one child studied at Reading, aged 1;2, the phrase *all-gone*, regularly said by the parent after each meal, was actually rehearsed by using the prosodic component only: the child hummed the intonation of the phrase first, viz. ⌐ ⌐, only then attempting the whole, producing an accurate intonation but only approximate segments ([ʌʔdʌ]). The phrase could be easily elicited after any meal, but it was not until a month had gone by that the child's segmental output became as stable as his prosodic. Menn's Jacob (1976: 195 ff.) also produced "proto-words" with a distinctive prosodic shape—the ones reported being used at 1;4 for a peekaboo game, an item with demonstrative function, and, later, a name-elicitor. Dore (1975) refers to the formally isolable, repeated, and situationally specific patterns observed at this stage as "phonetically consistent forms", whose "protophonemic" segmental character is complemented by a distinctive prosody, which is the more stable.

From a functional point of view, these prosodically delimited units can be interpreted in several ways—semantic, syntactic and social "explanations" have all been mooted. The latter view is perhaps the most widely held: here, prosody is seen as a means of signalling joint participation in an action sequence shared by parent and child. This view, emphasized particularly by Bruner (1975), is part of a developmental theory wherein vocalization is seen as one component in a communication activity alongside such non-vocal behaviour as reaching and eye-contact. In a peekaboo game, for instance, both the utterance and the activity of hiding-and-reappearing are obligatory, interdependent components (as the absurdity of attempting to play the game without either indicates). And when adults play these games, the lexical character of the utterance regularly varies ("Peep-bo", "See you", etc.) whereas the prosodic features display much less variation. Another example is in action sequences such as nuzzling the child or jumping him up and down, where there are parallel prosodic patterns. The development of "turn-taking" (see p. 198), either between parent and child (Snow, 1977) or between children (Keenan, 1974) also involves prosodic delimitation and interdependence. One Keenan twin, for example, would regularly take the prosodic character of the other's utterance and "play" with it. Another child, studied at Reading, marked the end of a jargon sequence with a distinctive two-syllable pitch movement (• ⌐), which was openly described by his parents as "their cue to speak".

Several attempts have been made to describe the social or "pragmatic" functions of such utterances, especially using the metalanguage of speech-act analysis (see p. 201). Dore, for example (1975: 31 ff.), argues that prosodic features provide crucial evidence for the development of speech-acts. Primitive speech-acts are said to contain a "rudimentary referring expression" (lexical items) and a "primitive force indicating device" ("typically an intonation pattern", p. 31), as in labelling, requesting and calling. The distinction between referent and intention is pivotal: "whereas the child's one word communicates the notion he has in mind, his prosodic pattern indicates his intention with regard to that notion" (p. 32). Likewise, Menn says about Jacob (1976: 26-7), "he ... consistently used certain particular intentions, so we can ascribe meaning to his use of those contours[10]".

As an alternative to a social approach, it is possible to see these prosodic frames—or primitive tone-units, to use the terminology above—primarily as having a formal or grammatical role. Bruner, for instance (1975), at one point describes the function of these frames as "placeholders": a mode of communication (such as a demand, or a question) is established using prosody, and primitive lexical items are then added. In a stretch of jargon, from around 12 months, it is often the case that we will recognize a word within the otherwise unintelligible utterance (cf. also several of the utterances in Keenan [1974]). And the transitional stage between one- and two-element sentences also contains uninterpretable phonetic forms which may perhaps be interpreted as remnants of a primitive prosodic frame[11]. Dore et al. (1976) in fact suggest seven transitional stages at this point:

(i) prosodically un-isolable, nonphonemic units ("prelinguistic babbling");
(ii) prosodically isolable, nonphonemic patterns ("prelinguistic jargon");
(iii) prosodically isolable, nonphonemic units ("phonetically consistent forms");
(iv) conventional phonemic units ("words");
(v) word plus "empty" phonetic forms in single prosodic pattern ("presyntactic devices");
(vi) chained conventional phonemic units forming separate intonation patterns ("successive single-word utterances");
(vii) prosodically complex patterns ("patterned speech").

The phonological and phonetic details of the development of these frames into determinate tone-units with a definable internal structure are, however, not at all clear, so little empirical work having been done. In particular, it is unclear whether tonicity or tonal contrastivity develops first, or whether they emerge simultaneously. The suggestion that the development is simultaneous is based on the observation that tonicity contrasts are early evidenced in jargon sequences (in which sequences of rhythms are built up which resemble the intonational norms of connected speech), whereas tone contrasts are early heard in the use of lexical items as single-word sentences. Menn, for instance, finds her child's semantic control of certain tones on "babble carriers" and their contrastive use on words to be almost simultaneous (1976: 186). If we ignore jargon, however, as being both less central to communicative development and less systematic in its patterning, then it would seem that tone develops before tonicity. Polysyllabic lexical items at this stage tend to have fixed tonic placement (Atkinson-King, 1973), though they may vary in

---

[10] The difficulty with all such approaches is empirical verification of the notion of "intention". As has been argued in other areas of child language, the fact that parents interpret their children's prosody systematically is no evidence for ascribing their belief patterns to the child's intuition. At best, we can argue, as does Menn (1976: 192), that "consideration of adult interpretation of intonation contour on vocalisations does give us information about what the child *conveys*, if not what he/she *intends*". See further Crystal (1979: 41).

[11] Cf. Dore, Franklin, Miller and Ramer (1976: 26), Bloom (1973).

terms of pitch direction and range, *e.g. dàda* (said as daddy enters the room), *dáda* (said when a noise was heard outside, at the time when daddy was expected). Of the two, range seems to become contrastive before direction, especially high vs. low, but also wide vs. narrow. Most of the contrasts noted by Halliday (1975), for example, involve range rather than direction—mid vs. low first, later high—*e.g.* the distinction between seeking and finding, signalled in his child by high vs. mid-low range, from around 1;3. Eight pitch range variations are in fact used by Halliday in his transcription (very high, high, mid high, mid, mid low, low, wide, narrow), as well as four directions (level, fall, rise, rise-fall). The notion of high vs. low register is discussed further in Konopczynski (1975), and a great deal of early child data can be interpreted in this way[12].

An analysis of early tonal development—the contrasts involving both direction and range—suggests the following eight steps:

(i) Initially, the child uses only *falling* patterns. Menn states that—except for imitations of adult rises—her child used rises on words only after these words were first used with falls (195). Halliday's range contrasts are all on falling tones (148).

(ii) The first contrast is *falling* vs. *level* tones (high level in Halliday [150-1]), the level tone often being accompanied by other prosodic or paralinguistic features, *e.g.* falsetto, length, loudness variations.

(iii) This is followed by *falling* vs. *high rising* tones, the latter being used in a variety of contexts. Menn's special study of rising tones brought to light a large number of contexts between 1;1 and 1;4, including offering, requesting, attention-getting, and several "curiosity" noises (*e.g.* when peering). Several of these notions, moreover, are complex—for example, "request" includes requests for help, recognition, permission to obtain an object, etc., all of which are distinguishable in the situation (186 ff., 198-9). The "natural" distinction between fall and rise is characterized as "demanding" vs. "requesting/offering" (193). Halliday's high rises are first used in association with falls as compound tones (151).

(iv) The next contrast is between *falling* and *high falling* tones, the latter especially in contexts of surprise, recognition, insistence, greetings. Halliday reports a high falling contrast between 1;1 and 1;3, and further distinguishes a mid fall.

(v) A contrast between *rising* and *high rising* tones follows: the Reading study suggested a particular incidence of high rises especially in playful, anticipatory contexts. Menn notes the latter mainly in "intensification" contexts: the child gets no response to an utterance with a low rise, and repeats the utterance with a wider contour—the extra height, according to Menn, is the "essential information-carrying feature" (193-4). Halliday's mid vs. high rise emerges at 1;3 to 1;4.

(vi) The next contrast is between *falling* and *high rising-falling* tones, the latter being used in emphatic contexts, *e.g.* of achievement (as in saying *thêre,* when an extra brick is placed on a pile) or impressiveness (*e.g. bùs* vs. *bûs,* the former being used by one child to refer to "any" vehicle, the latter to a *real* bus). Menn reports a mid-high-low

---

[12] For example, Keenan (1974), Menn (1976). The subsequent analysis of development is based on a synthesis of Menn (1976) and Halliday (1975), to which page references are given, work on the acquisition of tone languages (Hyman and Schuh 1974, Li and Thompson 1977, Tse 1978) and a study by the author.

contour at 1;4; Halliday has a similar contrast from as early as 1;1, but regularly from 1;3.

(vii) Next appears a contrast between *rising* and *falling-rising* tones, the latter especially in warning contexts, presumably reflecting the *be câreful* pattern common in adults; *cf.* Halliday (154), between 1;4 and 1;6.

(viii) Among later contrasts to appear is that between high and low rising-falling tones, especially in play contexts.

These features appear on isolated lexical items to begin with, and for a while cannot be distinguished from prosodic idioms (*i.e.* invariant prosodic patterns accompanying a fixed lexicogrammatical structure, as in a nursery-rhyme line). Only later, when the same lexical item is used with different prosodic characteristics, can we talk with confidence about the patterns being systemic and productive. At this point, too, the tones come to be used in juxtaposition, producing the "contrastive syntagmas" and prosodic "substitution games" reported by several analysts[13].

Particularly with the intonational studies, we must remember that the situational interpretations used cannot be taken at face value. In much the same way as has been argued for syntax and segmental phonology[14], it is necessary to free the mind from the constraints of adult language analyses, where situational notions such as "question", "request", "permission", etc. are normal. As already argued, it is insufficient to show that adults can differentiate these patterns and give them consistent interpretations, as several studies have succeeded in doing (*e.g.* Menyuk and Bernholz, 1969): as Bloom points out (1973: 19), this is no evidence of contrastivity for the children. Detailed analysis of both the phonetic form and the accompanying context of utterance, moreover, readily brings to light instances of contrastivity which have no counterpart in the adult language. Halliday's child, for example, for a while used rising tones for all "pragmatic" utterances (those requiring a response, in his terms), and falling tones for all "mathetic" utterances (those not requiring a response [29, 52]). Menn's child between 1;0 and 1;8 used a class of non-adult rising tones, *e.g.* between 1;1 and 1;3 he used a low rising tone (peak 450 Hz) to "institute or maintain social interaction" (the "adult-as-social-partner" function) and a high rising tone (peak 550 Hz) for "instrumental use of the adult" ("obtaining an object or service") (184). In the case of a child studied at Reading, the falling-rising tone was initially used only in smiling-face contexts, with a generally "playful" meaning, and never to express doubt or opposition, as it frequently does, with frowning or neutral face, in adults.

These are all examples of a relatively familiar form conveying an unfamiliar function. The converse also applies. Throughout this stage of development, the range of phonetic exponents of the prosodic frame increases markedly, to include contrasts in loudness, duration, muscular tension and rhythmicality, not all of which are used in the adult language. At around 1 year, contrasts have been observed between loud and soft, drawled and short, tense and lax, and rhythmic and arhythmic utterances. Halliday (1975) noted, in addition to the pitch direction and range contrasts already described, several other prosodic and paralinguistic

13 For example, Weir (1972), Carlson and Anisfeld (1969: 118), Keenan (1974: 172, 178).
14 For example, Howe (1976), Lenneberg (1967).

features: slow, long, short, loud; sung, squeak, frictional and glottalized. Contrastivity involving two or more non-segmental parameters emerges, *e.g.* the use of a low, tense, soft, husky, spasmodic voice (a "dirty snigger"). Carlson and Anisfeld (1969) distinguish loud and soft, and staccato and drawled articulations, amongst others. Other examples are the use of marked labialization, falsetto voice for whole utterances, and spasmodic articulations (lip trills, "raspberries", etc.). It is regrettable that a more comprehensive phonetic description of this stage of development does not exist.

Stage V. Tonic contrastivity (or "contrastive stress", as this area is often called) appears as sentences get more complex syntagmatically, with the appearance of two-word utterances at around 1;6[15]. The general developmental process seems clear. Lexical items which have appeared independently as single-element utterances, marked thus by pitch and pause, are brought into relationship (whether syntactic or semantic need not concern this chapter). At first, the lexical items retain their non-segmental autonomy, with the pause between them becoming reduced, *e.g. dàddy/ . gàrden/.* Often, long sequences of these items appear, especially repetitively, *e.g. dàddy/ gàrden/ sèe/ dáddy/ dáddy/ gàrden/ dàddy/ gàrden/ sèe/.* (Such sequences, of course, defy analysis in terms of the usually cited grammatical-semantic relations.) The next step is the prosodic integration of sequences of items, usually two, into a single tone-unit. How general a process this is is unclear, but in several English combinations studied, it was the case that one item became more prominent than the other; it was louder, and had an identifiable pitch movement. There was a rhythmic relationship between the two items (anticipating the iso-chronous rhythm of English), and intervening pauses became less likely in repeated versions of lexical sequences. This step is considered to be of central theoretical importance, because it is claimed to be the main means employed by the child for formally expressing grammatical-semantic relations within a sentence—"the simple concatenation under one utterance contour of the words which interact to create a compositional meaning that is different from the meanings of the two words in sequence" (Brown, 1973: 182). Unfortunately, the process of concatenation is not so "simple" as Brown suggests. All the following sequences have been observed (·, -, – referring to pauses of increasing length):

dàddy/ -- èat/	dáddy/ -- èat/
dàddy/ - èat/	dáddy/ - èat/
dàddy/ . èat/	dáddy/ . èat/
dàddy/ èat/	dáddy/ èat/
daddy èat/	dáddy eat/
dàddy eat/	dáddy èat/[16]

It is accordingly often difficult to decide whether we are dealing with one sentence or two—especially if the context is unclear, *e.g.* the child is looking at a picture. In the

---

[15] See Bloom (1973), Clark, Hutcheson and Van Buren (1974: 49). A single-word polysyllable in principle allows for a contrast *(e.g. DAddy* vs. *dadDY),* but there is no evidence of such forms at this stage (Atkinson-King 1973).

[16] A compound tone-unit, such as this, is in fact singled out by some analysts *(e.g.* du Preez 1974) as an important transitional stage.

above example, the subject-verb relation, so "obvious" to the adult observer, may motivate one set of decisions. However, in the following examples (each of which may be found with any of the above twelve patterns), the "compositional meanings" are by no means so clear:

dáddy/ càr/   (child is looking at daddy in a car)
dáddy/ mùmmy/   (child is looking at a photograph of both)
dáddy/ nò/   (daddy has left the room)
dáddy/ dàddy/   (said while being held by daddy)

Non-segmental phonology, it seems, cannot be used by the analyst as a primitive discovery procedure for semantics or grammar—just as it cannot be in the adult language. It is one factor, and only one, in the simultaneity of language, behaviour, situation and adult interpretation which constitutes our analytic datum. In certain settings, non-segmental factors will be a primary determinant of meaning; in other settings, it will be discounted. The way in which these factors operate upon each other in these various settings is however by no means clear (see further, Eilers, 1975).

However it is arrived at, it is plain that around 1;6 in most children, two-element sentences within single prosodic contours are used, and tonic prominence is not random. In the adult language, the prominence in a sentence consisting of one tone-unit is in 90 per cent of cases on the last lexical item[17]. Bringing the prominence forward within the tone-unit is possible, for both grammatical and semantic reasons, as we have seen (p. 63). In the former case, we may be constrained by rules of cross-reference within the sentence (*e.g. Jack saw Jím/ and hè said . . ./*); in the latter case, we may be making a (referential or personal) contrast between lexical items *(e.g. the rèd dress/not the gréen dress/).* The presuppositions and attitudes of the speaker also promote marked tonicity *(e.g. I wànt a red dress/, he isn't coming/).* However, at the two-element/three-element stage in children, there will obviously be little to note in relation to the prosodic marking of grammatical or lexical relations—such contrasts are likely to be more apparent when clause sequences appear.

Once grammatical patterns and lexical sets develop, then the tracing of non-segmental patterns becomes a much more straightforward task. What is important is to remember the central role prosody has in the adult language in relation to the delimitation and integration of such structures as questions, relative clauses, coordination, adverbial positioning, direct/indirect-object marking, etc.[18]. Very little research seems to have been done on the later development of such patterns in production, but it is probable that this kind of learning continues until puberty (and, in terms of the development of our stylistic control over non-segmental phonology—*e.g.* in dramatic speech—into adult life). Similarly, the comprehension of these features continues well beyond the preschool period; for example, Cruttenden's (1974) study of certain aspects of intonation in a restricted class of coordinated

---

[17] See Chomsky and Halle (1968: 17 ff.) for a theoretical statement; Crystal (1969: 263 ff., 1975: 22 ff.) for a statistical one.
[18] Cf. Quirk, *et al.* (1972), Menyuk (1969), Wode (1980).

utterances (football results) showed that awareness of the rules involved was in the process of development between 7 and 10 years. Comparatively late is the awareness of coreferential pronouns in certain contexts of coordination, *e.g. John gave a book to Jím/ and he gave one to Frèd/* vs. *John gave a book to Jím/ and hĕ/gave one to Frèd/*[19]. Here too research is needed. But for most clinical purposes, the more relevant kind of information about non-segmental phonology relates to the earlier period of intonational development, described above, and here sufficient data is available to establish useful guidelines for assessment and remedial work.

Non-Segmental Disability

The speech pathology literature makes little reference to the possibility of disorders of non-segmental phonology. The most general reference is to the notion of *dysprosody*, but this is usually given a phonetic, and not a phonological interpretation (*cf.* p. 60). The discussion of disorders of pitch or loudness, for example, is generally found in the context of voice disorders or hearing impairment[20]. Voices characterized by excessive pitch height/depth/monotony/width, etc. are well-recognized, but these are viewed as phonetic disorders, the consequence of an organic or psychogenic disturbance, and have no necessary implication for the linguistic system. Prosodic disability, in the sense of the present chapter, is however a phonological disturbance: it is the *linguistic* use of pitch, loudness, etc. which is affected, and not the phonetic ability to use these variables. On the one hand, there is the phonetic study of pitch and its disturbances, and this is carried on under the heading of voice disorders; on the other hand, there is the study of the linguistic use of pitch (intonation) and its disturbances, and this is carried on under the heading of prosodic disability. Similar distinctions would hold for disturbances involving the other attributes of sound sensation—loudness, duration, rhythm, etc.

There are several ways in which the clinical importance of this distinction can be illustrated. For example, presented with a patient whose speech is characterized by abnormal non-segmental effects, the first question which must be asked is whether the abnormality is a consequence of an underlying condition which operates regardless of the language he speaks (or is attempting to speak), or whether it is a consequence of disturbed learning (or relearning) of that language. P may speak at an abnormally high pitch level, because of an underlying organic or psychogenic condition: the point is that, given this condition, the high pitch level will result, *regardless of his language.* The disturbance affects P's basic sound-making abilities, and is thus a phonetic disturbance. By contrast, he may fail to use one of the English nuclear tones in an appropriate manner (*e.g.* mixing up rises and falls, and thus fail to distinguish clearly between statement and question): this disturbance hits at his ability to communicate meaningfully in English, and is thus a pho-

---

[19] See Chomsky (1969), Maratsos (1973).
[20] For example, Greene (1964), Berry and Eisenson (1956), Travis (1957).

nological disturbance, which will not necessarily have any direct parallel with cases of prosodic disability that present in French, Welsh, German, etc.

Here is a more detailed example of the importance of distinguishing between phonetic and phonological disturbance in non-segmental effects. Let us consider three voice patients, one with a normal pitch range, one with an excessively high range, and one with an excessively low range. These may be illustrated as follows (where the thick parallel lines represent the upper and lower bounds of pitch range within a voice register):

'normal'   'high'   'low'

We may now relate to this model such distinctions as that between falling and rising tones, both high and low varieties, as discussed above (p. 64). If these three patients are solely voice problems, they will all be able to express the contrasts involved in these distinctions, as follows:

'normal'   'high'   'low'

There will undoubtedly be some phonetic modifications introduced, as the "high" and the "low" speakers attempt to express the full range of tones. The "high" speaker may find that to make a clear contrast between low and high rising tones, for example, he needs to switch into a falsetto register for the high tones, or make them extra loud. Similarly, the "low" speaker may find that to make his contrast clearly, he needs to add some extra phonetic feature to his low tones, such as a creaky or husky voice. These falsetto, husky, etc. effects will sound as if they are characteristics of the voice disorder, and of course they are—but with the difference that their motivation is phonological.

These are the clear cases. Analysis becomes more difficult when patients present with a mixture of phonetic and phonological problems. Using the above model, an example of this situation might be as follows:

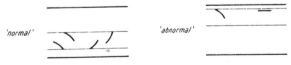

'normal'   'abnormal'

Here we have a patient who speaks in a high range, and within this only two tone contrasts are distinguishable in his speech. Some sentences end with a high falling pitch movement; others with a high level pitch. The question is: how can we decide which of the following phonological analyses is correct:

(a) \ is his high fall, and ⁻ is the realization of a rising tone, which for phonetic reasons he is unable to produce well;

(b) \ is his low fall (despite its apparently high position) and ⁻ is an attempt at a high fall (which he cannot reach, again for phonetic reasons);

(c) \ is a (completely deviant) realization of a low rising tone, and ‾ is his high rising tone (flattened, again for phonetic reasons).

In real life, there may of course be other possibilities, for I have selected only four tones for the purposes of illustration here. The \ or the ‾ may be realizing any of the range of tones English has available.

In all these cases, only an analysis of the tones' functions in speech can provide a solution. By studying the distribution of the tones with reference to grammar and semantics, it may be possible to arrive at a satisfactory analysis. For example, as we know that falling tones generally express statements, and rising tones questions, then if we see P using \ whenever he is apparently stating, and ‾ whenever he is apparently questioning, we would be motivated to analysis (a) above. On the other hand, if he uses \ for both questions and statements, this analysis would not work; we would then have to see whether there was any common factor in his use of ‾, e.g. whether he used it in attempting to signal new information (or emphasis, or surprise, or any of the other functions associated with the high falling tone in English). It will be apparent that the cogency of either analysis will depend on our confidence that P was intending his sentences to be used as statements, questions, emphatic, etc. Often, of course, it is not possible to be sure.

Given this kind of problem, it should be clear why the traditional term *dysprosody* is inadequate as a general label: it is usually unclear whether a purely phonetic sense is intended, or whether disturbances in phonological contrastivity are to be subsumed under it[21]. And the same problem is raised by other commonly used characterizations of non-segmental disturbance—such phrases as "distorted melody", "erratic rhythm", and so on. For example, one characterization of Broca's aphasia refers to it being "uncertain, monotonous, with defective intonation", and to Wernicke's as containing "false intonations and accent, monotony and disorders of rhythm" (Critchley, 1970: 218 ff.). Now, regardless of the empirical issue here (*i.e.* whether these syndromes are monotonous, uncertain, etc. in *fact*), there is the theoretical issue, as to whether a phonetic or a phonological difficulty is being postulated, or both. Quite different therapeutic strategies would be involved (*cf.* below). It is thus to avoid ambiguity that the framework on p. 60 was introduced.

It should be appreciated that the range of possible distinctions outlined in Table 9 is to some extent a programmatic one: not all of the distinctions it represents have been researched, and not all of them may turn up in practice. But there are several types of phonological problem which are recognizable under the headings of intonation and stress, and it is these which will provide the basis for the classification below. A wide range of other effects has however been noted, primarily in the context of psychiatric disturbance. An important review of this field is to be found in *Approaches to Semiotics*[22], where a considerable range of abnormal prosodic and paralinguistic effects are cited in relation to the study of anxiety states, schizophrenia, and other conditions. Some patients whisper, nasalize, speed up, etc. on certain words or at certain points in sentences. Their ability to use their voices

---

[21] For example, Eisenson (in Travis [1957: 443]) seems to include both phonetic and phonological phenomena in his discussion of the notion in aphasia. Cf. also Berry and Eisenson (1956: 403).

[22] See Sebeok, Hayes, and Bateson (1964), especially the papers by Ostwald, and Mahl and Schulze.

normally in other circumstances may be evident, so there is no ground for a discussion in terms of voice disorders. There may also be an apparent correlation between the incidence of the abnormality and the meaning of the language being expressed (*e.g.* always whispers when using first person pronouns, always nasalizes when embarrassed), and the phonological status of the problem is thus suggested.

The majority of the problems routinely encountered in clinical work, however, involve intonation. This is not surprising, if we recall the wide range of patterns subsumed under this heading, and the importance of intonation in signalling grammatical boundaries and variations in emphasis, as well as the quasi-linguistic contrasts of attitude and emotion. What this does mean, though, is that the notion of a single category of "intonation disorder" has to be replaced: to refer to "abnormal", "distorted", "defective", "exaggerated" (etc.) intonation, without further specification, is as useless as to refer to "abnormal" articulation, or "defective" grammar. We must ask instead such questions as: how much of the intonational system has been acquired? Which part of the intonational system has been disturbed? Specific problems can be located under each of the three main structural features of intonation identified above (p. 63): tone-units, tonicity, and tone.

Tone-Units

There are two main categories of abnormality in the use of tone-units: too few tone-units are used, compared with what would be expected for normal speech; and too many are used—again, when compared with what would be expected in normal speech[23]. Too few tone-units gives the impression of someone speaking "without paying attention to punctuation". The speech may be very rapid, as with clutterers, or some receptive aphasics, or it may be slow and ponderous, as in some cases of mental retardation or expressive aphasia. Here is an example of the first type, from a receptive aphasic man of 34:

we weren't wòrking the 'next 'day/ . no 'that day it 'raining the 'whole day it ràining/ . so I 'went to erm 'working on the 'yesterday and in the 'afternoon I had to 'fill up a hòle/ . yes 'very 'hard a 'lot of stùcky/ .

In this case, we would normally expect to have tone-unit boundaries at each of the main clause boundaries, and after the social minor sentences *yes* and *no*. The second type is illustrated by this extract from the retelling of a fairy-tale by a 10-year-old educationally subnormal girl:

'Goldilocks - 'sit - 'mum's - 'mum's 'chair - 'too 'hard - 'break . 'it . nòw/ -- 'sit . 'daddy chair - 'just 'right . 'no 'break chàir/ ---

Here, there is a general lack of definite pitch movement and rhythm: each lexical item has more or less the same loudness and level tone, and it is difficult to be sure if and when a non-segmental unit is being used, except at the main change-points in

---

[23] Cf. Crystal (1969: 256 ff.). The average length of tone-unit in the adult conversational data described there was 5 words.

the story's action, when the pitch level sometimes drops (shown twice in the above example). A similar uncertain, erratic pitch sequence occurs in much deaf speech, and also in many neurological patients.

In its extreme form, overuse of tone units is most noticeable in the speech which emerges as if "a word at a time", with each word being given a deliberate and careful pronunciation—an intonation commonly heard when children are heard reading aloud at an early stage in their learning. The following monologue was heard in the case of a language delayed child of seven, who had painstakingly learned the following construction, and who was being given a production exercise in it (each sentence corresponds to a new picture stimulus from T):

thé/ mán/ ís/ rùnning/
thé/ mán/ ís/ fàlling/
thé/ mán/ ís/ jùmping/
thé/ gírl/ ís/ éating/ á/ càke/

In more advanced cases, where an attempt is made to group words into some kind of tone-cum-rhythm unit, two main types of pattern can be identified: those where the insertion of extra tone-unit boundaries follows the grammatical structure of the sentence; and those where it does not. The former case may be illustrated by the following sentence, produced by an expressive aphasic:

T   'what's the 'man dòing/
P   the mán/ . is kícking/ . the bàll/

In this case, the Subject, Verb and Object of the sentence are each given an intonational identity, which presumably reflects the way in which the patient is processing one grammatical "chunk" at a time. But in the following response, the parallelism between intonation and grammar is not preserved:

P   the mán is/ . éating a/ . àpple/

This pattern, observed for example in the speech of the adult aphasic analyzed in Crystal, Fletcher, and Garman (1976: 177-8), is particularly disruptive, and can lead to deviant structures being produced. For example, when attempting to produce an intransitive verb, the rhythmical pattern of the above example carried over and motivated the following:

P   the mán is/ . físhing a /

Apart from the question of the number and location of tone-units in a sentence, there are several other ways in which abnormality can be manifested. For example, a stereotyped (or "idiomatic") tone-unit pattern may be used—an identical rhythm and pitch contour for every sentence uttered (or the majority of sentences). One familiar kind of stereotyping occurs normally when children recite their "tables":

'twenty-five thìrty/ . 'thirty-five fòrty/ . . .

Another is the prosody of nursery rhymes or limericks. Outside of such ritualized contexts, this degree of intonational predictability would sound extremely odd. It is however a fairly common phenomenon in clinical situations. It has been often noticed within the pattern of recovery from aphasia: something that is grammatically and lexically a stereotype will almost certainly be prosodically stereotyped as well[24]. Examples from adult patients where this was the case include:

you sèe thát/ ... I 'mean to sây/ ... as a màtter of fáct/.

Similar examples can be found in children, such as:

you 'know whát/ ... I don't knôw/ ... I wónder/ ... can't remèmber/.

The opposite kind of effect would be noticed where the grammar and semantics of the speech would normally require the repeated use of a single intonational pattern, and P fails to preserve the parallelism. For example:

that elephànt is 'lying on that/ . elephànt/
'I got a grèen dréss/ and I gôt a 'red 'jumper/

To what extent does the delay/deviance distinction apply to the field of tone-unit disability? Most of the examples discussed so far would have to be called deviant, in the sense of this book (p. 197). They are structurally anomalous, with respect to the accompanying grammar and semantics. In conversational exchanges of the kind illustrated above, neither adults nor children use the tone-unit patterns in question, and a judgement of deviance thus follows. The only cases where there might be grounds for talking about a "delayed" tone-unit development would be in relation to the earliest stages referred to above (p. 69), namely:
lack of any determinate tone-unit structure;
isolation of a tone-cum-rhythm unit within an otherwise indeterminate sequence;
juxtaposition of such units, with a clear phonetic boundary, such as silence;
a clearly identifiable lexical unit in a single prosodic contour, within an otherwise indeterminate sequence;
juxtaposition of two or more lexical items, within a single prosodic contour.

There may be more advanced stages of tone-unit structural development, in relation to grammatical development (e.g. whether the way in which a clause structure comes to be built up has any prosodic counterpart), but the research has not been done. There is thus relatively little to be gained by way of detailed assessment and remediation from operating with the notion of delay in this area.

What are the most relevant notions that might be extracted from this discussion of abnormal tone-unit structure and function? The following criteria seem especially important[25]:
(i) the proportion of incomplete to complete tone-units, with a separate tally being made of any indeterminate cases;
(ii) the number of stereotyped tone-units;
(iii) the use of a tone-unit that seems wholly the result of imitation of T's stimulus, e.g.

---

[24] See Van Lancker (1975: 120), Alajouanine (1956), Critchley (1970: 206).
[25] They provide the basis for the prosody profile in Crystal (1982).

T   he can sēe/ yōu/   (half-singing, joking)
P   sēe/ yōu/.

(iv) the grammatical structure of the tone-units, defined according to the terms of whatever model is being used elsewhere with the patient. For example, using the model discussed on p. 98, the following sentences would be analyzed thus:

he 'came in the mòrning/	1 tone-unit coterminous with a simple (1-clause) sentence;
the mán/ cáme/ in the mòrning/	3 tone-units, 2 coterminous with phrases, 1 with a word;
thé/ mán/ cáme/ ín/ thé/ mòrning/	6 tone-units, each coterminous with a word;
the 'man came in the 'morning and sat dòwn/	1 tone-unit coterminous with a complex (multi-clause) sentence.

Several more-complex cases will occur, such as:

the mán/ 'sat in a càr/ ... he câme/ in the mòrning/

where combinations of elements at different grammatical levels may need to be recognized.

(v) Tone-unit functions can hardly be given a systematic classification, given the present state of knowledge, and the indeterminacy of much of the clinical data. The best that can be done is to note the instances of apparently abnormal functions, *e.g.* P's use of a high rising tone to mark say, emphasis, without any questioning meaning involved, or P using a tone with an excessively wide range of functions, compared with normal language (*e.g.* the falling-rising tone being used for reservation, continuity and finality, as in the sample from Ian on p. 90). Any decisions about deviant prosodic function should however be viewed with great caution.

(vi) Lastly, the average number of words per tone-unit may be of some diagnostic value; but it is more likely that the qualitative measures will be of greater use than any simple measure of length (*cf.* Crystal, Fletcher, and Garman, 1976: 9-11).

Tonicity

The vast majority of tones in English are simple rather than compound in type (in a ratio of 9: 1, *cf.* Crystal, 1969: 225); hence problems of tonicity are generally going to be noticed only with reference to the former. Here there are two main ways of looking at what happens:

(a) items which are never normally tonic are made tonic by P;
(b) items which are normally tonic are not given any prominence by P.

A sub-classification may be made, under either heading, in terms of whether the item in question is grammatical or lexical (*cf.* p. 82). Examples of these errors are as follows:

norm:	I want to go to the cinema/	expected tonic, last lexical item: neutral interpretation

abnormal: (i)   I wànt to go to the cinema/   where there is no reason in the
                                                     context for P to be so insistent

       (ii)   I want tò go to the cinema/   where *to* would never normally
                                                     be prominent, under any inter-
                                                     pretation.

Other examples of abnormal (i), taken from various types of patient, include:

T   whìch 'man 'kicked 'that 'ball/
P   'this man 'kicked that bàll/   (where *this* should be tonic)

T   thìs car is cléan/ būt -   (prompt stimulus)
P   this câr is 'dirty/   (where *dirty* should be tonic)

P   me want a 'big 'red ràcing car/   (T hands him the middle-size of three
                                          red racing cars on the table)

   nǒ/   (P rejects it)
   me want 'big ràcing car/ (T hands him the biggest one, which he
                                          accepts; *i.e. big* should have been tonic)

Other examples of abnormal (ii) include:

P   I can dò that/ can Í/
P   ìt be 'raining/

P   'three hòrse/
T   hōrse   (prompt intonation, hoping to elicit plural)
P   'horse-ès/

The most primitive pattern in tonicity use seems to be one where only the last
lexical item in the tone-unit is made tonic: this would be the clearest case of delay,
with reference to this phenomenon. Here is an extract from a dialogue with Paula, a
six-year-old language-delayed child, where every multi-word sentence has final tonic:

P   she 'wash hàir/ -
T   'washing her hàir ís she/
P   yès/
T   m̂/ -
   hòw's she 'washing her 'hair/
P   [ə ɪ ɪ] . 'sit 'in chàir/
T   she's 'standing on the chǎir/ ---
   'what's she 'going to dò/
P   'wash hàir/
T   'wash her hàir/ -
   'in the bǎth/
P   yès/
T   yés/
P   [ɪ ɪ] too bìg/
T   'is she too bìg for the báth/
P   (*2 sylls*) she 'do . 'in thère/

T   in thĕre/
P   yès/ -
     'she wĕt/ -
     'she wĕt/

The next few multi-word sentences Paula uses are:

'wash 'her hàir/ . . . 'on . the flòor/ . . . 'no mòre/ . . . more bòok/ . . . 'me 'put awày/ . . .
'put . [ɪ ɪ] in thère/ . . . 'put it . on chàir/ . . . 'no 'fall dòwn/ . . . 'no 'fall dòwn/ . . .

and thus the pattern continues, producing an extremely predictable and generally a
somewhat boring pattern to the speech.

   A somewhat more advanced level of tonicity is illustrated by Stephen, a language-delayed boy of six. Here there are several cases where the tonic syllable has
been brought forward in the tone-unit, and each case seems well-motivated or at
least plausible, in terms of the semantic contrast conveyed:

P   'that's a càr/
T   that's ríght/
P   râcing 'car/ -   (points to big car)
     a little 'car/   (picks up small car)
     little 'car/
     little 'car 'there/
     a bòat/ --   (points to big boat)
     little 'boat/   (picks up small boat)
     Steve's - Stève's 'got a bóat/
T   háve you/
P   yèah/
     mĕ/ ---
     dàddy's 'car/
T   it's like dáddy's 'car/

   The main points to be noted under tonicity, for any profile of a patient's disability, would seem to be the following:
(i) whether any compound tones are being used; if so, whether the second element
of the compound is on the final item or not;
(ii) for simple tonicity, we would need to know whether the tonic item is final in the
tone-unit or non-final, and then, whether it is appropriately or inappropriately
tonic (as illustrated in the examples above);
(iii) the distinction between lexical and grammatical items is observed, in carrying
out this analysis, as the kind of remediation likely for a patient who consistently
stresses grammatical words is going to be different from that required if the wrong
lexical items are stressed. In the former case, a specific grammatical system is at
issue, *e.g.* *him* vs. other pronouns, or one preposition versus another, and the confusion engendered is usually easy to spot, being restricted to that system. With a
false lexical contrast, however, there is often an indefinite set of possibilities, and it
is usually much more difficult to pinpoint the error and do something about it.

(iv) lastly, if there are cases where an unexpected tonicity is due to P having imitated T's tonic structure, this might be noted under a separate category of imitation, *e.g.*

T he's 'using his 'fist to pùnch the 'ball/
P pùnch the 'ball/   (an apparently echoic response)

Tone

As there is clearer evidence of a developmental sequence in this area (*cf.* p. 70 above), the application of the notion of delay becomes more useful, and there are also several types of deviance which can be recognized. It is thus under this heading that the most important differential diagnostic statements can be made, regarding non-segmental phonological disability. Firstly, under the heading of apparently delayed tonal development, we may note the following three stages, each of which is frequently encountered in clinical analysis.

(i) *Indeterminate tone system.* In this, the earliest stage, there are few clearly defined tones: the dominant impression is falling tone, but this would seem to be no more than a reflex of the "innate|breath group" (*cf.* Lieberman 1967: 26 ff.), *i.e.* the natural tendency of the voice to fall at the end of expiration. Otherwise the pitch level is generally flat, with erratic features of pitch variation that seems not to correspond to any obvious semantic intention or contextual state of the patient. At the earliest stage, the tone-unit system is also indeterminate (*cf.* above), and it is therefore impossible to identify meaningful "chunks" at all in P's vocalization. The vocalizations seem to correspond to breath patterns, and have little or no superimposed prosodic structure. At a later stage, the vocalizations seem more restricted and controlled, within the overall duration of a breath, and display a shape whose identity is partly a matter of rhythm and partly a matter of pitch contour. At this point, we might expect a more determinate intonational structure to emerge.

(ii) *Systematic use of pitch range.* The more determinate structure initially takes the form of a systematic use of pitch range. Both a two-term and a three-term system of pitch range is common in patients at an early stage of speech development.

A two-term system represents the contrast between "neutral" and "high": the former is in the majority, being the range that P uses for routine utterances; P switches to high when something special happens, and there is an apparent expression of emphasis, excitement, frustration, or whatever. For example, the following extract from a severely educationally subnormal teenager illustrates this kind of system (I give only the relevant T stimuli, omissions being marked by . . .):

T   how òld are you/   *P's pitch range (cf. p. 75)*
P   fiftèen/   \
T   sixtĕen/
P   sixtèen/   \
T   . . . do you gó to 'school/
P   yès/   \
. . .

T   'what's thìs/
P   er -- màn/   ＼
T   ... 'what's the 'man dòing/
P   'leading the dòg/   ＿＼＿
T   ... 'where are they gòing/
P   for a wàlk/   ... ＼ ..
T   ... is 'that a 'nice pícture/
P   pīcture/   ‾ ‾ - ..
T   and 'what's hêre/
P   màn/ -   ＼ ..
     màn/   ＼
T   what's thàt 'man 'doing/
P   'smoking a cigarètte/   .. ＼

In the sample as a whole, the majority of tones are low falling, and these clearly constitute P's norm. In certain circumstances, however, P produces a tone which is
auditorily quite distinct from this norm, *viz.* a tone with extra height for the beginning of the fall, sometimes accompanied by a pitch "lilt" at the onset, sometimes by
additional loudness[26]. In one case there is a flat tone, which may be an echo of the T
stimulus, but which is difficult to hear, due to accompanying dysphonia. The
problem for the analyst is therefore to decide whether the phonetic contrast between high and low has any phonological significance: does P mean anything by it?
The only way to find out, in such a patient, is to scrutinize each context carefully, to
see whether there is any evidence to support a systematic interpretation. In the
present case, there is some evidence, but it is not totally clear. We might hypothe-
size that the instances where P switches to high range seem to relate to where he
begins a new task, and that as his attention wanders or he loses interest, his pitch
level falls to low. This reasoning could explain an almost cyclical pattern of
low→high→low→high range throughout the session—but with the highs being of
short duration, and becoming less common as the session proceeds, as T finds it
increasingly difficult to generate novel and stimulating situations from the material
being used.

   In the three-term pitch range system, the same procedure of analysis applies,
but in this case there seems to be evidence of a "high"—"mid"—"low" contrastivity,
with "mid" usually being the norm. In one five-year-old language-delayed patient, a
system of this kind seemed to operate: high range seemed to be used in a manner
very similar to the patient above, in contexts of excitement, surprise, etc.; low range
was used when P was playing by herself, or apparently talking to herself, and also
when talking to T in a teasing manner; mid was used elsewhere (*i.e.* for all responses,
for routine descriptions of what she was doing, what had happened, and so on).

   It should be noted, in all such cases, that the phonetic realization of the phonological contrasts between "high" and "low" (and "mid", where used), while usually

---

[26] There is a certain amount of phonetic variation in the low falling tones also, not all of which
would be transcribable with certainty without supplementary acoustic analysis. It is accepted that there
may be some arbitrariness about the high/low distinction in such cases, and the risk of reading too
much intonational structure into the data must always be borne in mind.

involving pitch movement, may also involve other phonetic parameters. For
example, the high falling tones of one patient were sometimes uttered in a falsetto
register, sometimes with a strong breathy quality. The low falling tones of another
patient were very low indeed, and were often produced with creaky or husky qualities. There may also be a component of loudness as part of the contrast, *e.g.* high
tones may be much louder than low tones, or the other way round. The phonetic
shape of the tone may also be affected. For example, the low tones in one patient
were all flattened at the end, *viz.* ＼＿ . In another patient, the high tones were
generally turned into rising-falling patterns. In a further case, there seemed to be no
"control" over the pitch directions used by P in producing her high contrast. Her
system looked like this:

low	mid ＼ –	high ＼ ＼" ＼ ∧ "∧ – ／ ∼ [27]
＼＼＿ – "＿		

It is possible that with a more detailed statistical analysis of the phonetic variations,
some kind of sub-system might emerge within the range of high tones used; but it
was difficult to see from the sample analyzed what this might be. None of the high
variants seemed to correlate in any regular way with changes in P's behaviour or
environment; they did seem genuinely to be in free variation. In some cases, in fact,
a straightforward spontaneous repetition of a word was produced, as P pointed out
something she had noticed in a picture first to T and then to her mother: the intonation fluctuated considerably between these utterances.

An important analytical point should be stressed here. Given the phonetic
range of pitch movement encountered in, for example, the patient just described,
the initial impression that she might give is of someone whose prosodic system is in
fact quite advanced: there are, after all, several of the more advanced pitch movements heard in the sample (such as the rise-fall-rise). But this variation is not
phonological in character: it seems to lack any kind of systematic, meaningful contrastivity, and this gives it a rather different status from variation used by patients at
a genuinely advanced level of prosodic development, where their use of, say, fall-
rise and high fall would convey a range of meaning similar to that used by normal
children or adults. Putting this another way, when the more advanced patient uses a
high rise, he "means" to question, echo, etc.; whereas when the patient above uses a
high rise, there seems to be no intent on her part to question, echo, etc.—the rise
seems inappropriate and random. A similar impression is of course given when we
listen to the sometimes quite wide range of pitches heard in babbling.

(iii) Tonal contrastivity. As the need to express a wider range of attitudes, speech acts,
etc. increases, patients will be encountered who have begun to introduce the range
of tones listed on p. 64 in a stable and systematic way. Research has not yet established the detail of how this process takes place, *e.g.* whether there is a pattern in the
way in which a new tone comes to "settle down" into a certain pitch range, or how
the repercussions of a new tone affect the other tones constituting the system. Such
points have been much discussed in the context of segmental phonology[28], but not

---

[27] " used in transcription refers to extra stress on a syllable.
[28] For example, Trubetzkoy (1939), Chao (1943), Martinet (1949).

in the non-segmental field. The patient illustrated on p. 82 above is an example of a child who seems to be about half-way through the process of acquiring the English tone system. The phonetic range of his first 30 utterances looks like this:

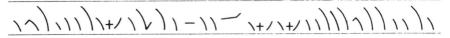

Here, the tonal contrasts are generally easy to contextualize. The falling-rising tone, for example, seems quite appropriate: it is used on *me, they crashed,* and, as fall-plus-rise, on *watch him* (twice), all of which are quite normal adult intonations. What is missing in this system, apparently, is the range of simple rising tones. In only one sentence is there a nuclear tone that seems to have a rising element, and this is very narrowed. Of course, it might be argued immediately that the context was one which did not require simple rising tones, and indeed, this kind of argument has got to be taken into account. There is only one way of really deciding the matter, of course, and that is to make other samples in other contexts where the rising tones might be more expected, *e.g.* a question-and-answer dialogue. But it must be pointed out that it is very difficult to think up an everyday speech context in English where simple rising tones are unlikely or impossible. There is usually a considerable number in conversational settings of any kind, and in children's play settings they are certainly common. Even in monologues: the verbalization of a normal child while he is playing contains a significant number of rising tones, of various sorts; and thus the above argument would not seem to be valid, in the present example.

Here is a case where the need to take other contexts into account *did* prove to be important, before an accurate decision about the quality of the patient's prosodic system could be made. The first line of the transcription illustrates a 5-year-old's prosody while retelling *The Bus Story*, by Catherine Renfrew. The second line gives the prosody of the subsequent conversation, when T begins to talk about P's holidays:

The first line has a reasonably varied set of tones, but an apparently limited (low) pitch range; the second line belies this interpretation. In impressionistic terms, the voice becomes much more animated, and indeed some quite complex meanings are expressed in some of the sequences, *e.g.* various degrees of doubt, puzzlement and exitement.

More detailed patterns of intonational development can be plotted using the guidelines from language acquisition presented on p. 70 above. The sequence falling→rising→rising-falling→falling-rising→compound would seem to be the most usual, and could be used as the basis of an assessment profile and also as part of a remedial programme. What is unclear is how range and loudness variables interact with pitch, during this sequence. At the very least, any developmental profile would have to recognize the importance of extra pitch height, extra loudness, widening and narrowing in pitch, but it is not yet possible to suggest an ordering of these for remedial work.

Lastly, any account of tonal disability must recognize the possibility of deviant tones, in the sense that their phonetic realization lies completely outside the normal range of English speech. Several types of pitch abnormality are quite common, in fact:

(i) *flattening*, in which attempts at rising or falling tones emerge with a strong level component, accompanied by a slight initial or final lilt, *e.g.*

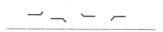

More bizarre flattenings can be heard in the speech of neurologically disordered patients, such as

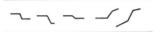

(ii) *widening*, in which the whole or most of the voice range is used in realizing the tone; there is often a change of register involved (to falsetto), and sometimes chant-like characteristics may be heard. A transcription of such tones would look typically like this (with F indicating a register-shift to falsetto):

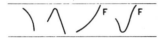

(iii) *diminishing*, in which the tones of a patient in connected speech progressively diminish in pitch range (for instance, in cases involving neuromuscular deficiency or poor respiratory control). A characteristic transcription would be as follows:

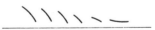

(iv) *laryngeal*, in which an abnormal state of the larynx disallows the normal range of vocal cord vibration, as in the various kinds of dysphonic speech. In such circumstances, the phonetic realization of nuclear tones may involve such variables as breathiness, huskiness, and whisper, as well as alterations in the resonance of contiguous cavities. Such variations are unfortunately unable to be conveniently transcribed, because of their multivariate character[29].

Combinations of these effects in the speech of individual patients are not uncommon. The following transcription of a tone sequence produced by a patient suffering from Parkinson's disease illustrates the way the tones are affected by flattening and diminution as he speaks; the whole sequence was uttered in a very low and husky voice:

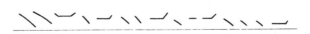

---

[29] And also because their constituent parameters are little understood. See Laver (1980).

Interaction of Tone-Unit, Tonicity and Tone

While many patients, especially the most severely language delayed, can be simply
analyzed in terms of one or other of the above three variables, there are many
others where the intonational disability is more complex, P having difficulty with
all three at once. I have never been in a position to trace why such severe intonational difficulties arise, but they are common enough, especially in patients who
have a fairly complex, but disturbed grammatical system, and perhaps fluency and
word-finding problems as well. This combination of factors is certainly present in
the speech of Ian, aged nine:

P and erm - and erm - I 'I . I 'I wa͞nt . I wa͞nt erm a bíngo/ gǎme/[30]

T a whát/

P a "bìngo/

T bǐngo/

P yèah/

T m̀/

P ha . 'have be 'lots of mòney . 'in/

T it has 'lots of ↑mòney in/

P yèah/

T dóes it/

P and - and erm . [ə] we 'have a *(4 sýlls)/* . and erm . a 'set dǐce/ and 'guess
 which nǔmber/ - and erm . and erm - [a] 'you [a] 'you mǒve/ abou͞t -- [a]
 óne or/ twó or/ tén/ tíme/

T *m̀/

P *and erm . [a] 'when . [a wə a] 'when you 'get . s . 'something - 'on the
 mǎn/ . [ə] 'have to ↑read thǎt/ [ə] be 'what 'this sǎy/

T what ìs it/
 a cǎrd/ -

P nò/
 [ə] be 'like erm --- [ə] be 'like a ↑bòok or 'something/

T *m̀/

P *and erm - [əə] (whāt) 'this 'say/ --   (? wōrds)
 hów/ - hów/ mǎny/ . tǐme/ are 'you have to 'move tèn/

T m̀/
 I sée/ .

P and erm . [ə] gǔess/ -
 and erm - 'after 'you . 'having 'got a prǐze/ - [ə] 'you - [ə] 'you cǎn/
 - mǒve/ a'bout ↑ten ↑tìme/

T I sèe/ --
 and 'who's 'going to bùy this 'for you/ --

P Nàn is/

T Nàn is/

P and . and erm -- 'I 'want - erm --- erm -- a s . a sáddle 'bag/

T a whǎt/

---

[30] ¯ over a segment indicates abnormal lengthening; ˘ abnormal shortening; ↑ a high onset to a
tone; * indicates overlapping speech.

P   a sàddle 'bag/
       'help you 'put all your fòod in/ --
T   'all the ↑fŏod/
P   yèah/
T   m̀/
P   [ə] be 'want 'one of 'them from Sănta/ . and erm . [ə] me . [ə] me 'want
T   "Ì 'want/
P   'I 'want - Stéve/ -   (pron. [tiːɣ])
T   ↑m̀/
P   Stève/ -
T   tĕeth/
P   nò/ .
       Stève/ -
       a 'six 'dollar màn/
       Stève/ --
       [ə] knów/
       'what we 'saw him [ə] .
       [ə] be with 'some a bi'onic . hànd/
T   Ì knów/
       Stève/
P   Stève/
T   'Steve Àusten/
P   yèah/
       'Steve Àusten/ -
T   'why do you 'want one of thòse/ -
P   sēe/ -
       [ə] be 'by elèctric/ . hìm ís/
T   ↑m̀/ --
P   er hìm/ er hĕ/ 'can jŭmp/ hìgher/
T   he càn/ -
       he can 'jump vèry high/
P   yéah/
       and . and erm - [ə] be a↑nòther mán/ -
       he biŏnic/
       [ə] 'fight Stĕve/
       and erm . Stĕv̄ie/ bóy/ . do . 'throw that 'other măn/ - and erm . [ə] 'all
       them - pòwer/ 'go òut/

...

       [ə] 'when you 'lift thát/ - 'all the smóke/ . and the 'number . do 'count
       ŏut/ and [ə] "blow ŭp/ . *and
T   *and it 'blows ŭp/ -
P   yĕah/
       'right ŭp/

...

       a 'doctor sǎy/ -- [ə] my . [ə] m . [ə] 'my căt/ -- mìght/ 'might 'feel bètter -
       sóon/

. . .

        and erm . a . dŏctor/ . dĭd/ [ə] *(1 syll)* 'try to - 'ease this pàin awáy/
T   m̊/
P   and 'pain have gŏne/
        [ə] but 'still hùrt a 'bit/

. . .

T   do you 'give him a cŭddle/
P   yèah/
T   m̊/
P   I be 'hope 'so . [ə] be my 'cat 'get 'better n . [ə] be 'when it . 'is Chrìstmas -
        tíme/

. . .

        [ə] my - [ə] 'my nǎn/ - sǎy/ - [ə] 'my cǎt/ can . 'go 'in . 'my bĕd/ - and
        n . and nǎn/ - and nan will . 'sleep 'downstǎirs/ . and 'me go 'in her bèd/

An analysis of this sample shows all aspects of Ian's intonation system to be affected. Tone unit structure, most obviously, is displaying an erratic and deviant relationship to grammar. In that part of the sample which is continuously transcribed
(up to . . .), Ian produces 63 complete tone-units. Excluding the stereotyped cases
(*[ə] knów/* and *sēe/*), the 7 cases of social minor responses *(yeah, no),* and the two cases
of possible imitation (*Steve* and *Steve Austen*), the grammatical structure of the
remaining 52 tone-units is as follows:

complete clause   19
complete phrase   7
word   15
clause partial   11

The way in which tone-units fragment the grammar is clearly indicated, both at
clause level *(e.g. you can/ move/ about ten time)* and at phrase level *(e.g. how/many/time/).*
The other extracts listed illustrate further examples of the abnormal tone-unit
divisions which characterize Ian's speech.
    The other main characteristic of his disability is in his use of nuclear tones. We
may compare the frequency of his use of tones with the expected frequency reported on p. 64 above:

Ian   \ 17   / 12   \/ 20   \+/ 2   − 1

Expected distribution of tones for an adult sample of 52 tone-units:

        \ 26   / 10.5   \/ 4   \+/ 4   − 2.5

The reversal of frequency for the falling and the falling-rising tones is striking, and
is certainly the dominant impression on the tape. A permanently dubious, cautious
tone of voice is the consequence, and while this is sometimes appropriate (*e.g.* in the
comment about his cat possibly feeling better soon) it is usually not (*e.g.* when he is
explaining the instructions about the dice game). Nor can we explain his use of the
falling-rising tone in grammatical terms—for instance, by its being simply a more
emphatic version of the rising tone that might be used to mark non-final structure.

There are too many cases where Ian *ends* utterances with fall-rises. This, as a consequence, adds to the problem T has in understanding him: it is often not clear whether Ian has stopped talking and is waiting for a reply, or whether he is about to continue, after a non-fluent pause. His use of rises and fall-rises in utterance-final position breaks a major semantic expectancy for this dialect of English[31].

Other Considerations

In all that has been said so far, the implication has been that non-segmental disability poses a problem which is in principle independent of the other kinds of linguistic disability. And indeed, the examples above illustrate many cases where the primary or only difficulty is located at this level—in other words, where segmental phonology, grammar and semantics are developing along lines which, if not normal or near normal, are certainly incommensurate with the non-segmental abilities demonstrated. But at the opposite extreme, there are also many cases where the non-segmental limitations are plainly no more than a consequence of what has happened elsewhere in the patient's linguistic system. To take an obvious case, if a patient is at the one-element stage of grammatical development, it would hardly be fair to point to his lack of tonicity contrast (which presupposes at least two words). Less obviously, to refer to the hesitant intonation and rhythm of an expressive aphasic as illustrating a non-segmental disability is to miss the point: a hesitant intonation is entirely appropriate for someone who is unsure of his ability to express grammar and lexicon. Likewise, the often over-confident intonation of the receptive aphasic, giving the impression of full control and comprehension where none may exist, is not a non-segmental disorder as such: it is the confident attitude which is inappropriate, not the intonation which (accurately) reflects it. There are indeed many intonational problems, both of expression and comprehension, in aphasia, but these must be carefully defined, and not subsumed under a single blanket impression of the speech pattern as a whole. But this whole question of the balance of the linguistic components which constitute an abnormal condition is in need of further study[32].

There have been several other limitations to the account of non-segmental phonological disability presented in this chapter. Chief among them has been the restriction of the topic to intonation, with only passing reference to stress, rhythm and pause. This restriction I think is justified, partly on empirical grounds (where a wide range of disability can be shown to operate, and useful differential diagnoses made) and partly on theoretical grounds (there being considerable evidence for the

---

[31] There are dialects where this rule does not apply, *e.g.* in N.E. England, N. Ireland, N. Wales.

[32] The only case where it is useful to talk of the *total* non-segmental effect of the speech is in patients whose altered system is liable to be a source of confusion to others about their social, regional or psychological identity. The case reported by Monrad-Krohn (1947), where the Norwegian speaker could be taken to be German, is a clear example; but less dramatic instances of changes in the non-segmental features of regional accent are common enough.

status of the tone-unit as a [?the] basic unit of neural encoding in speech)[33]. But it does ignore the evident relevance of other non-segmental variables (of stress, duration, pause, and especially rhythm) to the expressive organization and decoding of speech[34]. Secondly, within the field of intonation, our attention has been focussed on the internal structure of the tone-unit and its relation to other levels of linguistic description. This too I think is justified, given the present state of research, but it does ignore the existence of broader types of intonational disability than those described here, *e.g.* deviant patterns of tone-unit sequence. The relevance of both these limitations can be briefly illustrated from one receptive aphasic patient whose clause sequences were made largely incomprehensible due to a failure to reinforce the important information by appropriate prosodic means. If the sentence were, *e.g.*

so 'now they've 'gone and 'bought a hóuse/ 'near where I live you sée/

P would produce the main clause in a rapid, mumbling, quiet, low-pitched way, and then suddenly increase in loudness and range for the subordinate clause. The effect was that the listener heard clearly only "... near where I live you see". Repeated frequently throughout a discourse, this pattern is considerably disruptive.

Thirdly, nothing has been said on the important influence T's intonation can have on P's responses. The role of tonicity is particularly crucial in this respect: to alter the placement of the tonic syllable can give a quite different "shape" to an utterance, and it is therefore not surprising that patients' abilities to recall, comprehend, repeat and respond are much affected by this variable. Examples of errors

---

[33] See the review in Laver (1970: 69 ff.), and the evidence from the tongue-slip data (tongue-slips rarely crossing tone-unit boundaries or affecting tonic placement: cf. Boomer and Laver [1968: 8—9], Fromkin [1973]). The neurological evidence concerning prosody is not entirely clear, due once again to a failure to keep clearly apart phonetic and phonological information in the various investigative procedures (*e.g.* dichotic listening and tachistoscopic tasks, split-brain and hemispherectomy studies). There is evidence that non-segmental effects are processed bilaterally and subcortically (cf. Van Lancker 1975). The right hemisphere is normally superior for several effects, especially when attitudinal function is involved (see, *e.g.* Blumstein and Cooper [1974]); the left hemisphere is normally superior for certain other effects, including some tone language features (for Thai, at least: see Van Lancker and Fromkin [1973]) and certain rhythmical features (see Zurif and Mendelsohn [1972], Robinson [1977]). Unfortunately, the studies deal with both speech and non-speech (*e.g.* music, laughter) sounds, in both naturalistic and artificial (*e.g.* filtered) contexts, and methodological differences abound. It is therefore difficult to draw firm conclusions; but there is a growing body of opinion that (in left-hemisphere speech dominance) the left hemisphere is superior for phonological contrasts in non-segmental effect, and the right hemisphere for phonetic contrasts. Cf. Van Lancker's conclusion (1975: 166—167): "the types of pitch contour most likely to be processed in the dominant hemisphere would be those that carried grammatical distinctions rather than emotional ones". If this is so, there is an important consequence for those approaches to the treatment of language-disordered adults and children which aim to use musical or quasi-musical input (*e.g.* Sparks and Holland 1976): they will need to be supplemented by a more sophisticated set of phonological procedures than has hitherto been the case, in order to handle the problem of the hierarchy of intonational form (cf. p. 62), and the integration of intonation with syntax.

[34] For stress, see *e.g.* Goodglass (1968), Blumstein and Goodglass (1972); duration, Marckworth (1976); pause, Lasky, Weidner and Johnson (1976). The importance of rhythm as a primary device to promote a patient's sense of grouping, which must underlie tone-unit development, is a major theme of Van Uden (1970); see also Robinson (1977). For the importance of rhythm in language acquisition, see Allen and Hawkins (1978).

induced in patients by T's tonicity are common enough. One example is the following sequence:

T   there's a càt/
     it's a lìttle cat/
P   there lìttle/

Another example came from a drill sequence being used by T, of the following
form:

T   it's a NÒUN/
     whát is it/
P   it's a NÒUN/ .

After several instances of this exercise, T switched to

it's an ÀDJECTIVE NOUN/   (*e.g.* it's a rèd car/)

to which P replied

it's an ÀDJECTIVE/   (*e.g.* it's a rèd/)

the tonic syllable evidently being the main conditioning factor. A third example is
the conflict that can be produced if the item which is the focus of a remedial task is
not given tonic reinforcement; for example, if T is working on verbs, and says

'what's that màn 'doing/

a conflict between the demands of the grammar (which requires a verb) and the
demands of the intonation (which emphasizes the noun) may well be set up. One
child responded with *a dustman* (a correct identification from the picture), and this
was taken by T to be a comprehension error (*who* for *what*)—but it could simply have
been interference from the non-segmental structure of the sentence[35].

Lastly, it may be of interest to raise one intriguing question concerning the non-
segmental patterns T uses in remedial work. It is generally accepted that in doing
structured work with a patient, we should provide P with stimuli which are a step
ahead of his current linguistic level—but not too far ahead. The futility of speaking
to language-disordered children or adults using normal adult grammar or vocabulary is well-recognized—let alone using a *wider* range of grammar or lexicon than
would normally be encountered in conversation. But the non-segmental (and
especially the intonational) range used in remedial dialogues is invariably just that—
an exaggerated prosodic style quite unlike normal conversation, and much more
varied even than the widened pitch contours mothers use to children during their
period of grammatical learning. The contrast is often extreme, as can be seen by
comparing the tones used by the teacher to the ESN teenager illustrated on p. 83.

---

[35] See further, Goodglass, Fodor, and Schulhoff (1967), Wheldall and Swann (1976), Bonvillian,
Raeburn, and Horan (1979).

The reason for this exaggerated style is an obvious one: it is a natural attempt to produce a degree of interest and involvement on the part of the patient in activities which are often repetitive and dull. But the question must at least be asked as to whether T's varied prosodic output might not under some circumstances be a hindrance to the patient, distracting him from the other features of the utterance to which he should really be attending. Would structured work proceed more satisfactorily if T's intonation was more compatible with the level P uses? Clearly, this argument cannot be taken too far, but the fact that there is an argument at all is worth appreciating.

4 Grammar

Theoretical Background

An immediate problem with the term "grammar" arises out of the variety of its popular and scholarly interpretations. To carry out a grammatical analysis of a patient, or to talk of a grammatical disability, can mean different things to people of different backgrounds. Most of these variations, however, can be explained with reference to four main themes which characterize the history of ideas in the study of grammar.

(i) Traditional grammar. This phrase is an attempt to summarize the range of attitudes and methods found in the pre-scientific era of grammatical study. The term "traditional", accordingly, is found with reference to many periods, such as the Roman and Greek grammarians, Renaissance grammars, and (especially) the 18th and 19th century school grammars, in Europe and America[1]. Modern linguistics demonstrates a somewhat ambivalent attitude towards traditional grammars: on the one hand, their theoretical frameworks and descriptive statements have often been the source of ideas which are of importance to present-day linguists; on the other hand, the aims and attitudes underlying much of the early work run contrary to those espoused by the modern study. Several linguistic introductions to grammar have discussed this conflict, referring particularly to the need to avoid the impressionism, selectivity and prescriptivism of the traditional approach[2]. Comprehensiveness, objectivity and systematic descriptive statement, by contrast, are the principles which present-day linguists attempt to follow, in their work on grammar.

(ii) Pedagogical grammar. A pedagogical (or "teaching") grammar is a book designed specifically for the purposes of teaching or learning a foreign language, or for

---

[1] See, for example, Nesfield (1898). For a historical review, see Robins (1967).

[2] Examples of the prescriptive approach (*i.e.* the attempt to establish rules for the socially or stylistically correct use of language) may be found in Palmer (1971: Ch. 2), Crystal (1971: Ch. 2).

developing one's awareness of the mother-tongue. The standard "grammar books" used in English or modern language classes in schools are the main examples, and as much of traditional grammar had a pedagogical aim, most of the grammars in current school use display the biases characteristic of the earlier approach. Such grammars have little or no clinical applicability, however. They are largely based on the study of the written forms of language (especially of literature), and concentrate on topics which are too sophisticated or marginal for most clinical purposes. The study of the reality of modern spoken English, and of the regularities which under-lie it, is a major premiss of a systematic approach to assessment and remediation, but for this, alternative notions of grammar must be found[3].

(iii) Descriptive grammar. This notion constitutes an important area within contem-porary linguistics, and is historically in contrast with the prescriptive approach of traditional grammarians. A descriptive grammar is, in the first instance, a systematic description of a language as found in a sample of speech or writing. Descriptive studies of little-known or previously unresearched languages are often quite short, it sometimes being difficult to obtain large quantities of material from native-speakers. Descriptive studies of languages such as English, however, are usually very large, given the enormous amount of research that has taken place into this lan-guage, and the ready availability of data. When such studies have comprehensive-ness as their aim, they are sometimes known as *reference grammars,* or *grammatical handbooks*[4]. From a different theoretical point of view, grammars which go beyond the description of restricted samples of data, and which aim to make statements about the language as a whole, may be said to be "descriptively adequate"[5].

(iv) Theoretical grammar. This notion goes beyond the study of individual languages, using language data as a means of developing theoretical insights into the nature of linguistic enquiry in general, and into the categories and processes needed for sucessful linguistic analysis. In recent years, the study of theoretical grammar has become a major field of linguistics, and several models have been proposed, the most well-known deriving from the work of Chomsky and his associates[6]. Partly on account of the broad sense of "grammar" used in this approach, most of the insights it has produced are of considerable relevance to other areas of language analysis than those reviewed in the present chapter, and they require a separate and more general discussion (*cf.* pp. 97—98). On the other hand, *any* attempt at a grammatical description, even in a narrow sense (see below), presupposes that the analyst has made up his mind about certain theoretical issues; and unless these issues are made explicit, it is difficult to guarantee consistency or comparability when the descrip-

---

[3] There are however signs of progress in the mother-tongue field, reflecting the progress which has for several years characterized work in foreign-language teaching. The emphasis of the Bullock Report (H.M.S.O. 1975) is in this direction, and grammars which pay proper attention to speech have been written (*e.g.* Mittins 1962). But their influence on most pedagogical practice is still marginal.

[4] For example, Quirk *et al.* (1972), Jespersen (1909—1949).

[5] Chomsky (1964). See the discussion on p. 17 above. In this approach, the notion is seen as a pre-dictive account of a speaker's competence.

[6] See Chomsky (1957, 1965, 1975). Examples of general notions deriving from this approach in-clude the distinction between deep and surface structure, or the notion of grammatical transformation. For other theoretical models, see Lepschy (1970), Dinneen (1967), and for a general discussion, Matthews (1981).

tions come to be made. Distinctions such as syntax and morphology, sentence and clause, grammatical form and grammatical function, and the like, are not without controversy; and any clinical use made of these notions needs to be an informed one, if their theoretical strengths are not to be obscured.

The Scope of Grammatical Analysis

In a restricted sense (the traditional sense in linguistics, and the usual popular interpretation of the term), grammar refers to a level of structural organization in language which can be studied independently of phonology and semantics (cf. p. 19). In this sense, it could be loosely defined as the study of the way words, and their components, combine to form sentences and sentence-sequences. This is the way in which we shall be using the term later in this chapter; but this narrow sense must be contrasted with a general conception of the subject, where grammar is seen as the entire system of structural relationships in a language—including, in other words, the levels of phonology and semantics (which would now be referred to as the "components" of the grammar, along with the study of sentence structure, or *syntax*). This usage can be seen in the titles given to many of the major theories of language, such as stratificational grammar, systemic grammar, or generative grammar[7]. According to Chomsky, a grammar, in this sense, is a device for generating a finite specification of the sentences of a language. Insofar as a grammar defines the total set of rules possessed by a speaker, it is a grammar of his competence (a "competence grammar"); insofar as the grammar is capable of accounting for only the sentences a speaker has actually used (as found in a sample of his output), it is a "performance grammar"[8].

Such considerations take us well beyond the range of the present chapter, as conceived, and they have to some extent already been discussed (pp. 17–18). At this point, the focus on terminology becomes less useful, as despite the differences of approach, in the end everyone is paying attention to the same set of phenomena. Whether we label these phenomena as "grammar" or "syntax" is perhaps a side-issue, unless there are empirical differences which emerge as a consequence of the adoption of one or other of these terms. As far as clinical investigation is concerned, the kinds of difficulty manifested by patients can be usefully classified into grammatical (or syntactic), phonological and semantic (cf. p. 19). It is too soon to say whether there is anything to be gained, in terms of clinical insight, by integrating these factors into a single analytical framework (whether organized generatively, or in some other way). The present author's inclination is to adopt a fairly narrow view at the outset, in which the complexity of grammatical disability is studied without reference to phonological and lexical factors. It may be that, in due course, this assumption will be shown to be wrong—in other words, that to create such

---

[7] For stratificational grammar, see Lamb (1966), systemic grammar (Halliday 1967), generative grammar (references above).

[8] For the competence/performance distinction, see above, p. 18. The study of performance grammars, in a psycholinguistic context, goes beyond this, attempting to define the various psychological, neurological and physiological states which enter into the production and perception of speech.

divisions in fact complicates the statement of disability. But in view of the insights already achieved by working on the basis of this assumption, the narrow approach, if not correct, is certainly not a waste of time.

We shall, then, in the rest of this chapter (and in the book as a whole) talk about grammar as if it excluded phonology and semantics. Within the domain of grammar, several theoretical distinctions can now be made. One fundamental distinction, well-motivated by clinical practice, is that between *syntax* and *morphology*. Given the definition of syntax above, as the study of sentence structure and sequence, many grammatical models limit this study to combinations of words. Syntax, in this view, is the study of the rules governing the way words are combined to form larger units, such as phrases, clauses and (above all) sentences. The study of the structure and form of words is conceived as a separate enterprise, under the heading of morphology. Morphology thus deals with the way words vary to show grammatical relationships (the "inflections" of words) and how they can vary in terms of their lexical construction (the field of "word-formation")[9]. The minimal grammatical units into which words can be analyzed are referred to as *morphemes*, in the linguistics literature. The neuropsychological and remedial significance attached to the notion of "word" is well-attested (*cf.* Lesser, 1978: 34 ff.), and justifies its recognition as a main structural level in grammatical analysis.

But apart from *word*, what other specific notions need to be recognized, in order to proceed with grammatical work? The fundamental status of *sentence*, as the main unit of grammatical organization, is plain from the above, and is not controversial. Rather more problematic is the question of how many other levels of grammatical organization to recognize between the levels of sentence and word, and whether there are higher levels than the sentence that need to be taken into account. The approach used in this chapter operates with two main levels between sentence and word: that of *phrase* and *clause*. The distinctions are illustrated in the following sentence:

SENTENCE

after	the man	went out,	the dog	bit	the cat,	and	the cat	howled

CLAUSE	CLAUSE	CLAUSE

PHRASE	PHRASE	PHRASE	PHRASE	PHRASE

Word	Word	Word	Word	Word	Word	Word	Word	Word	Word

From examples of this kind, it can be seen that:
(i) within a sentence, there may be several recurrent patterns of comparable complexity, some of which have the ability to stand on their own as sentences in their own right *(e.g. the dog bit the cat)*; it is these which are referred to as clauses;
(ii) within clauses, several structural positions can be distinguished, corresponding to such notions as "who did the action", "what action took place" and "who or what was acted upon". These semantic constituents of a clause are given a formal defini-

---

[9] In English, inflections are limited to word-endings, such as *-s, -ing, -er, -ed*. Examples of word-formation include compounds *(e.g. blackbird)* and the use of prefixes and suffixes *(e.g. de-valu-ation)*. For an introduction to morphology, see Matthews (1974).

tion as *elements* of clause structure—the *subject, verb, object* of the clause, respectively[10]. The range of meanings "when/where/why/how . . . did the action take place" is subsumed under the *adverbial* element of clause structure.

(iii) clause elements may consist of single words (*bit* and *howled* in the above sentence), but they may also consist of groups of words, and it is to this possibility that the notion of *phrase* applies *(e.g. the man, the dog)*.

(iv) clauses may be connected in various ways (*e.g.* by the conjunctions *and* and *after* above), and this sequencing property at this level of grammatical analysis is referred to under the heading of *connectivity*.

There are several standard references which expound this kind of approach in detail, and discuss problems in its application[11]. As it is an approach to grammar which I have found helpful in clinical investigations, I shall continue to use it here, as a frame of reference. But the existence of alternative ways of analyzing such sentences as the above must be recognized. For example, we might dispense with the notion of clause, as an independent level, and see each of the units under (i) above as being based on structures which are sentences in their own right; or again, we could dispense with the distinction between single words and multi-word structures, referring to both as types of "phrase". We might give primacy to the formal elements of sentence/clause structure, and dispense with a statement in functional terms (*i.e.* not using such notions as "subject" and "object"); or we might do the reverse, and give primacy to the functional elements, without bothering too much about their formal realization. All of these positions are represented in the theoretical literature, and each could be insightful in the analysis of clinical material. Which approach we use will be partly a matter of personal training and taste, and partly a matter of pragmatics—the approach that seems to handle the data of disability most directly. It is unlikely that we will be convinced solely by referring to the theoretical arguments in linguistics, which do not produce a consensus as to the overall viability of one or other of the above approaches.

Misconceptions

There are certain characteristics of the grammar of a language which all of the above approaches would be in agreement about. Two of these characteristics in particular need to be mentioned, as they function as a corrective to traditional misconceptions about the nature of grammar often encountered in clinical studies.

The length of a structure. Since the early years of this century, the length of a structure has been cited as an efficient index of linguistic complexity[12]. Sentences in particular have been studied in this way: the longer a sentence gets, the more complex it

---

[10] There is no simple correspondence between elements of clause structure and their semantic function, *e.g.* Subjects usually "do" the action, but not always—they may "experience" or "receive" it, as in *John saw a book, The window broke,* or *John was kicked.* See further, p. 161.

[11] See Quirk, *et. al.* (1972), and Crystal, Fletcher and Garman (1976) for its clinical applications; cf. Roberts (1956), Strang (1968), Halliday, McIntosh and Strevens (1964). For the alternatives referred to below, see Huddleston (1976), Matthews (1981). For clinical applications using other models, see Lee (1974), Morehead and Ingram (1973), Dever (1972).

[12] See the review by McCarthy (1954). For a critique, see Crystal, Fletcher and Garman (1976: 9–11), Minifie, Darley and Sherman (1963), Rees (1971).

must be. However, the fact that there is no simple correlation between sentence length and sentence complexity can be easily illustrated, by taking two sentences of the same length (as measured in terms of words, or morphemes, or syllables) which are widely different in terms of their internal complexity. For example, the sentences *there is a cat and a dog and a horse and a rabbit* and *the man who fell over had been drinking heavily since the pub opened* are identical in length, in terms of number of words used; but the second is intuitively much more complex than the first. The relationships between words, and the number of levels of organization within a sentence are plainly far more important than any single quantitative index; and it is accordingly the qualitative studies of grammatical structure which have been the focus of attention in recent clinical applications. A similar point would apply to other length measures (*e.g.* phrase length, utterance length) and counts (*e.g.* part of speech ratios).

Parts of speech. The classical tradition of grammatical analysis handed down by the Greeks viewed language in terms of parts of speech, such as *noun, verb, adverb* and *conjunction.* In describing a language, the aim was to identify the part of speech a word belonged to, and then to study the way parts of speech were used in sequence to form sentences. This emphasis permeated the whole of the traditional grammatical study of English, and it is reflected throughout the field of grammatical development and grammatical disorders. But this orientation, by itself, is an inadequate account of grammatical ability or disability. Grammar is far more than an ordered collection of parts of speech, and parts of speech constitute a very minor aspect of grammatical analysis and description when compared with the various processes of sentence construction referred to above. The reason is that the very definition of the various parts of speech depends on these other processes. If we ask "What part of speech is the word *round?*", for example, the answer has to be: "It depends on the grammatical context in which the word is used." In the sentence *he went round the corner*, it would be called a preposition; in *it's your round*, it would be a noun; in *he rounded the bend*, it is being used as the base of a verb; and so on. Only after we have studied the context can we draw a conclusion about parts of speech (or *word-classes*, as linguistics texts tend to call them); and this means that the initial focus of attention in any grammatical analysis must be on the processes of sentence construction as a whole[13].

Grammatical Acquisition

Research into the development of English morphology and syntax in normal children made rapid progress in the 1970s. A large number of naturalistic and experimental studies came to be published, and several important syntheses of their findings were produced[14]. The clinical use of these findings was twofold. Firstly, the detailed look at the acquisition of individual structures, such as question forms or negation, provided the clinician with a set of guidelines for the assessment and remediation of these structures in cases where they were absent or in error. Second-

[13] See further, Crystal, Fletcher and Garman (1976: 7—9), and the papers in the special volume on word-classes (Lingua, 1967).

[14] One of the earliest was Brown (1973). More recent textbooks include Dale (1976), Cruttenden (1979), de Villiers and de Villiers (1978), Fletcher and Garman (1979: Part II).

ly, the syntheses motivated the construction of descriptive frameworks which aimed in principle to incorporate all aspects of the grammatical learning process, particularly for the period where this learning seemed to be most noticeable—between one and five years. Of course, as soon as we try to develop a comprehensive framework, the many gaps in our knowledge become immediately apparent: there are still several topics in morphology and syntax where information about norms of acquisition is totally lacking. But the existence of gaps does not invalidate the framework as a whole. As long as the framework contains a sufficiently large and wide-ranging set of grammatical variables about which developmental information is known, it is capable of being used in a positive and discriminating way for clinical purposes, and this is what has happened (see p. 108 ff.).

To achieve their results, the clinical studies have had to rely not only on the empirical findings of child language research, but also on certain theoretical principles which have guided work on grammatical acquisition in recent years. Chief amongst these has been the principle of *stages* of development. It is postulated that the emergence of grammatical structure, in either production or comprehension, is stable and predictable, and that within the developmental continuum it is possible to isolate discrete stages, capable of definition in formal linguistic terms. It is important to note that different kinds and numbers of stages are proposed by different authors, depending on the level of generality at which they make their observations. Bloom and Lahey (1978: Ch. 5), for example, discuss the development of semantic-syntactic structure in terms of four broad stages: single-word utterances, successive single-word utterances, linear syntactic relationships, and hierarchical syntactic relationships. Crystal, Fletcher and Garman (1976: Ch. 4) operate with seven syntactic stages in their LARSP profile:

Stage I Single-element sentences, *e.g. daddy, there, more;*

Stage II Two-element sentences, defined in terms of clause elements *(e.g. daddy go, kick ball)* or phrase elements *(e.g. big car, mummy's bag);*

Stage III Three-element sentences, defined in terms of clause elements *(e.g. daddy kick ball)* or phrase elements *(e.g. in the box);* the stage includes the beginning of hierarchical development, with phrase units being incorporated into clause structure (see further, p. 112); associated developments, such as pronouns and the copula, are thus placed at this stage;

Stage IV Four-element sentences, defined in terms of clause elements *(e.g. daddy kick ball window)* or phrase elements *(e.g. in the big box),* along with any associated developments *(e.g.* the development of phrasal coordination);

Stage V Complex sentence formation, defined in terms of clausal coordination *(e.g. the table is broken and the chair is broken),* clausal subordination (clauses as subjects, objects, or adverbials, *e.g. the chair broke when he sat on it)* and phrasal subordination (especially relative clauses, *e.g. the man who came in sat down);*

Stage VI Consolidation of the grammatical systems operating at the different points in phrase and clause structure *(e.g.* quantification structures in the noun phrase, more complex verb phrase and complementation structures); also, the gradual elimination of most surface morphological errors;

Stage VII Remaining structures, *e.g.* patterns of sentence connectivity, patterns of emphatic expression.

It should be appreciated that, while stages of this kind have empirical validity (they are based on a synthesis of findings about the order of emergence of the categories listed), they have no explanatory force. The LARSP procedure does not attempt to explain why, say, three-element sentences appear after two-element ones, or why the time-scale attributed to these stages of development takes the form it has. There are many possible reasons that could underlie the emergence of stages in grammatical development—they might be related to associated developments in cognitive skills, input, or of course to properties of complexity inherent in language. Bloom and Lahey's stages, by contrast, are firmly related to postulates about cognitive development, and this indeed is the dominant approach in the field[15].

Working with stage-based models of grammatical acquisition has undoubtedly proved illuminating in clinical contexts (see below), but the unidimensionality of these models is restricting. It obscures the fact, for example, that there may be several developmental processes simultaneously ongoing in the child, as he copes with the different demands of comprehension, production and imitation tasks. While there are certain parallels, there is no identity between the order of emergence of structures within these three domains[16]. It also does not permit a statement of the various strategies which the child experiments with as he gains control over a structure. If, for example, a child assumes that the first noun phrase in a sentence is always the doer of the action, he will make in due course several errors of comprehension and production; but while these might be noted as a feature of a particular stage of development, there is no easy way of incorporating onto a stages chart why the errors are there[17]. These points have undoubted clinical relevance, and indicate the need for a stages-based approach to be supplemented by a detailed analysis of the acquisition of individual structures in different linguistic settings, and of individual patterns of response[18].

A good illustration of this issue, which has particular utility for clinical work, is in the field of question acquisition. How children come to ask and respond to questions is an issue whose importance goes well beyond the task of grammatical learning, as it affects the whole nature of interaction between clinician and patient. Without questions to ask, what would one do! But which questions should be asked first, and what order of emergence should we anticipate? This was one of the first topics to be addressed in language acquisition studies, in fact (*cf.* Brown, 1968), and several stages have been proposed:

---

[15] See further, Slobin (1973), Levelt (1975). We must guard against too ready a correlation between cognitive and linguistic stages, however. See, *e.g.* Corrigan (1978).

[16] On imitation, see Bloom, Hood, and Lightbown (1974), R. Clark (1977), Folger and Chapman (1978). On recent studies of the comprehension and production of specific structures, see Slobin and Welsh (1971), Clark, Hutcheson and Van Buren (1974), Shatz (1978), Sachs and Truswell (1978), Emerson (1979, 1980), Benedict (1979). For an early statement of the problem, see Fraser, Bellugi and Brown (1963).

[17] For problems in the acquisition of element order, see de Villiers and de Villiers (1973), Kail and Segui (1978), Bridges (1980).

[18] On individual differences, see Ramer (1976), Furrow, Nelson, and Benedict (1979), Bridges (1980). On specific grammatical structures: verb phrase (Fletcher 1979), passive (Baldie 1976, Horgan 1978 a), conjunctions (Lust 1977, Ardery 1980, Lust and Mervis 1980), adjective order (Richards 1979); on later grammatical development, Karmiloff-Smith (1979).

(i) no formal grammatical marker, with intonation being used to signal a questioning attitude (*cf.* p. 61), *e.g.* ↑*dáddy* (="is that daddy?");

(ii) the use of a single question-word, or a question-word along with another element of clause or phrase structure, *e.g. where?, what that?, where daddy?;*

(iii) the development of this structure, with more than one clause element, but with the internal structure of the verb phrase being unaffected by the presence of the question word, *e.g. where daddy going?, what he is doing?;*

(iv) the use of inverted-order questions, *e.g. is he?, do he go?;*

(v) the incorporation of inverted-order structures into the question-word matrix, *e.g. where is daddy going?;*

(vi) the development of more complex question-forms, *e.g.* tag questions.

Stages of this kind are helpful as far as they go, but they are not sufficiently detailed to answer the clinical request above, and nothing has yet been said about differential patterns of acquisition. To investigate this, we need to reverse our direction of interest: instead of seeing question-forms as just one of the features of a composite profile of the child's usage, we need to focus directly on these forms, referring to other aspects of usage only when necessary, in order to explain anomalies. Several studies have adopted this line in recent years[19], and their results (for the main question-forms) may be summarized as follows:

Production

Smith, 1933	Tyack and Ingram, 1977	Savić, 1975 (Serbo-Croatian)
yes/no	yes/no	what
what	what	yes/no
where	where	where
how	why	who
why	how	how
when	who	why
	when	when

Comprehension[20]

Ervin-Tripp, 1970	Tyack and Ingram, 1977	Cairns and Hsu, 1978	Horgan, 1978
yes/no			yes/no
what	where-Intrans		where
where	why	who	
why	who-Subject	why	
who-Subject	where-Trans	when	
how	what-Object	how	
when	who-Object		
who-Object	when		
	how		
	what-Subject		

---

[19] See Smith (1933), Ervin-Tripp (1970), Savić (1975), Crosby (1976), Snow (1977), Tyack and Ingram (1977), Horgan (1978 b), Cairns and Hsu (1978).

[20] In these lists, —Subject and —Object refer to the clause roles of the interrogative item, *e.g. who is kicking?* (*who*-Subject), *who is he kicking?* (*who*-Object). Intrans = Intransitive verb in the interrogative

These studies have some important similarities and differences. On production, they agree that *yes/no* questions appear first (*cf.* the intonational questions referred to above), and these are followed by *what*-questions and then *where*-questions. Less clearly, *how*-questions may be said to precede *why*-questions. *When*-questions are plainly last of all, for this selection of forms; and *who*-questions remain unclear. In terms of comprehension, the earliest period seems to show a certain parallelism about order of development: *yes/no*-questions are correctly responded to first, and then *where*- and *what*-questions. The order of emergence here is not entirely clear, however, and one factor which complicates the statement is the apparent relevance of the class of verb to the decision as to when *where*-questions can be said to be comprehended. *Where*-questions involving an intransitive verb in the clause were in Tyack and Ingram's data comprehended well before those with transitive verbs in the clause. A similar complication affects the statement of the *why/who* sequence: *why*-questions seem to be comprehended before *who*-questions, for some of the studies, but there are different responses obtained for *who*-Subject and *who*-Object questions, the latter being later. *When*-questions are comprehended earlier than *how*-questions, the reverse of the production studies. And *what*-questions are surprisingly late, compared with the production studies—though here too a distinction between *what*-Subject and *what*-Object is required.

There is plainly no easy parallelism between the production and the comprehension data. In order to explain the discrepancies, it is thus necessary to look more closely at one side or the other. The production data are unhelpful, as it proves impossible to be sure how far the children were in full control of the comprehension of the forms they were using. As a result, attention has focussed on the strategies presumed to be underlying the comprehension data (results which were based on the errors in children's responses to questions about pictures). The patterns noted in the error-analysis led Ervin-Tripp to speculate about the strategies children might be using, and she proposed four criteria:
"(i) If you recognize the word, give a correct reply.
(ii) If there is a transitive verb, respond with the object of that verb.
(iii) If you are over three, and there is an animate subject and an intransitive verb, give a causal explanation.
(iv) For the remaining intransitives, give a locative or direction if it is missing."
These strategies predicted between 67% and 84% of the errors made. Tyack and Ingram, thinking along similar lines, were led to accept the first of these strategies, but proposed a replacement for the other three by a single semantic criterion:

"If you have not acquired the question word, respond on the basis of the semantic features of the verb."

They then added a further criterion, to handle some residual cases:

"Process a verb that ends a sentence as intransitive."

So, for example, if a child were asked *Where is the boy going to kick the ball?* (expected answer "into the goal"), we would expect an appropriate answer only under crite-

---

clause *(e.g. where is he going?)*; Trans ▬ Transitive verb in the interrogative clause *(e.g. where is he kicking the ball?)*. The groupings in Tyack and Ingram are made by them on statistical grounds.

rion (i) above. If the child did not know the meaning of *where*, in this context, criterion (ii) would predict that he would reply by saying something about the ball.

The findings are limited by the relatively small samples used in these studies.
There is still a great deal of individual variation in the responses, and several unclear
trends. But three important conclusions can be drawn:

(a) from the ages of the children studied (between 2 and 4 years in the production
studies, between 3 and 5$\frac{1}{2}$in the comprehension studies), it is clear that the learning
of question-words is not a sudden, "across-the board" exercise; there is a time-lag
between production and comprehension, not only in the experimental settings, but
also in the naturalistic situation[21];

(b) children's ability to respond to (and possibly also to use) question-forms may
depend in part on the verb's grammatical relationship to the rest of the clause, and
also on its position in that clause;

(c) likewise, their ability may depend on the verb's semantic features, *e.g.* a question
about an animate verb (such as *sleep*) may be interpreted as an animate question-
word, even if it is not (as when *What is he sleeping on?* is interpreted as if it were the
question "Who is sleeping?").

Further research will have to concentrate on these variables, to see if the effects
obtained so far can be replicated. It will also be important to broaden the data-base
of the enquiry, to include the wide range of question-forms available in English that
are morphologically more complex than the above, *e.g. what else, what sort, what about,
what for, who else, where from, how many, how long,* etc. It may well be that the way the
child uses some of these forms may affect his ability or motivation to use the
"central" items above—*what for,* for example, is in several respects a competitor of
why.

The implication that emerges from a review of research such as this is primarily
that future studies of grammatical acquisition are not going to be as autonomous or
as straightforward as was once imagined. Cognitive, semantic and social factors evidently exercise important influences on the development of grammatical patterns,
at every stage. It is presumably for this reason that explanatory models of acquisition which focus on grammar as a central principle are these days less popular than
they were in the 1960s[22]. However, at a descriptive level, the need to be able to
handle syntactic and morphological features is just as essential now as it ever was.
Apart from anything else, these constitute a far more "tangible" point of departure
than do the other areas mentioned: the variables are more determinate, in the
present state of knowledge, and better understood. And of course it does not follow
that because cognitive or social factors are being seen as primary, in an explanatory
sense, that formal linguistic factors should be ruled out altogether. On the contrary,
it is essential to develop an acquisitional perspective in which neither linguistic nor
non-linguistic factors are undervalued, if a realistic framework for clinical investigation is to be devised.

---

[21] Savić (1975) reinforces the point, showing the existence of an "incubation period" of 6 months
or more between the mother's use of these forms and the child's subsequent use of them (cf. also
Furrow, Nelson, and Benedict, 1979).

[22] See Fletcher and Garman (1979: 128—129); but cf. Erreich, Valian and Winzemer (1980).

Several other points of general significance emerge from the example given above. The intricate way in which comprehension and production factors interrelate is something which has often been overlooked in clinical investigations, which generally test the two abilities separately, and often on the assumption that the one (*i.e.* comprehension) must precede the other. That this is generally the case is undeniable, but increasingly studies are showing that there are many areas where this assumption is untenable—where grammatical production precedes comprehension, or where the two seem to be moving so closely in parallel that it proves impossible to disentangle them. The point has been noted both with reference to the early stages of syntactic development and to the more advanced stages[23]. Children have often been observed to use structures without fully comprehending them—a point which is felt not to be surprising in the learning of vocabulary, but which is often neglected in relation to grammar. A well-studied example is children's use of *because*, encountered as a connective from around age three, but not fully comprehended until age eight and after, as shown by examples such as *My father never got sick because he catches cold* and *Why do wolves bite? Because they are from Little Red Riding Hood*[24].

Why has the point about the late development of comprehension been neglected? Doubtless this is something to do with the difficulty of observing and measuring the phenomenon. A great deal of ingenuity has been used in recent years to bring the notion of comprehension under experimental control, and while this inevitably introduces a measure of artificiality into the settings, about which we should always be on our guard[25], the research findings are invariably helpful, when it comes to interpreting behaviour in (inevitably artificial) clinical situations. That comprehension problems are difficult to observe is illustrated in the following extracts from a series of tape-recordings involving a six-year-old. The child is in the kitchen while his mother is cooking the evening meal. The mother asks him to "go and ask daddy if he wants potatoes for dinner this evening". The child runs into the other room and says "Mummy says there's potatoes for dinner this evening". The father says "That's nice", and carries on reading the paper. The child runs back to the kitchen and says "Daddy says yes". Sometime later, while the family is having dinner, the father comments that "perhaps we could try rice with this next time, darling", and the dialogue proceeded as follows:

Mother: well yès/ but you 'said you 'wanted potàtoes/
Father: nò I dídn't/
Mother: you dìd/ I 'sent Mìchael to ásk you/ and 'you said you dìd/
Father: well I 'don't re'member thăt/
Mother: yès he díd/ you dìd go/ dìdn't you/ (to Michael, who nods)
Father: well 'I don't re'member 'any such thìng/ - I re'member him saying 'something about potătoes/ but he 'didn't 'ask me if I wànted ány/
Mother: well he shòuld have done/ because 'that's what I àsked him to 'do/ - (turns to Michael) 'why didn't you 'ask 'daddy like I tòld you to/ ...

---

[23] See fn. 16 above.

[24] Examples from Emerson (1979: 299). See also Kuhn and Phelps (1976), Corrigan (1975).

[25] See Donaldson (1978), Fletcher and Garman (1979: Part III).

The example need not be continued, for the source of the confusion is obvious to anyone who is aware of the problems of *ask* and *tell* (see, for example, Chomsky, 1969). But the point I wish to stress is how the fact of the child's confusion between *ask* and *tell* on this occasion would not even have been noticed, if the father hadn't happened to comment about the rice. If the meal had dealt with other topics, there would have been no issue.

This situation is by no means an atypical one. It was fortunate that, in this case, the interaction had been captured on tape; but intuitively, we can recognize that this kind of confusion happens a great deal. What this indicates, though, is that the occasions where we do notice that something has gone wrong are probably far outnumbered by those occasions where we do not, or where we have not time or opportunity (or inclination) to make the correction for the child. It is perhaps for this reason that so many grammatical topics take so long for their comprehension to become adult-like. The late learning of the meaning of the definite article (in all its contexts), the passive, relative clauses and conjunctions provides further examples[26].

Lastly in this section, it is important to stress the need to provide as full an account as is possible of the language production of the child, in order to arrive at a reliable grammatical analysis. This means, in particular, being on our guard that we do not read structure in to the child's utterances (*e.g.* the child says *I sitting there* and we transcribe "I'm sitting there")—something that parents regularly do, if asked to transcribe their child's utterances. It also means that we do not leave structure out, by ignoring phonological material that we see no reason for, or which we believe to be hesitation noise. Such apparently empty inserts may have developmental significance, in that they might be the first signs of a child's awareness of the existence of a structure in the adult language, or be an illustration of a transitional stage between one construction and another[27].

Of all the formal features of child utterance which get omitted from routine consideration, however, it is the prosody of speech that is the most significant. We have already seen the important role prosody has to play in identifying and integrating the grammatical structure of speech (p. 64), and its description ought to become a routine feature of child language enquiry, both in normal and remedial contexts. Being aware of such factors as intonation, rhythm, stress and pause in the delimitation of utterance is often the only way in which a decision can be made as to the status of an utterance as a sentence, a clause element, or whatever. The pair of items *man sleeping,* for example, can be uttered in three quite different ways, and result in three different grammatical analyses (in each case, T is showing a child a picture of a man in a bed):

(i) màn/ (child points to the page, then looks up at T, who says nothing; child refers back to the page)
slèeping/
(ii) man slèeping/ (child looks up)

---

[26] See Karmiloff-Smith (1979). On articles, see Maratsos (1976), Warden (1976); on the passive, Baldie (1976), Horgan (1978 a); on connectives Coker (1978), French and Brown (1977).
[27] See Dore, Franklin, Miller and Ramer (1976), Bloom (1973).

(iii) màn/ (child stays looking at the page, and after a short pause says)
slèeping/

In the first case, the definite intonation on *man*, plus the long pause and the accompanying non-verbal activity, would motivate our taking the utterances *man* and *sleeping* as two one-element sentences. The single tone-unit on (ii), however, would presumably warrant the opposite conclusion: that here we have a single two-element sentence. The third case is more problematic: if the intonation on *man* is rising, and the pause is not too long, then a similar decision to (ii) will be made; whereas if the intonation on *man* is falling, and the pause is fairly long, the decision will probably be to interpret it as (i). But such notions as "fairly long" and "not too long" are not easy to define, and there will plainly be many ambiguous cases—a point which in itself could be of developmental significance.

Decisions of this kind, involving intonation, can be encountered throughout the language acquisition period. At around age three, for example, similar problems arise over whether we take a sequence of clauses linked by *and* as a single (complex sentence) or as a series of *and*-initiated simple sentences. From age six onwards, there are problems over deciding whether a child's rearrangements of the word-order in a sentence are to be viewed as grammatical errors or not, and intonational evidence will be an essential factor to consider *(e.g.* his attempts at the thematic variations permitted by English clause structure, such as *Lucy my name is* or *it was outside school we said we'd meet)*[28]. Whatever the difficulties involved in familiarizing oneself with prosodic variables and their transcription, the risks of misconstrual are so frequent, and affect so many areas of grammar, that the aim of incorporating this information routinely into child descriptions must become a priority, both in normative research and in clinical applications.

Grammatical Disability

In view of the amount of attention paid by the present author and his colleagues to this topic in recent years[29], there is perhaps justification for a brief review of only the main findings of this work, as a preliminary to discussing current trends in the field. These findings may be summarized under three headings.

(i) The importance of grammatical levels. The view that a grammatical disorder is in some way a single of homogeneous phenomenon is replaced by a conception of grammatical structure in which four main levels are recognized, at each of which a type of grammatical difficulty can be located. These levels, deriving from the approach outlined on p. 98 above, are identified as *connectivity, clause, phrase* and *word.* Difficulties at each of these levels can be illustrated by taking a sentence and showing what might happen to it if produced by a patient with a disability at one or other of these levels:

---

[28] See Quirk, *et al.* (1972: Ch. 14). On the relevance of late intonation, see Cruttenden (1974), Chomsky (1970), and p. 73 above.

[29] Crystal, Fletcher, and Garman (1976), Crystal (1979 a), Crystal and Fletcher (1978).

normal sentence

the man broke his arm because the ladder slipped and he fell off

connectivity difficulties

the man broke his arm and the ladder slipped because he fell off
the ladder slipped because the man broke his arm and he fell off

clause difficulties

the man his arm and because the ladder and he off (Verb omission)
the man his arm broke because slipped the ladder and he fell off (element order)
broke his arm because slipped and fell off (Subject omission)

phrase difficulties

man broke arm because ladder slipped and he fell (no phrase development)
man the broke arm his because ladder the slipped and he off fell (word order in phrase)

word difficulties

the man break he arm because the ladder slip and he fall off (no inflections)
the man broking his arm because the ladder slippeding and he fells off (wrong inflections)

These are of course only some of the possible errors that this sentence might display. Also, the example is somewhat unreal, in that it is unusual to find a patient whose grammatical difficulties are neatly located at a single level. Far more usual are the "mixed" examples, such as:

the mans broked his arm and ladder slipped cos he fell

which contains a problem from each level.

While all possible combinations of difficulties can be found in patients, there are two patterns which are much more common than any others. The first is by far the commonest: it consists of a bias towards single word sentences, with a subsequent phrasal development; clause structure relations are largely absent. If the phrase bias is allowed to continue, connectivity may come to be used, still with the clause level development by-passed. The following selection of sentences was typical of one four-year-old language-delayed child, when he first presented for treatment:

hòuse/	on grăss/	nò/
window/	mê/	thère/
càr/	rùnning/	thàt one/
trèes/	grèen/	wàter/
in strèet/	flòwer/	mòre/
yés/	màn and/	mùmmy/
hère/	hím/	dò it/

Apart from *do it,* which illustrates a verb-object clause structure, all sentences are either single-word or two-element phrases. Moreover, there is little sign of the prerequisite for subsequent clausal development, namely verbs (apart from *running*). For various reasons this child received no structured therapy for several months, by which time his sentence structure had developed as follows:

lòrry/	in a strèet/	with hânds/
on tòp/	at a bùs/	hìm/
'very dàngerous/	thàt 'man/	in his hòuse/
yès/	'man and a làdy/	a 'big fàt/
mhm̀/	in thère/	gòne/
nò húrt/	'big hàt on/	mòre thére/

The greater complexity of the sentences is apparent, but there is still little sign of clause structure (apart from *more there* and possibly *no hurt*). The phrase-level bias is now quite marked, and is beginning to cause difficulties for those trying to communicate with him, a typical dialogue being:

T	'what's 'happening in the pìcture/	
P	'big hàt on/	
T	whò's got a 'big 'hat on/	
P	thàt 'man/	
T	'what's he dòing/	
P	hàt on/	
T	m̀/	(puzzled)
P	mòre/	(points at picture, but not clear at what)
T	whère/	
P	on tòp/	
	thère/	
T	is the 'man rŭnning/	(tries new tack)

Later still, as P's command over connectivity (especially *and*) developed, the length of his utterances increased dramatically; but far from this being a promising sign, it turned out to be a cause for concern. In the above extract, the effect of P not expressing clause relations (making it clear who was doing what to whom, etc.) was alleviated somewhat by T's sharing of the context with P, and the fact that his sentences were fairly short. Monologues such as the following, however, produced problems of a quite different order:

T   'what did you 'see on tèlevision last 'night/
P   a còwboy/ . and . and . the 'best 'gun in the wèst/ . and he . a 'fire for the gròund/ . 'all gòne/ so the 'other 'cowboys and the báddy/ a 'big fíght/ and . and . he dèad/

This is doubtless the inevitable effect of an uncorrected phrase bias in a child of reasonable initiative and intelligence, and a rapidly developing vocabulary.

The opposite effect is also common in language-delayed children: it again begins with a bias towards single-word sentences, but with a subsequent clausal development; there is little or no development of phrase structure, and word structures also tend to be absent. As clause structure develops, the speech sounds increasingly "telegrammatic". Elizabeth's first sample (age 4) produced the following sentences:

shòes/	twò/	twò on thére/
nò/	drèss/	blúe/
bùtton/	ôh/	in thère/
thère/	yès/	anòther one/
hìding/	tàble/	sìt/
lòok/	rêd/	'that at hòme/

The sample does not look very different from the first sample taken from the previous child; indeed there seems to be a corresponding phrase bias. But there are certain differences: the phrases are "emptier" of meaning (because of the use of deictic forms: see p. 120), and there are three verbs in the sample. A later sample (again, no structured therapy having intervened) thus looked very different from that taken from the previous child:

'is hìding/	dò 'that/	'me hìde/
'what thàt/	'one mòre/	nò/
ôh/	'where shĕ/	dàddy/
gòt óne/	'I 'not hìding/	shòe todáy/
thère/	yès/	lôok/
anòther one/	I dò it/	'you gò/
'listen mè/	thère she ís/	'where mán/

In this case, there is a considerable amount of clause structure at the two element stage (subject-verb, verb-object, and combinations involving adverbials), and there are even some three-element clauses (*I do it, there she is*). There is a limited indication of phrase structure developing within clause structure (*I not hiding, is hiding*). Unfortunately, this phrasal development did not continue, and at a later stage (immediately prior to the child being referred for structured therapy) sequences using connectives had begun to build up, *e.g.*

'see 'man and pùsh him/
'I get 'that and 'give you and you hìde it/
'bicycle 'gonna thère nów/ cos it it . 'chained ùp/ sée/ and 'boys fìnd it/ wòn't/

Sequences such as *boys find it won't* indicate that P is aware of the meaning that needs to be expressed, but lacks the phrasal ability to structure it correctly. It is interesting to speculate what might have happened if therapy had not begun at that (already extremely late) stage. I have not encountered a patient whose syntax is at a more advanced telegrammatic stage.

(ii) The interaction of grammatical levels. In contrast to the previous children, normal grammatical development shows a regular and parallel increase in structures operating at both phrase and clause levels. One 19-month-old, for example, was using the following:

CLAUSE	PHRASE
'want thàt/	my càr/
'see dàddy/	my dàddy/
'car thère/	in thère/
'look màn/	in càr/
'what thàt/	anòther one/

A little later, he began to use his phrases as exponents of clause elements, *e.g. want my daddy, car in there.* The importance of this stage has been stressed in the language acquisition literature, as it is the first evidence of the child's awareness of the hierarchical organization of sentence structure. It is perhaps not surprising, then, to find that it turns out to be a major stumbling-block in remedial work with language-disordered patients. Often, however, the effects of this stage of development have not been anticipated by the clinician.

A typical progression is as follows. T has been working on a language-delayed patient who has reached the two-element stage. A great deal of time has been spent on obtaining a fairly balanced profile, *i.e.* one where phrase-level and clause-level complexity are roughly equivalent. Clause element order and phrase word order are good. In short, the patient looks very much like the 19-month-old referred to above. From a developmental point of view, the next step is to get P to begin using his phrases as part of clause structure, and at this point things often begin to go wrong, as the following dialogue illustrates:

T   (having already elicited *red ball* and *yellow ball* in response to *what's the man kicking,* and *kick* in response to *what's the man doing*)
      'what's the 'man dòing/   (makes man kick red ball)
P   'kick bàll/
T   thàt's ríght/
      he's 'kicking a bàll/ ìsn't he/
      he's 'kicking the 'red bàll/
      whát's he 'doing/
P   'red bàll/   (presumably tonicity influence, *cf.* p. 93)
T   yès/
      it's the 'red bàll/
      but 'what's he dòing to the 'red 'ball/
P   he kìck it/
T   thàt's ríght/
      he's kîcking the 'red 'ball/
      'you tèll me/
P   'kick bàll/
      'red bàll/
T   'kicking the -   (prompt)
P   'red bàll/
T   he's ---   (prompt)
      he's -
      'go ón/
      'you tèll me/

P   'kick - 'ball a rèd/
T   'kicking the 'red bàll/
P   'red 'ball kìck/
T   ṁ/   (puzzled)
P   'red bàll/
     he kìck it/

It seems clear from this sequence that while P has no trouble producing either the verb or the noun phrase in isolation, as soon as he attempts to integrate them, his syntax begins to collapse—even to the extent of his apparently losing the word order ability previously painfully established. No wonder T seemed puzzled! What has to be appreciated is that putting an extra element into a drill (adding an adjective, in this case) may do far more than just increase the length of the sentence by one. It may, as here, add a whole new dimension to the psychological complexity of the sentence for the patient, so much so that in being asked to focus upon it, P loses control over other aspects of sentence structure. Under such circumstances, the introduction of phrasal complexity would need to proceed with great caution, using vocabulary that is more well-established (colours had only recently been taught, in the above example), avoiding open questions (of the *what's he doing* type), providing better intonational reinforcement, and so on.

The kind of difficulty which this example illustrates is by no means restricted to the two- to three-element stage of language development. It may appear at almost any stage of development where P's psychological or linguistic limitations are being stretched. An example of this temporary regression from a much more advanced patient took place when T switched from *where*-questions (which P was familiar with) to *when*-questions (which had only recently been introduced). The *where*-question produced the answer *the children went to the seaside;* the immediately following *when*-question produced the answer *in summertime they go seaside/ the children.*

The developing interdependence between linguistic levels can present a patient with major problems of comprehension or expression, as these examples show. The problem may involve phrase/clause integration, as above, or phrase/word integration (*e.g.* inserting a morphologically complex word into a phrase), and, in the more advanced patients, connectivity might be seriously affected by residual difficulties from earlier stages of phrasal or clausal development. A frequently occurring example of this latter type arises out of a poor command of auxiliary verb and copula usage[30], which, if still present when P is attempting complex sentence structure, can lead to sequencing difficulties. That these problems can affect adults too is illustrated by the following ambiguous sentences, taken from the speech of an expressive aphasic:

she 'come to the 'house and 'car rèady/ (*i.e.* she came to the house when the car was ready)
at 'home a nìce cháir/ and 'sit in it èvenings/ (*i.e.* I intend to buy a nice chair so that ...)

---

[30] Auxiliary verbs are illustrated in *he* is/**was**/**has been** *going, he* **may**/**might**/**can** *go.* The copula is a form of the verb *be* when it is the only verb in a clause, *e.g. he* is *happy/a boy.* See Quirk *et al.* (1972: 820), where the notion is also applied to verbs with a similar linking function.

(iii) The importance of a comprehensive description. The need to develop a clinical grammatical awareness—the main theme of this chapter—means that observations about a patient's grammatical usage need to be much more systematic and comprehensive than has traditionally been the case. A selective commentary on the most noticeable features or errors is of limited value—for example, pointing to the omission of certain grammatical words, such as *the* or *of,* to errors in pronouns or in word-order. Assessment on the basis of such an impressionistic inventory is bound to be unreliable, as there is an inevitable tendency for the clinician to pick out those features of syntax and morphology which are the most easily describable, and there is no guarantee that T will notice what P has *not* been using. Almost by definition, there will be far more features of grammar omitted than present, in a clinical sample; and the need to think systematically and comprehensively about the absent structures is thus paramount.

"Comprehensiveness" means, in the first instance, that *all* the instances of grammatical construction, in a sample from a patient, should be accounted for, no matter how incomplete or anomalous they may seem. There are several clinical grammatical procedures where the patient's attempts at sentences are discounted, and only his complete versions analyzed. But while this may give an idea about the patient's level of achievement, it does not help explain his underachievement. Only an analysis of the sentences he is leaving unfinished, or avoiding altogether, will indicate those aspects of sentence construction which he is finding particularly difficult. For example, we might expect a patient who is having problems with verb tenses to stop mid-sentence before he arrives at the verb, especially if he is attempting to express a meaning that demands syntactic resources which he has not yet mastered. Some incomplete sentences from one such patient were:

so 'later on we -- we 'all --- and 'then at hôme/
if he júmp/ he [kə dɪ] --- he 'fall dòwn/

The attempts at auxiliary verbs here might well be put down to nonfluency, especially if there were any associated articulation problems, but the reason for the difficulty is almost certainly grammatical. Here is a more complex example, taken from a child of 2¹/₂ whose "normal nonfluency" was at times quite severe[31]. To analyze only this child's fluent sentences (*i.e.* 95% of his total output) would produce a clear picture in terms of the grammatical stages given on p. 101. Examples of his clause structures were:

Stage I yès/, nò/, crâsh/, rèd/, lòok/, wátch/, òh/;
Stage II 'got sòup/, 'just in thère/, I cân't/, gò ón/, I'm fàlling/, on hòliday tomórrow/, it ìs/, I hàven't/, 'might see grándpa/;
Stage III it's in thêre/, yòu 'find it/, 'what's thât/, 'where (="who") shall I sèe/, 'do that nōw/, 'me have to 'cut my nàils/, 'can we 'go outsìde/, I 'got no wàter/, 'that is mỳ 'cup of 'tea/, 'I want òrange/;
Stage IV 'you have lòok in 'there/, he's 'naughty 'boy nǒw/, that's 'blue 'house and rèd 'house/, we gó on hòliday 'then/;
Stage V 'cos it's gròwing 'time/, and 'mummy 'woke ùp/.

---

[31] Cf. the discussion in Dalton and Hardcastle (1977: 69 ff.).

The child had a fairly balanced profile down to Stage IV, and was beginning the task of building up Stage V sentence sequences. Now let us look at the examples of non-fluency produced in the same sample as the above:

(i) did did . did wàsh it/

(ii) cos - [kə kə kə] cos . [bə]' Bev - [bə bə] erm couldn't Ni - 'Nicholas - was - bàd 'boy/ (*i.e.* Bev couldn't do the ironing because Nicholas was a bad boy)

(iii) erm . erm . erm . li 'like . [bə] 'Bev - [gə gə . gə gə] erm - [gə gə gə] got gòt one thóse/

(iv) 'all [fɔ:] . 'flowers . go gò/ . [g] gò/ . gròw/

(v) erm [æ:æ:] and . when it's . sùmmer [tam] . tìme/ . and - [əə] 'alway . [ma] 'make sòapy 'water/ 'when it's sùmmer 'time/

(vi) [kʊ kʊ] could 'make . [kə] 'cup of tèa/

(vii) [də] 'there yours [dɪ] drínk/ . [də də] 'there you āre/

(viii) [m m] erm - what's erm . 'make a - [wə] ràinbow/ . erm . [lʊ] Lùcy [reɪ] . 'make a 'rainbow/ [æ] at . hers . at hers [kə kɑ́:snum]/ (*i.e.* classroom)

(ix) erm - 'you mùst 'do/ erm - [pə pʊ pʊ] put me will erm just . just 'put them in còrner/

There are several apparent reasons for the non-fluency. Example (iv) seems to be a clear example of phonological difficulty, as the child attempts /fl-/ and /gr-/ clusters. But this is also an attempt at a future tense form (the context being that the flowers will grow when the seeds mummy has planted come up). As the child has produced both *flowers* and *grow* correctly elsewhere in the sample, the simple phonological explanation is called into question. Evidence that the child is still having trouble with auxiliaries is to be found elsewhere, both in the omissions made in the fluent sentences above (*e.g. we go on holiday,* where the "habitual" sense is not appropriate), and in the pattern of the non-fluency: *cf.* examples (i), (vi), (ix), in particular, and also (ii).

Examples (ii), (iii), (v) and (viii) illustrate a different kind of grammatical difficulty for the child, related to his attempts at handling Stage V constructions. The previous context to (ii) had produced the observation from the child that Nicholas had been smacked, to which the mother had responded with "Why?" The immediate use of "cos" in the response shows that the child understands the point of the question and the causality notion involved, but he then gets tangled up in the syntax, the order-of-mention in his language failing to correspond to the sequence of events that took place. Putting this another way, (ii) is an attempt to produce two responses simultaneously to the *why* question: *Bev couldn't do the ironing* and *Nicholas was a bad boy*—a possibility that English permits, but only at the cost of having to use fairly complex syntax. A similar "blend" of constructions is illustrated in the other examples. In (iii) the two "underlying" sentences seem to be *(I can see something) like Bev's got* and *Bev's got one of those:* these are "run into" each other, and a syntactic blend is produced[32]. (v) may be a problem over handling multiple and competing time expressions in the single sentence—the generality of *always* and the specificity of *when it's summer time.* (viii) may be an attempt at a *what*-Subject construction *(what makes a*

---

[32] For syntactic blends, see Bolinger (1961). For order-of-mention, see Hatch (1971), Clark and Clark (1977: 129, 506 ff.), Coker (1978).

rainbow is . . .)—an extremely advanced construction, but one which the child has attempted elsewhere, using a less complicated construction *(what you do . . .).* The intonation on the word *rainbow* suggests continuity rather than sentence-end. But (viii) is altogether more awkward to explain, due to the simultaneous occurrence of an articulation difficulty (an *r/w* substitution) and a problem from a quite different area of syntax that the child was currently working on (the form of possessive pronouns—*hers classroom;* cf. *yours drink* in [vii]).

While there is plenty of scope for interpretation in such examples, the general point being made seems clear enough—that an analysis of the "performance" errors in a sample can lead to important insights concerning the nature of the difficulties P is facing, at any given time. A great deal would be missed by failing to analyze such errors—not only in cases of non-fluency, but in any context where it might be felt that the language used by P was in some sense discountable (*e.g.* his tendency to be echolalic, to use jargon). If a grammatical analysis is truly comprehensive, it will be able to cope with every syntactic and morphological feature of P's performance, in the sense that it will force T to consider each example systematically and to assign it to a category. Only then can a reliable explanatory process begin.

The Role of a Grammatical Profile

Examples of the kind discussed above force us to think again about the aims and means of carrying out grammatical analyses. A procedure such as LARSP (Crystal, Fletcher and Garman, 1976) is sometimes characterized as a grammatical analysis. It would however be more appropriate to refer to it as a first approximation to a gram-matical analysis. Despite its apparent complexity (for those unfamiliar with the task of grammatical analysis), it is in fact a massive simplification of the grammatical facts of English. Its role is twofold: firstly, to direct T's attention to the range and diversity of grammatical structure in the language of clinical interaction; and secondly, to provide specific indications of areas of strength and weakness in a patient, through the analysis of a sample of his output, or a sample of a clinician's input. Working through procedures such as LARSP may sometimes indicate a solu-tion to an assessment or remediation problem, but more usually their main role is to sensitize the clinician to the existence of a problem, and to make suggestions as to its more precise definition. Further, more detailed grammatical analysis is then required, before the situation can be resolved[33].

We can see this process operating by following up a profile analysis where the initial statement was quite unclear. A language-delayed boy of five had consider-able ability at the two- and three-element stages of clausal development, and had a fair command of the associated phrase structures, but his use of auxiliary verbs and verb endings was apparently erratic. This can be seen by the following sample of data, in which the relevant verb phrases have been listed as they occurred in a five minute exercise describing the events in a picture-book.

---

[33] Cf. the notion of micro-profile, introduced in Crystal (1979 a).

'man wàlking/   'man 'eating dìnner/
'man is 'fall dòwn/   'man sìtting nów/
'man smìling/   'man rùnning/
'man 'kick bàll/   'man 'is jùmp/

At no point did P produce the correct forms of the present tense—*man is walking*, etc. The profile chart was accordingly somewhat confusing, with approximately equal numbers of correct vs. incorrect uses of auxiliary and -*ing*. In order to clarify the problem, an obvious first step is to list the sentences on the basis of their formal characteristics—as if they were different word-classes in a foreign language:

man walking/   man is fall down/
man smiling/   man is jump/
man eating dinner/
man sitting now/   man kick ball/
man running/

The next step is to scrutinize the groupings to see whether there is any formal or semantic reason for the patterns being the way they are. For example, there are many verbs in English that do not normally take an -*ing* ending *(e.g. seem, know, like)*—but these do not seem to be the ones. Perhaps it is something to do with phonological structure—say, monosyllabic verbs allowing -*ing*, polysyllabic verbs not—but again, there is nothing obvious that we might say about one group that did not also apply to the others. From a semantic point of view, is there perhaps something in common between *walk/smile/eat/sit/run* which distinguishes them from the verbs in the other groups? At this point, in dealing with the interrelationship between grammatical and semantic categories, it is important to be aware of any hypotheses which have been proposed in the psycholinguistic or language acquisition literature—especially the latter, where studies may have brought to light systems of grammatical classification and interpretation which are not those normally used in the adult language, and which might otherwise be missed by the process of normal adult introspection. One such system seems particularly relevant, namely, the way in which many children make a distinction in their use of verbs based on the salient characteristics of the activities involved—in particular, whether the action in question involves a change of state of the entities involved in the action or no such change of state. Activities such as "fall over", "kick" and "jump" are all clearly change of state activities, whereas "activities" such as "think", "look" and "breathe" are not. Unfortunately, the picture-book presentation of the stimuli tends to reduce the potential of this distinction, in all but the most dramatic cases: pictures of people eating, running and jumping are invariably static—people frozen in mid-air, or with a fork half way to their mouths. There would be very little to choose between the running and the jumping in this respect.

But the idea of the mode of activity is a good one, and has frequently been referred to in language acquisition studies[34]. Perhaps there are other characteristics of change of state verbs which might attract the attention of a child learning language? There are presumably three main possibilities: activities which have a

[34] See Antinucci and Miller (1976), Macrae (1976), Fletcher (1979), Smith (1980).

discrete starting-point; activities which have a clear limit to their duration; and activities which have a clear finishing-point. For the present sample of data, these distinctions are relevant indeed: there are no grounds for using the first (when the person in the picture starts to walk is just as unclear as when he starts to kick), but the other two criteria provide a relevant basis of contrast: *walk, smile, eat, sit* and *run* are of indeterminate duration, whereas *fall down, jump* and *kick* have a more momentary duration; and whereas the former have no clear end-point, the latter have a definite end-point. There is a clear end to the activities of kicking, falling down and jumping, whereas there is no comparable definiteness about the finishing of the other activities.

This analysis now becomes a hypothesis against which to measure the usage of the patient. There is of course no way of knowing in advance why the patient may have chosen to classify his verbs in this way; on the other hand, it should be pointed out that, if he is going to classify his verbs at all, there are a very limited number of logical paths available for him to follow. P may choose any one of six possible interpretations for the use of *is* vs. *ing* in relation to this classification:

(1) he may think that the way English marks end-point verbs is by using the morpheme *is,* with *ing* or zero being used for other verbs; if he speaks according to this hypothesis, he will produce

| man is fall over/ | vs. | man walk(ing)/ |
| man is kick ball/ | | man eat(ing)/ |

(2) he may think that the way English marks end-point verbs is by using the morpheme *ing,* with *is* or zero being used for other verbs; if he speaks according to this hypothesis, he will produce

| man falling over/ | vs. | man (is) walk/ |
| man kicking ball | | man (is) eat/ |

(3) he may think that the way English marks verbs without end-points is by using the morpheme *is,* with *ing* or zero being used for other verbs; if he speaks according to this hypothesis, he will produce

| man is walk/ | vs. | man fall(ing) over/ |
| man is eat/ | | man kick(ing) ball/ |

(4) he may think that the way English marks verbs without end-points is by using the morpheme *ing,* with *is* or zero being used for other verbs; if he speaks according to this hypothesis, he will produce

| man walking/ | vs. | man (is) fall/ |
| man eating/ | | man (is) kick/ |

(5) he may think that the way English marks end-point verbs is by adding the morpheme *is,* and verbs without end-points by adding the morpheme *ing;* if he speaks according to this hypothesis, he will produce

| man is fall over/ | vs. | man walking/ |
| man is kick ball/ | | man eating/ |

(6) he may think that the way English marks end-point verbs is by adding the morpheme *ing,* and verbs without end-points by adding the morpheme *is;* if he speaks according to this hypothesis, he will produce

man falling over/
man kicking ball/   vs.   man is walk/
                                     man is eat/

Given this range of possible interpretations, it would seem from the data listed on p. 117 above that P is operating according to the fourth hypothesis. The point can be checked immediately, by introducing a wider range of verbs in the next remedial session, and seeing whether we can predict P's behaviour, on the basis of the hypothesis. If we are right, he ought to say *man swimming* and not *man swim* or *man is swim*, for example. If we are wrong, the exercise has not been wasted, for it has eliminated a possibility, and suggested a promising direction for further thinking. It may be, for instance, that the general line of reasoning is correct, but that we were wrong to restrict the field to *be* and *ing* in the first place. Several other factors may need to be followed up and eliminated before a solution to P's problem is found.

Working routinely with grammatical profiles leads us inevitably to intricate detective-work of the above type, where the aim is to think predictively about P's behaviour (*cf.* p. 8). The initial grammatical statement, concerning P's use or misuse of structure, is only a starting-point, which sensitizes us to areas of grammar worth investigating in greater detail. It should be noted, also, that any such follow-up involves repeated reference to vocabulary, and to the context in which the structures were elicited. In most cases of grammatical disability, micro-analysis leads us inexorably in the direction of semantics.

Grammatico-Semantic Problems

It is not difficult to isolate instances of grammatical disability which are unaffected by semantic factors, *e.g.* a straightforward failure to use the correct word order, or to make a verb agree with its subject, where it is plain that P knows what he means to say and is fully in command of the vocabulary involved. There are also equally clear cases of semantic disability, where grammar remains unaffected, *e.g.* a straight-forward (sic) lexical retrieval problem (see Chapter 5). The distinction between grammar and semantics is clear in principle, as the following quotation suggests: "Our general principle will be to regard grammar as accounting for constructions where greatest generalization is possible, assigning to lexicology constructions on which least generalization can be formulated (which approach, that is, the idiosyncratic and idiomatic)."[35] But language presents many cases which fall between these extremes, as the authors of this quotation acknowledge, and it should not therefore

---

[35] Quirk *et al.* (1972: 11–12). An alternative way of making the distinction is to refer to grammar as constituting the study of "closed systems" of contrasts in language (*i.e.* finite sets of mutually defining and mutually exclusive entities, *e.g.* singular vs. plural, the pronoun system, the tense system), whereas the lexicon deals with "open sets" of items (*i.e.* sets which are in principle extendable, and which lack the rule-governed interdependence characteristic of the above, *e.g.* items to do with movement, food, vehicles, etc.).

be surprising to find areas of linguistic disability which can be resolved only with reference to a combination of both grammatical and lexical factors. In fact, such areas are quite common in the early stages of remediation, as can be seen from a consideration of the phenomenon of *deixis* in this context.

Deixis, from the Greek word for "pointing", is a term which has been used in linguistics with increasing frequency in recent years. Under this heading would be subsumed a whole range of grammatical and lexical items and categories which refer directly to temporal and spatial characteristics of the situation in which an utterance takes place. According to Lyons, whose account of deictic language is seminal, we are here dealing with "the location and identification of persons, objects, events, processes and activities being talked about, or referred to, in relation to the spatiotemporal context created and sustained by the act of utterance and the participation in it, typically, of a single speaker and at least one addressee"[36]. Essentially, therefore, it is language whose meaning is contingent on factors in the face-to-face situation in which the utterance is used. Taken out of this situation, the language becomes unclear and ambiguous. For example, in the following sequence between therapist and patient

T   'where shall I 'put the cár/
P   thère/

without further explanation about the situation, P's utterance is uninterpretable. It is not totally meaningless, for the general notion of directional location has been expressed; but unless T has kept full contextual notes, or has an extraordinarily good memory, listening to a tape of the session afterwards will be of little value, in attempting to determine P's intentions or achievements concerning that utterance.

There are in fact several types of deictic expression in a language, which would all cause the same or similar problems. Chief amongst these in terms of frequency in English are the personal pronouns—*I, you, he, him, mine, yours*, etc.—though it must be remembered that some of these (as well as some of the other deictic items below) have a non-deictic as well as a deictic use[37]. Further important deictic categories include the definite article, certain adverbials *(e.g. here, there, now, then, yesterday, today, this way, DISTANCE away, TIME ago)*, other pronouns *(e.g. this, that, one)*, and a wide range of spatial expressions *(e.g. in, out, inside, up, down, left, right, front, back, top, bottom, edge)*. Tense can also be viewed as a deictic category: the choice of a tense-form such as "past" needs to be interpreted with reference to the time of speaking *(e.g. he was here* presupposes that he no longer is, from the viewpoint of the speaker). And several other verb contrasts also require the viewpoint of the speaker to be taken into account: *come* and *go*, or *take* and *bring*, for example. *He is coming* means basically

---

[36] Lyons (1977: 637). See also, Fillmore (1971), Clark and Garnica (1974), Lyons (1975), Webb and Abramson (1976) and Wales (1979).

[37] Compare: *He's badly dressed* (pointing to a man) and *A man came up. He was badly dressed.* The first sentence is a deictic use of *he*, because its interpretation is wholly dependent on the non-linguistic situation. The second sentence is a non-deictic use of *he*, as it refers back to the phrase *a man* from the previous sentence. Its function is therefore one of linguistic cross-reference (an *anaphoric* function, as it is usually called). Because of the very different linguistic functions involved, it would not necessarily follow that a patient's ability to use pronouns deictically would mean he could use them anaphorically: indeed, the reverse is usually the case.

"moving in the direction of the speaker", whereas *he is going* means "moving away from the speaker".

Reliance on deictic language seems to be a predictable feature of the early stages of language acquisition, as illustrated by such common sentences as *there, that, gone, mine*. Indeed, insofar as the earliest stage of acquisition seems wholly situation-dependent, it is possible to argue that deixis is a foundation for later development, and that deictic uses of language always precede non-deictic. However, it is not normal for children, even at the earliest stages, to be wholly or even predominantly deictic (see Nelson, 1973, Benedict, 1979)[38], and while deictics are commonly introduced into early syntactic structures (Brown, 1973), it is evident that by around two years, children do not rely so much on deictic expression. An example of the clash between adult and child expectations in this respect, at around this age, can be illustrated as follows:

Parent (downstairs, hearing crash from upstairs):
  Jòhnny/
  'what was thàt/
Child it 'fell dòwn/
Parent whàt did/
Child thàt did/
Parent 'what's thàt Jóhnny/
  whàt fell 'down/
Child 'that 'table thère/

Interactions of this kind are presumably a main means of teaching the child that deictic language is inappropriate when the participants in the conversation do not share the same context.

This basic rule of conversational interaction is however often broken by patients in the early stages of language development. It is a familiar clinical experience to have a conversation proceeding relatively smoothly as long as the subject-matter relates to the "here and now" of the patient, but as soon as topics outside the room are introduced, the smoothness disappears. The reason is usually that the success of the conversation is largely dependent on the patient's use of deictic forms, and a readiness of the clinician to "do the work" of expanding and making explicit the intent of the communication whenever P is unclear. A particularly clear case of reliance on deictic expression can be seen in the following extract from a language-delayed boy of 4½:

T   do you 'want to 'take the 'lid off that bóx/   (giving box of
       and 'see what's in thère/ -   miniature furniture)
    'then we can 'put it in the hòuse/ --
    'what can you sèe/ ---

---

[38] A similar point applies to maternal input language: between 18 months and 2½, around 70% of speech has immediate reference (Cross 1977: 169), a considerable proportion of which is deictic (especially using *that, there* and *the*), with gestural support (*e.g.* pointing). But by 2; 6, maternal reliance on gesture and deixis is much decreased, and more explicit language is predominant (see Bridges, 1979). On the general issue in language acquisition, see Macrae (1976), Clark (1978), Clark and Sengul (1978), Charney (1979), and the review in Wales (1979).

	'open the pácking/ -	(P looks in box)
	'that's ríght/ -	
	ôoh/	
	'what's in thère/	
P	lòok/	(pointing)
T	yês/	
	it's thère/ -	
	'what's thàt/	(P picks up table)
P	'that tàble/	
T	is 'that a tăble/	
P	[dì]	
T	'what's thàt one/ ---	(P picks up cooker and opens drawers)
	âh/	
	is there 'anything insíde/	
P	nò/	
T	is 'anything in'side thàt one/	
P	nò/	
T	I 'wonder if we could pùt 'something in'side/ -	
	lôok/	
	we could 'put thàt in'side/ -	(pointing to pan)
	thère/ --	
	'will it go ĭn/ ---	(P puts pan in cooker)
	thàt's ríght/ -	
	shall we 'put it in our hòuse Cíeron/	(P puts cooker on table)
	--- Cíeron/	
	shall we 'put it in our hŏuse/	(P puts cooker in house)
P	thère nów/	
T	'that's ît/	
	it's thère nów/ -	
	what èlse is 'in that 'box/ ---	(P picks up lamp)
	shall we 'put thàt in the 'house/ as wèll/	
P	lòok/	
	('that way thère)/	
T	yès/	
	'where does the tàble 'go/	
P	'up thère/	(puts table in bedroom)
T	'up thĕre/	
P	up thère 'then/ -	(takes table out and puts it in another room)
T	'put the 'table in the bédroom/	
P	nŏ/ -	
	not ín/	(puts lamp on house floor)
T	'that's the lìght/	
P	lòok/	
T	ôh/	
	'what's thàt/	

P	lòok/	(P picks up TV)
	lòok/	
T	'what ìs it 'Cieron/	
P	[aʔ ʔaə]	(puts TV in house, upside-down)
T	'does it go thàt wáy/ --	
	'shall we 'turn it rŏund/ --	(P turns it round)
	thàt's ríght/	
	'good bòy/ --	
	'what can you 'see thère/	
P	lòok/	(P picks up kettle)
	'look thère/	
T	'put the 'kettle upstáirs/ --	
	we could 'put the 'kettle on the còoker/	
P	'not (on) thĕre/	
T	nòt on 'there/	
P	nò/	
	'up thère/	
	nò/ [bə̀ mĭ:]/	
T	'put the 'pan on the còoker 'then/ ---	(P puts pan on cooker)
	thàt's ríght/ -	
	'going to 'put it in the hŏuse/	
P	[ì ba də]/	
	up thère/ nòw/	
	lòok/	(there is an egg in the pan)
	a ègg/	
T	'what's in thère/	
P	a ègg/	
T	an ègg/	
P	'here ègg/	

An analysis of the whole of this sample (which was, incidentally, felt by his mother to be very typical of P's speech) brought to light several interesting features. P produced 342 sentences altogether, of which:

88 were unintelligible;
54 were *look* or a phrase beginning with *look;*
51 were *yes/no* or equivalent.

Of the remaining 149 sentences, 124 were wholly or largely deictic in form. The flavour of this dialogue can be seen in the above transcript—a pattern which continued consistently throughout the sample, sometimes in relatively long sentences:

'not going ìn nów/
'me got a bìg one/
'not 'going bàck on thére/ the bíg one/

Two particularly interesting sequences were:

(referring to an object under a cooker)
that thère ís/ . thàt is/ . thère thére is/

(referring to his own shoes)
thère 'got them/ (*i.e.* "I've got them")

Several sentences have a deictic "pivot", *e.g.*

'there my shòe/
'no wànt thát/
that ègg/ thát is/
Hèidi got 'that/

There are only 25 sentences in the sample (one fourteenth) which lack deictics of any kind[39], and almost all of these are heavily dependent on the context of the previous speaker's speech, *e.g.*

pàn/	my dàddy 'does/	'not lie dòwn/
mèat/	'not got lìd/	Hèidi 'have/
a ègg/	a bèd is/	'we got dòg mý 'house/
bàby/	'two chàirs/	and my mòney/

In short, P is using a semantically "empty" language, for the most part, and gives a spurious impression of grammatical advancement. On a LARSP profile, analysis of all the sentences would place P at Stage III approaching Stage IV; omitting the sentences containing deictics from consideration leaves a picture of a developing profile at Stage II, with only an occasional use of later structures. P seems to have picked up a few later clause and connectivity structures, but these remain undeveloped with reference to either phrase structure or semantically "full" lexis.

   This observation suggests that the initial remedial aim with this child is to develop his phrase structure at Stage II, with the aim of integrating this immediately into Stage II or Stage III clause structure (*cf.* p. 112). For example, Stage II phrases involving Adjective+Noun, Noun+Noun or Preposition+Noun might be elicited, and then used to replace the deictics in clause structure, *e.g.*

big car		me got that⟶me got big car
mummy's bag		mummy's bag
etc.		etc.

For this aim to be achieved, however, several factors would need to be borne in mind.

(a) Replacing a deictic by a noun phrase or prepositional phrase can be a considerable strain on P's linguistic abilities, as it simultaneously adds lexical, grammatical and phonological (both segmental and non-segmental) structure. Thus it would be desirable to begin by using less advanced clause structures, familiar lexical items, and items which are within his phonological range.

---

[39] If *have* and *got* are analysed as deictics, this total is almost halved.

(b) A formal strategy will be needed to focus P's attention on the point in structure to be expanded, such as a forced alternative question. For example, instead of

P   me gòt thát/
T   whàt have you got/
P   thàt/

T might use

    whàt have you got/
    a 'big cár/ or a 'big brùsh/
P   'big càr/

(though when this strategy was used, it in fact took P some time to stop using *that* even here).

(c) Formal strategies of this kind need to be reinforced wherever possible by an expansion strategy from T and, perhaps, from P's parents. As we have seen, deictic use is a very natural style of speech when playing with children, and the above extract shows T in a remarkably deictic vein (*what's in there, what's that, we could put that inside, will it go in,* etc.). Obviously, this style will have to change, if P is to be provided with better models, *e.g.*

'what's in the bòx/
'what's thàt/ - is it a cóoker or a càr/
we could 'put the 'car 'in the bòx/
will the 'car go 'in the bóx/

T will have to be careful, to avoid making her sentences too long and complex, possibly exceeding P's short-term memory limitations (*cf.* p. 205). A guideline here might be obtained by looking at P's sentences which are non-deictic. These were around Stage II in clause structure. Thus if T operates a little ahead of this, at the three-element stage, she might best facilitate P's responses. On the other hand, to use a stimulus such as

will you put the car in the box
    S   V   O   A

will very likely be too advanced, with its four main clause elements. It would also be advisable not to expand all elements of structure at once. For example, if the sentence had a Subject+Verb+Object form, then T might keep a Pronoun as Subject, and concentrate on expanding Object, following normal developmental expectations[40].

The "deictic patient" seems to be a very general phenomenon, and is by no means restricted to children. The following extract is taken from a 44-year-old predominantly expressive aphasic, about five months following a stroke. T had asked him to go through the months of the year, but he had been unable to begin, despite prompting:

---

[40] Cf. Limber (1976), Crystal, Fletcher and Garman (1976: Ch. 6).

P   á/ -- erm -- yèah/ I 'know sóme/ but I 'don't 'know them 'very wèll I
    ex'pect at the *móment/
T   *m̀/
P   I'd I'd 'probably 'do them in the ĕnd/ but it would 'take rather a 'long 'time
    to *tèll you/
T   *m̀/
    that's alrìght/
    that's fìne/ -
    *was your 'wife
P   *a 'few I 'know ŏf/ but
T   your 'wife was ìn this 'morning to sée you/ wàsn't she/
P   ôh 'yes/ yès/ yès/ yès/
    ôh 'yes/ -
T   did she 'stay lŏng/
P   hòur and a hálf/ --
    hòur and a hálf/   .
    yès/ -
    she had she had . sòmething like thát/ -
    only she 'had to 'go and 'see .
    pèople came 'round this mórning/ you sée/
T   oh ýeah/
    'what péople/
P   erm -- 'people came 'round to see mè/ -
    she was she both . she 'came alóng and we 'both did it togèther you sée/ -
    but at 'this móment/ I 'think I'm doing alrìght nów/
    I can ma . 'manage it on mysèlf you sée/
T   *yés/
P   *if you can 'do it withòut mé/ there's 'no point in 'doing (it) on your òwn/
    ìs there/
T   nō/
    nō/
P   and I had a 'big . big chàt with him/ on my ŏwn/
    we had a 'very 'interesting er --- tàlk to stárt with/
    'very ìnteresting áctually/
T   was 'this the dôctor/ . the consûltant/ . 'coming róund/ on his wârd round/
P   dòctor/
    dòctor/
T   dòctor/
P   dòctor/
T   'what did he sây/
    'what did you tâlk a'bout/ .
P   wèll/ . the 'thing ìs/ I 'know nŏw/ at the mŏment/
    I 'know ex'actly what is 'coming thròugh the 'whole 'thing/
    so it's 'quite èasy you sée/ --
    know ex'actly what's 'going ŏn/
    so it'll be àlright thén/ you sée/

T   'that's grêat/   (loud noise nearby)
     'sorry about *the (   )*
P   *(   )*
     erm nò/
     it's 'just a'bout we were tàlking abóut/
     so we're alrìght thén you 'see/ -
     but the 'trouble 'is wi with mě you see/ at the mŏment/ I 'lose 'one or two
     ǎrguments/ . cos I have to 'get 'back the sìgns which are 'lost you sée/
T   ḿ/
P   it 'takes a little 'while to sort of come bàck at *tímes/ you knów/
T   *ḿ/ -- ḿ/
P   'this is the trŏuble/
T   ḿ/
P   but it's 'getting 'better than it wǎs/ -
     where 'as you 'know befòre/--
T   mûch 'better/

The "emptiness" of this kind of speech is largely due to P's reliance on deictic items
that relate to elements of meaning that he has internalized but not expressed. T is
unable to share this "internal context" with him, and consequently takes a while to
work out what he must be referring to.

The Ambiguity of Grammatical Error

When a patient makes a grammatical error in his speech, it is traditional clinical
practice to isolate the error and assign it to a category, such as "omission of the
article", "word order inverted" or "wrong form of the pronoun". Sometimes, this is
an easy and unambiguous process: a patient who says *him is doing it* is presumably
doing no more than using the wrong form of the pronoun, for reasons that have
been well discussed in the acquisition literature. However, the vast majority of
patient errors are not like this. The isolation of the error poses no problem, but its
identification does. For example, the following sentence was written by a partially-
hearing child: *Mr. Smith's dinner time four o'clock.* There is evidently something wrong
with this sentence—but what, exactly? Did the child "intend"

Mr. Smith's dinner time was at four o'clock.
It was Mr. Smith's dinner time at four o'clock.
Mr. Smith's dinner time was four o'clock.

The more deviant the sentence becomes, the wider the range of possible interpretations which might underlie it. For instance, how many errors should be identified in
the following sentences, and where should they be located?

the car wouldn't go can is was muddy
the boy is tired up the stone
he wore blue and star

This kind of output poses a major problem for the clinician. Such sentences would usually be regarded as *deviant,* in the sense of Crystal, Fletcher, and Garman (1976: 28-9), *i.e.* sentences that would not only be inadmissible in an adult grammar of the dialect in question, but would also fall outside the normal path of grammatical acquisition, insofar as this is known. Being deviant in form, there is therefore very little help to be had by considering them in terms of the stages of grammatical development used earlier in this chapter. So what can be done?

An essential initial step is to establish from the patient, as far as it is possible to do so, what his intentions were in respect of the sentence in question. What did he intend to say? This might seem like stating the obvious, but it is not usually done. Few teachers have the time and opportunity to go into individual detail on the background to every sentence in their pupils' written work. And the deviance encountered in taped sessions is often missed while the session is in progress, it being only afterwards that T realizes the need for further information. The value of obtaining guidance from P as to his intentions is however crucial, as can be seen from the following example. P wrote *Mr. Gump sat there couldn't,* referring to the picture of a man sitting in a car stuck in the mud. T assumed that the word order was wrong, and that P meant either *Mr. Gump couldn't sit there* (because the car would sink in due course) or (with a negation and auxiliary error) that *Mr. Gump was sitting there.* The sentence was corrected accordingly, but this provoked P to sign that what he meant was *Mr. Gump sat there. The car couldn't move.* The error, in other words, was quite different: it was not simply a matter of word order, auxiliaries or negation, but a more fundamental problem of sentence conflation, with omission of the subject of the second sentence.

What P conveys, in other words, is often very different from what he intends; and if T finds it impossible, for practical or theoretical reasons, to establish what was intended, he must exercise great caution before coming to a decision as to the identity of an error. Even quite "simple" constructions are affected. If the child says *a cups broke,* is this to be analyzed as an article error (for *the* or zero), a number error (plural for singular), or, conceivably, both (the child wanting to say not only that a particular cup [or cups] is broken, but that cups do break when you drop them)? If he says *the boy was ate the cake,* is this to be analyzed as a tense error (for *the boy ate the cake*) or aspect error (for *the boy was eating the cake*), or, again, both? If a decision cannot be made on empirical grounds, then the fact that there is ambiguity must be preserved in the descriptive statement about the patient. It might then be that in due course, as more examples of the error range accumulate, it would be possible to draw some conclusions as to what is happening. For example, if error 1 can be referred to three possible explanations (A, B, C), and error 2 to three possible explanations (A, C, D), and error 3 to three possible explanations (A, B, E), then the fact that explanation A is repeatedly turning up will very likely have some significance.

The analysis of deviant speech or writing, in other words, often takes the form of code-breaking, in which we search for as many possible patterns to account for the data as we can find, and then check each of these out with reference to those features in the data which have not been problematic. Here is an example of this procedure in operation. P wrote:

The bird is sat on the nest
The boy is climbed up the rock

The question is should these be corrected to *sitting on/climbing* or to *has sat on/ climbed*—the present tense vs. the present perfect interpretation, respectively? The pictures being used were of no help: in the first case the bird is shown sitting on the nest, whereas the previous picture had shown her in the air; in the second case, the mountaineer is nearly at the top of a mountain. To decide between these alternatives, the first thing to do would be to see if there were instances of the correct use of either *ing* or *have* (in its auxiliary use) elsewhere in the data. If one of these were being used correctly, it would suggest that the child's attempt to produce the other was the source of the problem. (If both were being used correctly, then we would either have to consider a third hypothesis for correction, or, alternatively, look for an explanation along the lines of the verb end-point analysis above, p. 118.) In fact, neither form was used elsewhere in the data, so the question remained open. The next step is to see whether P is attempting to express the meanings of "present-ness" and "past perfect-ness" using alternative means. If he believes, for example, that present tense in English is signalled by *the*, then we would expect to find lots of examples of the type *he the walking, he the swim*, and we could then conclude that he was attempting to do something different with the sentences above. This time, there was some evidence to suggest that P *was* using alternative means to express present perfect time—the word *just*. He used it quite often, in fact, in sentences such as *he just came in, the car just crashed*, and always with an appropriate meaning of "recent past with current relevance"[41]. This leaves us with the suggestion that P is thus attempting a present tense form of expression. As he regularly uses the unmarked form elsewhere (*he go, he sleep, he jump*, etc.), he must therefore be attempting to express something special about the activity, such as its duration, or his expectancy that something is about to happen. The remedial goal would thus seem to be the introduction of *ing* into such contexts, taking into account the range of meaning with which this form is associated.

In this example, it is not obvious why P chose to develop his syntax in the way he did. In many other cases, the analysis of the deviant speech or writing produces perfectly good reasons for the abnormal development. It would not need a sophisticated analysis to show that the reason for the deviance in much deaf speech or writing is that P has not heard the omitted features, or has heard them intermittently. On the other hand, the residual hearing of most deaf children is sufficient to rule out any simple explanation of this kind. Other possible explanations could be semantic or cognitive in character (see further p. 191). Or there may be a straightforward grammatical reason, such as the overgeneralization of a wrongly-learned pattern, as in the following examples:

Bill held carefully a nest
He saw in the town a car

where the Verb+Adverbial sequence seems to have been generalized from sentences of the type *he ran quickly*. Unfortunately, very little analysis of deviant

---

[41] See Twaddell (1960), Palmer (1974).

grammatical structure has taken place. The above examples are thus of largely pro-grammatic importance, and in no way constitute a typology. But I hope they are sufficient illustration of the main principle: that grammatical error is a complex phenomenon, and, in the way it focuses our attention on those areas of linguistic structure which the patient is currently finding problematic, is a positive index of immediate remedial objectives[42].

---

[42] For more on error analysis, in second language learning, see Svartvik (1973).

Semantics 5

Theoretical Background

Semantics is the study of meaning in language. Introduced into English in the late 19th century, the term has since competed with such other terms as "semasiology", "semology" and "semics" to identify a possible science of meaning. It is now the most widely used label for such a science, despite the popular pejorative sense which has developed in everyday speech (as in "That's just semantics", *i.e.* quibbling unnecessarily over word meanings, or deliberately using language to mislead or confuse). Semantics is one of the main components, or levels, of linguistic analysis (*cf.* p. 19). Given that the communication of meaning is the central function of language, we might thus expect semantics to be the most well-developed branch of linguistics. But semantic studies have lagged behind most other aspects of linguistic investigation, partly because of linguists' preoccupation with phonetics, phonology and grammar, and partly because of fundamental difficulties in subjecting the notion of "meaning" to successful analysis. In the 1960s and 1970s, however, the subject attracted increasing attention in linguistics, so that there are now several introductory texts available[1] and several advanced reviews of the field[2]. There is as yet no orthodoxy in semantics, but certain common themes have emerged in this literature which can help to distinguish linguistic semantics from other, more well-established approaches to the study of meaning—in particular, those which take their rise from philosophy and psychology.

Traditional Semantics

Discussion of the nature of meaning in language formed an important part of the writings of Plato and Aristotle, and since that time, a strong philosophical tradition for the study of meaning has developed, most recently under such headings as

---

[1] For example, Palmer (1976), Leech (1974), Lyons (1977).
[2] For example, Fillmore and Langendoen (1971), Steinberg and Jakobovitz (1971).

"semiotics" and "the philosophy of language"[3]. Several important theoretical issues have been elucidated, within this tradition. An early example was the Greek debate over whether the relationship between words and things was fundamentally natural (a word's sound or shape in some way reflecting the characteristics of the reality to which it referred) or conventional (the link between word and thing being arbitrary). The essential arbitrariness of the relationship is a major tenet of modern semantics, especially since de Saussure's emphasis on the point—though there is still much to be discovered about the cases where one might plausibly argue the reverse view (onomatopoeic words, and sound symbolism generally)[4].

The history of ideas in traditional semantics shows a tendency for theories of meaning to fall generally into two main types. Both types take observable linguistic behaviour (referred to variously as "sounds", "words", "acoustic image", etc.) as a given, but differ as to the other "worlds" which relate to it. The first type postulates a direct correspondence between linguistic behaviour and the (in principle) observable entities, events, states of affairs, etc. of the external world (the world of "reference"). Such theories, interpreted psychologically, will be behaviourist in character. By contrast, the second type insists on the mediating role of individual consciousness in relating linguistic behaviour and reference. Interpreted psychologically, these will be mentalistic in character. Terminology again varies considerably in labelling this intermediate stage ("thought", "concept", "sense", etc.). Both types of theory have attracted criticism: for example, critics of the former theories point to the very limited amount of language whose meaning can be established with reference to observable properties of the external world; critics of the latter point to such problems as the difficulty of operating with introspection to define clearly what personal concepts are. However, most linguistic semanticists these days find it possible to discuss the analysis of meaning quite profitably without committing themselves to either one of these general positions[5].

There are several emphases in "philosophical" semantics[6] which distinguish it from the "linguistic" semantics reviewed below. In particular, the philosophical approach has been concerned to establish the conditions under which linguistic expressions can be said to be true or false, in relation to the external world, and the nature of the factors which affect the interpretation of language as used. Of central significance here is the study of the meaning of expressions in the idealized terms of logical systems of analysis, or calculi, so that we can determine their status, as expressions—for example, whether an expression is internally consistent, or contradictory, or whether one expression implies another, in some strict sense. For analyses of meaning carried on in these terms, the labels "logical"/ "pure"/ "formal" (semantics) will be found. For some linguists, a logical frame of reference provides an indispensable foundation for semantic analysis; for others, the idealized con-

---

[3] For example, the work of Charles Peirce, Rudolf Carnap and Alfred Tarski; see the review in Lyons (1977: Ch. 4).

[4] See Ullmann (1973), Stankiewicz (1964).

[5] For behaviourist semantics, see Osgood (1953), Bloomfield (1933) and the review in Lyons (1977: Ch. 5); for mentalistic semantics, see de Saussure (1916), Ogden and Richards (1923) and the review in Lyons (1977: Ch. 4).

[6] For example, the work of Ayer (1936), Strawson (1971), Wittgenstein (1953).

trasts debated in this literature are too removed from everyday language to be anything other than marginally relevant (cf. below).

In addition, apart from these studies of the internal structure of linguistic expressions, the philosophical tradition has focussed attention on the evaluation of the various uses to which language may be put, and to the several factors which contribute to the total interpretation, or signification, of a message. These factors—the "meanings of meaning", as they are sometimes called—have been variously labelled; and while it is impossible to generalize about usage (in view of the different technical senses these labels have in various theories), labels do cluster around three major themes. When the emphasis is on the relationship between language, on the one hand, and the entities, events, states-of-affairs, etc. which are external to the speaker and his language, on the other, terms such as "referential meaning", "denotative meaning" and "extensional meaning" are used. Secondly, when the emphasis is on the relationship between language and the mental state of the speaker, two types of terminology are used: the personal, emotional aspects are handled by such terms as "affective meaning" or "connotative meaning"; the intellectual, factual aspects involve such terms as "cognitive meaning" or "ideational meaning". Thirdly, when the emphasis is on the way variations in the extra-linguistic situation affect the understanding and interpretation of language, terms such as "social meaning", "interpersonal meaning" or "situational meaning" have been used. Broad distinctions of this kind are often made as part of linguistic studies of meaning (for example, in classifying children's utterances into general functional types)[7], but many linguists remain sceptical of the possibility of achieving a precise account of meaning at such an abstract level, and prefer to operate with a more restricted application of these concepts, in precisely delimited experimental or naturalistic settings (cf. below).

Within traditional language studies, semantics would generally be thought to involve two areas of study. First there is the study of meaning in historical terms, the description and classification of the changes of meaning which affect the words in a language. Tracing these changes back to the earliest known appearance of a word in any language ("etymology") is one of the oldest traditions in the study of meaning. Secondly, there is the provision of an inventory of the forms and meanings of a language, in dictionaries and thesauri. The compilation of dictionaries ("lexicography") is again a long-standing tradition in the history of language study[8].

Linguistic Semantics

This term is often used to distinguish the study of meaning from the viewpoint of linguistic science, as opposed to the philosophical, psychological or traditional language studies referred to above. But the distinction (between "linguistic" and "non-linguistic" semantics) is not clear-cut. Indeed several linguists have attempted to develop a broad conception of the subject, in which linguistic analyses of meaning

---

[7] For example, Rodgon, Jankowski and Alenskas (1977); see further, p. 175.
[8] See Collinson (1981) for a historical review.

hin a philosophical, psychological or social frame of reference. For
? of the earliest discussions of semantics by a linguist, Leonard Bloom-
tes the influence of behaviourist psychology, in his attempt to restrict
meaning to only observable and measurable behaviour. It was in fact
primarily due to the pessimism of this approach, which concluded that semantics
was not then capable of elucidation (*i.e.* in behavioural terms) that the subject came
to be so neglected in post-Bloomfieldian linguistics. Indeed, semantics as a branch
of linguistics became a serious area of enquiry only in the early 1960s. Since then,
the most ambitious attempt to provide an integrated view is the two-volume Lyons,
1977: this book sees linguistic semantics as part of a frame of reference constituted
by communication theory, semiotics, philosophy, logic and the study of society[9]. I
do not doubt that such views will one day be of considerable value in clinical
studies: a comprehensive approach to the analysis of meaning, of the sort provided
by Lyons, may well assist in circumscribing and distinguishing the various types of
central language disturbance, particularly in the study of aphasia and of psychopathological conditions. But it would be premature to attempt an application at this
level of generality, until the relationships between the various components of the
approach have been more fully investigated, and the empirical consequences of the
various theoretical decisions more fully tested. Of far greater value to clinical
studies, at the present time, is to focus upon the range of specifically linguistic concepts and methods which have been introduced in recent years, and which constitute the characteristics of a linguistic approach to the study of meaning. In my view,
there are five main characteristics which identify the linguist's contribution.

(a) He stresses the need for synchronic description, as well as the diachronic study of
meaning (the latter providing the sole emphasis of traditional language studies).

(b) He is primarily concerned with the properties of natural language (as opposed to
"logical" languages), and with the semantic characteristics of naturalistic everyday
speech (as distinct from the carefully constructed contrasts found in philosophical
discussion or in the experimental situations of psychology).

(c) A major focus is the relationship between meaning and other levels of analysis
(especially phonology and grammar) as part of the aim of providing an *integrated*
theory of linguistic behaviour[10].

(d) He is much involved with comparative study—investigating the similarities and
differences in the way meaning is structured across different dialects, styles, languages and cultures; these days, there is increasing involvement with semantic *universals*—those properties of meaning manifested in the linguistic expression of all
languages.

(e) Above all, he is concerned with the establishment of the minimal units of
semantic description, through the detailed analysis of sets of words and of the lin-

---

[9] Other broad conceptions, which emphasize the relationship between linguistic and philosophi-
cal/logical theories of meaning, are illustrated by Fillmore and Langendoen (1971), Leech (1974) and
Keenan (1975).

[10] Note, in this respect, that linguists see "meaning" both as a datum and as a criterion of analysis.
Linguists study meaning, and also use meaning to study other aspects of language, through such
notions as "contrastivity" and "distinctiveness".

guistic contexts in which they occur; this concern is reflected not only in empirical studies of vocabulary (the *lexicon*), but also in several conceptual and terminological refinements, some of which will be introduced below.

Other Senses of "Semantics"

There have been many applications of the term "semantics", in the past 50 years, other than those reviewed above, and it may perhaps be helpful to refer to some of the ways in which other contributory disciplines to speech pathology have used the term differently. Firstly, in psychology, the notion of "semantic differential" (as introduced by Osgood, Suci, and Tannenbaum, 1957) refers to a technique for establishing the emotional reactions of speakers to words, and thus suggesting the main affective dimensions in terms of which a language's concepts are organized. It "measures" the meaning of words by plotting the associations they carry within a two-dimensional hypothetical "semantic space", so that, for example, a word such as *conservative* can be judged in terms of whether it is strong/weak, beautiful/ugly, active/passive, and so on. This approach has little in common with the linguist's analysis of meaning, though some linguists have occasionally used this method of investigation in their work (*e.g.* in analyzing intonational attitudes). Another psychological distinction is that between "semantic memory" and "episodic memory" (Tulving, 1972), differentiating between a person's knowledge, on the one hand, and his store of experiences, on the other.

Secondly, in semiotics, the notion of "semanticity" is used as a very general defining property of a semiotic system: it refers to the system's ability to convey meaning, by virtue of the associative ties which relate the system's signals to features of the external world (*cf.* Lyons, 1977: Ch. 3). For example, the system of a policeman's traffic-signalling has semanticity, as it can be conventionally interpreted. The notion thus applies to far more than language.

In speech pathology itself, the term has sometimes been used in a restricted sense, in relation to classifications of aphasia. "Semantic aphasia", in the terminology of Wepman and Jones (1961) refers basically only to nominal aphasia, or anomia; in Brown (1977), it is contrasted with nominal aphasia, being used to describe deeper disturbances in the process of moving from thought to speech; in Head (1926), Luria (1964), and Jakobson (1964), the term refers not to the meaning of single words, but to disturbance in the ability to make logical connections between words, combining separate details in the construction of larger linguistic units. Other such narrow interpretations can be found. However, given the development in the importance of semantic studies since the 1960s, so that it now ranks as a major component of most models of language structure, alongside grammar and phonology, it would seem sensible to reserve the term for its broad sense, as described earlier, and this is the way in which "semantics" is used throughout this book.

Lastly, it is important to stress the difference between semantics, as outlined in this chapter, and three other notions with which it is often confused: conceptualization, comprehension, and reference. Firstly, semantics should not be identified with the topic that is variously labelled conceptualization, cognitive skills, concept-formation or concept development. Such notions are used as part of the psychologist's attempt to understand behaviour and its development, and can be specified in more detail using such notions as object-permanence, decentration, conservation, and so on[11]. The contrast that needs to be made is that cognitive or conceptual skills are not the same as semantic skills. Depending on your view of cognitive studies, language may be seen as one aspect of cognition, or excluded from it ("language and cognition"): either way, the properties of cognition plainly extend well beyond whatever is needed to account for linguistic behaviour. Semantics, being only one level of linguistic organization, cannot be equated with cognition either[12]. While certain semantic properties of a language may presuppose certain cognitive skills, and while semantic similarities between languages may suggest that there is a parallel between certain cognitive and certain semantic skills, it would seem wrong to equate the two (as is often done, when writers talk about "semantic/cognitive" in their discussion of child development). On the contrary, it is far more illuminating to stress the differences between, on the one hand, such tasks as are carried out in the Piagetian paradigm, which can be used on and get the same results from children of whatever language background, and on the other hand the business of semantic analysis, which is patently language-specific. Putting this another way, French, English and Chinese children may all develop object permanence at around the same time and in the same way, but the manner in which they express their awareness, using the lexical/grammatical/phonological resources of their language, will differ. It is the business of the linguistic semanticist to study the way these resources are organized, and relate the linguistic structures he discovers to those conceptual structures, or schemas, postulated to account for behavioural development in general. In some cases, there may be a 1-1 correspondence, but it is more usual not to find a simple correspondence: a "simple" concept such as "movement" may be expressed in many ways, using lexicon *(run, arrive, ascend...)* or grammar (using prefixes, verb endings), and these will vary between languages. The distinction between conceptualization and semantics thus needs to be kept clearly in mind—or at least (for I am by no means sure of the theoretical status of the former), in clinical linguistics we may proceed to a study of semantic structure without tying ourselves to a particular model of conceptualization, or to any particular cognitive theory.

Secondly, semantics must not be confused with comprehension. Comprehension, or lack of comprehension, is a feature of a person's performance with reference to language: he understands, or fails to understand, the meaning of language. It is not to be identified with meaning, which needs to be specified separately. This distinction is made at other language levels also. We may specify phonological units and structure without reference to how efficient a person is at producing or understanding (*i.e.* discriminating) them; we may specify grammatical units and structure again without presupposing how well a person can express or comprehend them; and likewise with semantics, we can specify semantic units and structure

---

[11] Cf. Piaget (1926), Donaldson (1978).
[12] For a development of this view, see for example Bloom (1973: 20 ff.), Schlesinger (1977, 1979).

without reference to the ability of an individual to comprehend or produce them. Put like this, the point is perhaps an obvious one; but it is nonetheless common to find clinicians who, having carried out a comprehension test, will assume that they have thereby done a semantic analysis. On the contrary: comprehension tests involve grammatical, phonological and semantic information; and the selection and grading of the semantic features of the test needs to be independently evaluated.

Thirdly, semantics must be distinguished from the direct study of the objects, entities, events, states of affairs, etc. in the external world—the province of chemists, geologists, historians, and others. Rather less obviously, neither is semantics primarily concerned with the study of the way language is used to refer to these states of affairs (the "reference" of language). To understand the domain of linguistic semantics, a basic distinction has to be drawn between the study of reference and that of *sense*. The primary business of semantics is to study the latter—how people make linguistic units (words, sentences, etc.)[13] relate to each other, and thus how they "make sense" of them. The "internal sense" of most conversations is appreciated without any direct reference to the external world at all—for obvious reasons (such as that we can point to what we are talking about for only a tiny fraction of what we want to say). Usually, the sense of an unknown word will be clarified by the speaker using other words (as in the whole process of dictionary definition); the sense of an obscure sentence will be clarified by providing an alternative formulation of the sentence (a paraphrase of it). It is this internal sense structure which is the main focus of semantics—how words and sentences define each other—and this way of approaching the subject has accordingly come to be known as *structural semantics*.

The Structure of the Lexicon

One of the most promising approaches to lexical semantic analysis has come from the application of structuralist ideas. It will be recalled (*cf.* p. 21) that the structuralist view sees language as analysable in terms of an underlying network of relationships between elements, or units. There are, accordingly, two main questions for semantics: (a) what are the units of the semantic system? and (b) how are they interrelated? The answer to these questions will vary somewhat depending on the formal features whose meaning is being investigated (whether in phonology, grammar or vocabulary), but most attention has been paid to vocabulary analysis, and it is here that several important notions have developed that are directly applicable to clinical data. Perhaps the most fundamental point arises out of a consideration of whether the notion of *word* constitutes a valid unit for semantic analysis. Traditional language study would say that it was—but there are serious problems.

---

[13] The point of the phrase "linguistic units" is to draw attention to the range of linguistic structures which communicate meaning. It contrasts with a traditional view that all that is involved in semantics is the relationship between "words", or "names", and "things".

The ambiguity of the term *word* is routinely pointed out in introductory text-books[14]. Three main senses are usually distinguished (though terminology varies): (i) words are the physically definable units bounded by space in writing, and sometimes marked by pause and juncture features in speech; such "word-forms" are often referred to as "orthographic words" (for writing) and "phonological words" (for speech); they can be identified without any reference to the meaning they express. (ii) words are also units of grammar, which operate in strings in the construction of phrases, clauses and sentences, and which are themselves constructed out of morphemes; notions such as "word order", or measuring sentence length in terms of words illustrate this sense; this is also a formal notion, which does not rely on the meanings the individual words express.
(iii) in a more abstract sense, a word is the unit underlying a set of variant grammatical forms; for example, *walk, walks, walking* and *walked* are all variants of the "word" *walk*. There is obviously scope for considerable confusion here, if the term "word" is allowed both for the underlying form and its variants; and as a result, fresh terminology has developed to identify the underlying form. The term *lexeme*, or *lexical item*, refers to the underlying units involved, "word" being then reserved for grammatical use. Lexemes are thus the minimal units of vocabulary, and thus of semantics (*cf.* "phonemes" in phonology). It is lexemes which tend to be listed as the head-words in dictionary entries.

Throughout this chapter, accordingly, whenever problems of meaning arise at word-level, we shall be discussing semantic analysis in terms of lexemes and their interrelationships. While for the most part this corresponds to the popular use of the term "word" (*e.g.* "What's another word for …?" is equivalent to "What's another lexeme for …?"), there are many occasions where an important distinction will need to be drawn between the grammatical and lexical senses, *e.g.* the distinction between "word-finding" and "lexeme-finding" problems reviewed on p. 187. It should also be noted that there are many examples of lexemes which are realized by more than one word, *e.g.* prepositional units such as *near to* and *in accordance with*, or phrasal verbs such as *come in, switch on* and *come up to*, or idioms, such as *kick the bucket* (=die). These have unitary meanings, *i.e.* they are not decomposable into the sum of the meanings of the constituent words; and if they cannot be analyzed into constituent meanings, they must, accordingly, be minimal semantic units (lexemes), despite the fact that they consist of more than one grammatical word. The importance of having the term "lexeme" available in such cases is clear, as otherwise we would have no clear way of identifying the whole multi-word unit. To say "the word *kick the bucket* consists of three words" is odd, to say the least; to say "the lexeme *kick the bucket* consists of three words" is much more satisfactory.

Having identified a unit for structural semantic analysis, the general principle of the structuralist approach also needs to be borne in mind: in a structuralist network of relationships, the units have no validity apart from the relations (of equivalence, contrast, etc.) which hold between them, and it is this network of relations which constitutes the structure of the system (*cf.* p. 21). This view was originally developed for phonological studies, and later for grammar, and in these fields

---

[14] For example, Lyons (1968: Ch. 2), Palmer (1971: Ch. 2).

it is not difficult to demonstrate the concepts involved: for example, to ask "What is /p/?" is to ask a question which cannot be answered, without reference to the contrasts /p/ has with other units, and in the end it is the bases of contrast themselves (voicing, etc.) which turn out to be crucial. The units of phonology have no independent existence: they are identified solely by the relations they contract. We cannot ask "What phonemes has P got?" and then "Let us see how P uses them", for in order to identify the phonemes in the first place, we must examine their distribution. In the area of vocabulary, however, the structuralist concept is more difficult to grasp, because to say that lexemes have no independent existence seems to run against common sense. Lexemes, it might be argued, do have an independent meaning, because they can be applied directly to the objects to which they refer, as when we point to the cat and say *cat*. What is wrong with a view which sees lexemes as independent labels for things, events, etc. in the world and our experience?

What has to be appreciated is that this process of directly labelling an encountered object is an uncommon, primitive and altogether atypical activity. It is of some importance in the early stages of language acquisition, when an overt labelling of this kind often takes place (*e.g.* identifying objects in a picture book), and in some social contexts in later life (*e.g.* introducing someone by name). It is also an extremely common technique in clinical teaching situations. But rarely do labels come to be used in this way without amplification, *e.g.*

Teacher: Here's a picture of an elm tree. I want you to look carefully at it. How would you tell an elm? ... What's been happening to elms recently? ...

The normal state of affairs in language is for lexemes to be introduced, defined, interpreted, and so on, through the use of other lexemes. While it is possible (and sometimes desirable) to provide a definition by pointing to the object in question (an "ostensive" definition), or referring to it deictically (*e.g.* A. "What's an elm tree?" B. "There's one."), it is more usual to attempt a definition linguistically, referring to other lexemes to identify the form and function of the lexeme in focus, along the lines of the classical definitional method: "An X is a Y which does Z." That this should be the most normal form of exposition is not surprising: apart from impracticality (the relevant objects not always being around when we want to talk about them!), ostensive and deictic labelling is often ambiguous (*e.g.* if there were several trees in our line of vision, the reference to elms would require amplification, in terms of their size, shape, colour, etc.).

The dictionary, of course, is the place where the total dependence of lexeme upon lexeme is most apparant[15]. A complete dictionary of a language would be wholly circular, in the sense that all the items in the defining vocabulary for a lexeme would themselves be defined elsewhere in the dictionary. In poorer dictionaries, the circularity is vicious (as when X is glossed by Y, and Y is glossed by X), but usually this is avoided by the introduction of several intermediate stages between X and Y, involving an increasingly widening range of "associated" lexemes and illus-

---

[15] The introduction of encyclopaedic information, pictorial aids, etc. into some dictionaries, as an aid to immediacy of understanding, should be seen as a separate development, in principle distinguishable from the need to provide linguistic definitions throughout.

trations of usage. For example, in one dictionary, looking up the lexeme *benefit* involved reference to *advantage* and *profit* (amongst others); *advantage* led us to *gain* (as well as *benefit* and *profit*); *gain* led us to *increase, obtain,* and *profit; increase* to *rise* and *large;* and so on[16].

If we were to draw the paths through the lexicon in this way, the concept of a multidimensional network of relationships would quickly become apparent. The main aim of structural semantics is to describe these relational networks, and to establish a set of principles governing the lexical organization of language.

The fact that the lexicon is organized in certain ways is the main reason for the inadequacy and contradictoriness of the traditional measure of semantic development—vocabulary counting. Estimates of the number of words a person commands at any given time are notoriously unreliable, and rarely illuminating. The unreliability is due to several factors:

— uncertainty as to what should be counted as a word (*e.g.* is *I'll* one word or two?)
— should we be counting words or (what in this chapter we are calling) lexemes? for example, is *kick the bucket* to be counted as three items, just as *kick the cat*?
— should we include passive as well as active vocabulary (*i.e.* vocabulary understood, but not in active use)? if the former, how do we ensure that a word is in active use? does a single instance of a word suffice, or should a child have used a word several times? if the latter, how many times[17]?
— what do we do if a child uses a word half-correctly? for example, the child who called a picture of a *brontosaurus* a *pterodactyl* at least knew that it was something to do with dinosaurs, but he did not get it right—should this word therefore be included, or excluded from a vocabulary count?
— how representative are the samples of language anyway?
Because of differences in counting method, due to these uncertainties, estimates of the average size of vocabulary vary wildly: 5-year-olds, for example, have been estimated to have anything between two and ten thousand words[18].

But even if an accurate estimate of vocabulary size can be made, how illuminating will this be? The limitations here are several:
— there seems little point in counting forms without reference to the range of meaning that a person intends to express by their use; reference to any general dictionary will show that most words are polysemic (the commonest words most of all); a child learning a word, however, does not learn all of its potential meaning at once, but will learn it in certain senses only; perhaps it is therefore the senses of words that should be counted, if counting is to be done at all?
— counting words, or their senses, in isolation from grammatical context is misleading and often impossible; we often know the meaning of a word only by referring to the grammatical context in which it is used;
— knowing that a child uses a word is only the beginning of the story: more important is the question of how well he is using it, in relation to how many and what

---

[16] Dictionary examples throughout this chapter will be taken from the *Longman Dictionary of Contemporary English* (Procter, 1978).

[17] See for example the discussion in Bloom (1973).

[18] Most vocabulary counts are based on written language samples, whether for child (*e.g.* Edwards and Gibbon 1973) or adult (*e.g.* Thorndike and Lorge 1944).

kind of situations; for example, three children, A, B, C, may all use the lexeme *cold,* but if A uses it only for "water", whereas B uses it for temperature generally, and C uses it, in addition, for grim faces, it would not be reasonable to rate all three children as being "the same".

For such reasons, a clinical semantic analysis takes a lexeme inventory only as a starting point, and will place little store on the total number of lexemes counted, or the frequency of use of each lexeme. There are no norms against which to rate individual differences in lexeme use, which are very marked; and general comments about "poor vocabulary" are so vague as to be of little help. A lexeme inventory does have some general interest, in that it suggests something about the interest levels of the patient, and it will provide the analyst with clues about the viable semantic fields within which he will have to work (see below); but by itself it cannot provide meaningful information, either about assessment or about remediation. For this we need to investigate the structural relationships between the lexemes, and to work out the principles governing P's lexical organization.

Semantic Fields

An influential view of lexical organization is that based on the notion of semantic fields[19]: vocabulary is said to be organized into areas of meaning, within which lexemes interrelate and define each other in various ways. To take a much-studied example, the lexemes denoting colour define one semantic field: the precise meaning of a colour term can be understood only by placing it in relation to the other terms which occur with it in demarcating the colour spectrum. In the strongest form of this hypothesis, the *whole* of the vocabulary is seen as a single, integrated system of sense-related lexemes; in a less strong version, certain areas of the vocabulary are seen as being more clearly structured than others. The theory of semantic fields has in fact attracted considerable controversy, especially in the psychological form in which it was originally propounded, where the linguistic structuring power of the vocabulary was seen as a means of organizing the continuum of our conceptual experience. From a linguistic point of view, the postulation of a universal, neutral,

---

[19] See Lyons (1977: 250—261), Robins (1971: 66—69). For the original German ideas, see Trier (1934); for developments by American anthropologists, see the papers in Part 4 ("Cultural focus and semantic field") of Hymes (1964: 167—214). Much of the cogency of the original proposals lay in the illuminating comparisons of different languages or language states—demonstrating, for example, that lexemes were not totally equivalent in their domain of application between languages (see the discussion of the difficulties of translating *the cat sat on the mat* into French in Lyons [1977: 237—238]), or that there were gaps in the lexical expression of one language compared with another (well-discussed examples such as the range of words for "snow" in Eskimo, compared with English). In this chapter, the illustration will be wholly from English, and this comparative dimension will be only indirectly referred to.
It should also be noted that a different sense of "semantic field" is found in the neuropsychological use of the term by Luria, where it refers to the sound and meaning associations of a word with other words, as determined by the physiological measurement of orienting reactions. Lesser (1978) also prefers a more general sense for this term, using "semantic category" in its place.

conceptual continuum which is given structure by language would these days be seen as both unjustified and unnecessary (cf. Lyons, 1977: 260). It must also be accepted that there are great problems facing anyone who would try to formalize this theory, or who expects the neat analyses of, say, colour terms, to be replicated throughout the lexicon—much of the lexicon is far more indeterminate in its structuring than these analyses might lead us to expect. But despite these difficulties, the notion of semantic field is intuitively a very plausible one, and in those areas of the lexicon which have been systematically studied in this way, it has been possible to demonstrate underlying patterns.

From a clinical viewpoint, the analysis of these more determinate areas is of great interest. Clinicians have long worked with patients using a loose notion of semantic field—one might work on P's vocabulary for colour, body-parts, furniture, fruit, and so on. But usually the items within each field are seen as an inventory, not as a structure: there is no particular reason why a picture-naming task should commence with *chair* rather than *table*, or *apple* rather than *banana;* and at the end of such a test, when perhaps ten names of fruit might have been presented, we are left unclear why this particular selection of ten was made (might P have performed differently on an alternative ten, or on the same ten presented in a different order?), and whether there is a clear boundary-line to be drawn around fruit terms (as opposed to, say, vegetables). Plainly, if there are structural guidelines to be found, whereby some kind of hierarchical organization might be imposed on lexical items, this could be of value, in avoiding the arbitrariness of lexical stimuli (as in eliciting or testing), in assessing whether there is any pattern in P's developing or residual abilities, and in devising remedial strategies (*e.g.* teaching lexeme X before lexeme Y).

For the notion of semantic field to be clinically meaningful, the lexical range of each field must be identified in such a way that it corresponds to the levels of categorization and discrimination at which P operates. There would be little point, for example, in an assessment or remedial programme which divided P's lexicon into no more than a handful of very abstract fields, such as Roget did in organizing his thesaurus (viz. *abstract relations, space, matter, intellect, volition,* and *affections*). To work in terms of such fields would involve several thousand lexemes immediately, and we would need further principles of organization to see order within them. At the other extreme, there would be little point in assessing P in too narrow or specific a manner, *e.g.* his ability to use lexemes associated with ships, or cutlery. Such a restriction would be no guide to P's general lexical abilities, and would be too prone to the influence of personal factors, *e.g.* if P was once a sailor. Obviously, some level between these extremes has to be aimed for; but it is not easy to give this "middle-level" a theoretical definition, as can be seen by continuing further into Roget's classification. Roget divides his field of *affections* into five categories: *general terms, personal, sympathetic, moral* and *religious;* each of these is then further subdivided, *e.g. moral* into *obligation, sentiments, conditions, practice* and *institutions;* and there is still further subdivision, *e.g. practice* into *temperance, intemperance, sensualism, asceticism, fasting,* etc. A more everyday example would be from the field of *fauna,* which presumably divides into such categories as *animals/birds/fish/insects; animals* then divides into *zoo/domestic/farm/wild,* etc.; *domestic* into *cat/dog,* etc.; and for certain purposes it might be useful to go further, *e.g. breeds* of dog. The problem of deciding at what level of categorization to intervene is not one which is capable of *a priori* solution; presumably everything depends on the level at which P and his friends, relations, etc. talk to each other in routine conversational settings, and this will vary to some degree, along with interests, background, purpose, etc. (see further, p. 182).

On the other hand, it is equally evident that conversations do not proceed randomly, and that people have expectations concerning the level of generality at which a topic might be dealt with. Certain topics recur more frequently than others, and are dealt with using lexemes that recur more frequently than others. It is certainly possible to construct a list of semantic fields of intermediate generality, corresponding to the levels at which clinical conversations most generally proceed. The following list was constructed in just such a manner, based on the kinds of lexeme most commonly used by clinicians talking to both children and adults with language problems. It should be stressed that this is in no sense a complete list, being based on only a few hours of unstructured conversation with relatively severe cases (15-minute samples from 40 different therapists). But it is remarkable how much similarity there is between clinicians, and even between child and adult situations, in their use of semantic fields, and even of specific lexemes within these fields[20].

Twelve fields account for 55% of the total lexemes used: (in decreasing frequency of use) time, leisure, possession, people, cognitive activity, quantity, location, coming and going, sensory perception, animals, food and meals, house and furniture. Fifteen verbs account for 60% of all verbs used: *call, come, do, get, go, happen, have, know, look, make, put, see, tell, think* and *want*. The level of categorization chosen by T is largely concrete, and restricted to the "here and now" of the clinic, school, or P's personal background. This level can be illustrated from the following fields, citing only those lexemes that were used more than once and by more than one therapist in the data:

PEOPLE mother, sister, brother, mum, daddy, nan, granny, husband, wife, sister-in-law; girl, boy, baby, man, woman, friend, people; doctor, teacher.
PERCEPTION see, look, watch, listen, look at, cry.
COGNITIVE ACTIVITY know, think, want, suppose, mean, feel, understand, learn, forget.
TIME time, now, week, recently, last, next, ago, just, again, soon, today, morning, evening, yesterday, NAME OF DAY, still, minute, yet.
FOOD AND MEALS tea, bacon, ice cream, cake, egg, food, sausage, eat, cook, drink, breakfast, lunch, dinner.

Apart from the "empty" items, which constitute a great deal of T input (*what's happening,* etc.), the only abstract terms used more than once were language terms (*e.g. word, sentence),* names of school subjects (*e.g. maths, science),* and general dimensional terms (*e.g. colour, kind, time, shape, measure, different, same, place).* The only higher-

---

[20] It should perhaps be pointed out that only a small proportion of the data is relevant to this question, as the following statistics show: of all the words used by the clinicians, 55% were grammatical, 9% were social or stereotyped (in the sense of Crystal, Fletcher and Garman 1976), and 2% were proper names; which leaves only 34% for semantically "full" lexemes.

order substantives used more than once were *people, food, drink, clothes, game, animal, house* and *colour*. There was nothing at a more abstract level, and more specific notions were few (8%), these being handled by attributes rather than new substantives *(e.g. dog with spots on,* rather than *dalmatian)*.

This kind of information, limited as it is, is nonetheless helpful, in indicating the lines along which we should be thinking. On the basis of such an approach, for example, it would be possible to construct a list of semantic fields within which Ts generally work, extending it on logical grounds to make its coverage more systematic. One such inventory is the following:

FIELDS

General characterization	examples of 1st order abstraction	examples of 2nd order abstraction
HUMAN FORM	People	Family, Visitors; Male, Female
	Body and Parts	Face, Limbs, Frame
	Clothing	Inner, Outer, Accessories
HUMAN LIFE	Awareness	Possession, Affective, Judgement
	Food and Drink	Drink, Fruit, Meat, Vegetables
	Health	Illness, Medicines
HUMAN LIVING	Routines	Meals, Sleep, Toiletting
	Leisure	TV, Books, Art, Sport
NON-HUMAN MOTION	Movement	Processes, come/go, Momentary
	Movers	Road, Rail, Air, Water
	Fauna	Animals, Birds, Insects, Fish
DOMESTIC SETTING	Home	Rooms, Inside Features, Outside Features
	Furniture	Kitchen, Bathroom, General
	Flora	Trees, Flowers
UTILITIES	Tools	Home, Garden, Work
	Containers	Wholes, Parts of
	Machines	Factory, Domestic
	Fuel and Power	Electricity, Gas
SOCIAL SETTING	World	Space, Earth, Weather
	Buildings	Farm, Shops, Offices
	Institutions	Religion, Law, Government
DIMENSIONS	Extent	Size, Shape, Measurement
	Colour	Brightness, Primary
	Time	Day, Year, Frequency
	Location	Here-and-now, Absent

The amount of arbitrary decision-making involved in such an exercise becomes plain as soon as one attempts it. The role of context is not explicitly indicated in the above, and yet it is crucial in assigning lexemes to semantic fields. Most of the time, given this reliance on context, there would be little dispute, but there are many instances where no amount of context will resolve the difficulty. For example, (a) the boundaries between fields are often not as discrete as the above list may suggest, *e.g.* do we classify *tar, soup, porridge* as "liquid" or "solid"? is *door, wall, window* the "inside" or the "outside" of a house?
(b) the distinction between form and function means that many lexemes can be classified twice, *e.g. pan* is both "container" and "for cooking"; *see* is both "body-parts" (in relation to eyes) and "sensation";
(c) several lexemes cut across fields, *e.g. see* applies to both people and fauna, *break* to body-parts and machines;
(d) often, the primary function of a lexeme is unclear, *e.g.* is *book* "leisure", "language", "goods" ...? is *glasses* "clothing", "body-parts", "health" ...?
(e) often, there is uncertainty as to the best level of abstraction to use, *e.g.* is *shoe* "clothing", or should we specify "footwear"? is *brooch* also "clothing", or should we specify "personal ornaments"?
Analytical problems of this kind mean that we must always be extremely cautious before using a semantic field model in clinical investigation; but as long as we are aware of the danger of arbitrariness, it is still possible to make some fairly gross observations concerning P's ability, in terms of his use of specific fields, and to use the notion as a means of guiding remedial activities in teaching vocabulary (see further, p. 177). It is also possible to use the approach as a framework within which we can look at P's vocabulary to see if he presents *lexical gaps*, *i.e.* if he lacks a lexeme at a particular place within the structure of a field. For example, applying the male/female distinction within "people" produces a range of parallels which P may not fully control—he may, for instance, lack lexemes at the places marked X in the following:

boy	girl
daddy	mummy
husband	wife
brother	X
X	aunt

An important initial step would be to see whether P can operate with the notion of semantic field at all, a prerequisite for which would be his ability to distinguish relevant from irrelevant, when a theme is introduced. For example, in answer to the question "What do you know about Xmas?", P_1 responded with "holiday, mince pies, turkey, Jesus ...", whereas P_2 said "happy, Africa, boating ...". Such associations may be explicable, at some level of consciousness for P_2, but they are certainly eccentric, in terms of adult norms (*cf.* Postman and Kleppel, 1970). If the behaviour were random, other themes would be affected (*e.g.* "what can you keep in a fridge/wear on your feet/see at the zoo ...?"), and in such circumstances the only way to impose some control would be by operating within the semantic structure imposed by the language, which accounts for only a sub-set of all the associations a theme may have[21]. What, then, is involved in the notion of semantic structure?

Structural Semantics

As a first step in defining the structure of the lexicon, the relations between lexemes can be analyzed in terms of the complementary dimensions of syntagmatic and paradigmatic (see p. 21). From a syntagmatic point of view, lexemes are seen in terms of their potential to combine in sequences within a structure. From a paradigmatic point of view, lexemes are seen in terms of their potential to be selected for use at a given place in structure. The interdependence between these dimensions may be illustrated as follows:

The	fat	cat	sat	on	the	chair
	thin					mat
	ugly					table
	.					.
	.					.

Here, the relationship between *fat* and *cat, cat* and *sat*, etc. is syntagmatic; the selection of *fat* vs. *thin*, or *chair* vs. *mat* is paradigmatic. Most discussion in semantics has focussed upon the types of relationship implicit under the latter heading (see further below). The particular attraction of these dimensions for linguists is that it allows them to reformulate the principles of semantic field analysis, without any need to postulate some sort of underlying conceptual "substance". Lexical networks are seen instead in terms of specific relations of sense operating between individual lexemes, in the first instance. The question is no longer "What do these lexemes refer to in the (non-linguistic) world?" or "How do sets of lexemes parcel out experience?" but rather "How do these lexemes (or sets of lexemes) relate to each other?"

That sense-relations are stateable independently of our knowledge of their reference is easily demonstrable. I can inform you that, in the as yet undiscovered language of Liliputian, *clak* is the opposite of *bong*, that *clak* and *rig* have the same meaning, and that a *clak* is a kind of *trub*. Having told you this, you could now tell me several other things, *e.g.* that a *rig* is a kind of *trub* also, or that *rig* and *bong* are opposites. Whether we are talking about colours, or clothes, or whatever, will not emerge, but a great deal can be learned about the lexical structure of the language nonetheless. The clinical situation is not altogether dissimilar. Aphasic productions, for example, may bear an unclear relationship to the world of reference, but nonetheless be internally consistent in certain respects (for example, an identifiable

---

[21] A "theme", in this sense, does not constitute a semantic field: it is a non-linguistically motivated notion, which cuts across the notion of semantic field, and may use lexemes from several of them. For example, the theme "What can you see at the zoo?" could be correctly answered by *lion, tiger*, etc. (field: ANIMALS), *cages, cafe* (field: BUILDINGS), *boys, girls*, etc. (field: PEOPLE), and so on. Examples of other themes include the story-lines of novels, plays, fairy-stories, etc. To determine when P can determine a theme from a list *(e.g. queen... mirror... cottage... seven beds... dwarfs...)* is an interesting exercise, but it is not one directly involving semantic structure.

set of lexemes may seem to follow certain rules, *e.g.* animate nouns cooccurring with animate verbs [*man ... sleep ...*]).

Paradigmatic Relations

Only some of the lexical substitutions which can be introduced into a sentence warrant analysis in terms of sense-relations. A sense-relation is, as its name suggests, a relationship between sentences such that we perceive their lexemes to be in some kind of systematic correspondence. We intuitively see a connection between them. There is no such connection normally made between the focussed lexemes in the following two sentences, for instance:

I've just bought a new *car*.   I've just bought a new *pencil.*

By contrast, the focussed lexemes in sentence pairs such as the following *do* seem connected in some way:

I've just bought a new *car*.   vs.   I've just bought a new *bike.*
I've just bought a *new* car.   vs.   I've just bought an *old* car.
I've just *bought* a new car.   vs.   I've just *sold* a new car.
I've just bought a new *car*.   vs.   I've just bought a new *automobile.*

It is argued that there are only a small number of ways in which sentences can be brought into predictable relationships with each other. In fact, four main types of sense-relation are regularly cited in semantics, established on the basis of the different effects produced by substituting one lexeme for another, at a particular place in structure. The following classification follows Lyons (1977).

1. Synonymy

For this sense-relation to obtain, the selection of one lexeme rather than another has no effect on the meaning (in the sense of "denotation") of the sentence. For example, in response to the question "Do you like the wine?", one might reply using any one of several possible lexemes, *e.g. absolutely, certainly, definitely, surely, assuredly.* In this context, these could be said to be synonymous. The point to be emphasized is that it does not therefore follow that this range of lexemes will *always* be synonymous: in a different context, a subtle contrast of meaning might be apparent, or one lexeme might be preferred to the others, *e.g. Surely he won't do that* vs. *Certainly he won't do that.* The principle involved is a general one: synonymy can be decided only with reference to context.

There are several implications for clinical practice. For example, to ask P for a lexeme which "means the same as" another, without providing a context, could be a confusing exercise. "What's another word for *bad*" could elicit "evil, wicked, naughty, unjust, wrong, sinful, cruel ..."—even "good", if *good* were the lowest point on a scale (as in some systems of hotel classification!). For P to be given the impression that *bad* and, say, *naughty* are interchangeable could lead to problems—*naughty*

10*

weather, naughty mistake, naughty king...? There is plainly an overlap of meaning between these lexemes ("partial synonymy"), but no identity. Providing context also means taking into account stylistic differences *(e.g. kingly/royal/regal)*, regional differences *(e.g. pavement/sidewalk)* and emotional differences *(e.g. youth/youngster)*.

2. Hyponymy

For this sense-relation to obtain, one lexeme involved in the substitution must be seen as in a subordinate or superordinate relationship to the other. For example, *horse* is subordinate to *animal*, *car* is subordinate to *vehicle*. The relationship is one of entailment *(cf.* the notion of class-inclusion in logic): if X is a horse, it follows that X must be an animal. On the other hand, the relationship is one-way ("unilateral"): it does not follow that if X is an animal, X is therefore a horse. In dictionaries, hyponymy is represented by such definitional formulae as "An X is a kind of Y". The subordinate terms are referred to as "hyponyms" of the "superordinate" term. To say that X and W are "co-hyponyms" would mean that they are both included under the same superordinate term, *e.g. horse, cow, dog*, etc. are co-hyponyms of *animal*. From these examples, it can be seen that hyponymy is the main way of imposing a hierarchical ordering on vocabulary. A fuller example is provided by the following schematic outline of orchestral instrument nouns:

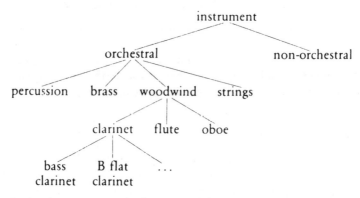

This is a fairly obvious example, because of the conventionality of the classification. It is more difficult to establish hierarchies among more abstract sets of lexemes, *e.g. noise, racket, din, uproar, tumult*. Is a *tumult* a kind of *uproar*, or an *uproar* a kind of *tumult*—or are both types of *din*? Also, it will often be the case that a set of lexemes will apparently lack a superordinate term, *e.g.* there is no single verb under which all and only verbs of motion *(come, go, arrive*, etc.) can be subsumed in English. It should further be noted that a lexeme may appear in several places in a hierarchy (thus permitting ambiguity). A good example is *animal*, discussed by Palmer (1976: 76-7): *animal* may contrast with *vegetable*, where it subsumes *birds, fish, insects* and *mammals;* but it may also be used in the sense of *mammals*, when it is then opposed to the other three; and under the heading of *mammals*, it may be used in yet a third sense, to provide a contrast between *animals* and *humans*.

A degree of hierarchical organization seems to be an essential feature of all areas of vocabulary. An important step in clinical investigation is thus to establish whether P can operate at different levels of abstraction, as defined in terms of lexical hyponymy. Several possible types of disability exist. For example, P may be able to operate with superordinates, but does not have the hyponyms available: pictures of dogs and cats may elicit a label such as *animal*—and if pressed, P may modify the superordinate term, perhaps referring to *barking animal*, and the like, a circumlocution which can be explained only with reference to the breakdown of the conventional hierarchy for this area of the lexicon. The converse case, where P can operate with hyponyms, but lacks the relevant superordinate term, is also well-attested in the aphasia literature (*cf.* Lesser, 1978: Ch. 6). Typical elicitation exercises for hyponymy are of two types: those where P is presented with a superordinate term and is asked to produce hyponyms; and the reverse, where he is given a set of hyponyms, and is asked for the superordinate term. Examples of (a) include:

Mr. Jones likes a drink in the evening. What sort of thing do you think he drinks?
I bought some fruit yesterday. What kind of fruit do you think I bought?
In a magazine, I saw a man wearing some nice clothes. What kind of clothes do you
    think he was wearing?

Examples of (b) include:

What do you call things like tables, chairs and sideboards?
What do you call things like cats, lions and horses?
What do you call things like the Daily Express and the Daily Telegraph?

An important point to note, in using exercises of this kind, is to ensure that there must be a genuine *linguistic* relationship between the lexeme in the stimulus and that in the anticipated response. We are testing P's awareness of hyponymy, not of sense association. For example, if T asked: "What sort of thing do you find on a farm?", and P replied "horses, cows, pigs", the response would not qualify as hyponymy (because horses, cows and pigs are not "kinds of" farm). P might have continued, "tractors, people", which illustrates the point. One P answered "my mother-in-law" to this question, which also proves a point. Most patients are able to provide a loosely associated list of lexemes, given enough patience and stimulation on T's part: the only semantic skill involved in this is recognizing that they all belong to a single semantic theme (*cf.* p. 146). To count as a sense relation within this field, far more stringent criteria are required.

3. Opposition (Binary Contrasts)

For this sense-relation to obtain, one lexeme involved in the substitution must be felt to be in some way opposite in meaning to the other. This is the sense-relation that has attracted greatest discussion—partly because of the traditional interest of logicians in contradictory and contrary terms[22]; it is consequently the area where there is the greatest terminological disunity. The problem arises from the existence

---

[22] In logic, contradictory terms are those where p and q cannot both be true or both be false, *e.g.* if X is *male*, X cannot be *female*, and vice versa: one cannot be both male/female or neither male/female. Contrary terms are those where p and q cannot both be true, but both may be false, *e.g.* if X is *hot*, X cannot be *cold*; but X may be neither hot nor cold, *e.g. lukewarm.*

of many different kinds of oppositeness. This point is often missed in clinical approaches, which follow the lead of traditional terminology, setting up a simple contrast between synonymy and antonymy: synonymy is identity of meaning between lexemes, and therefore antonymy is maximum difference of meaning between lexemes. In fact, there are many kinds and degrees of oppositeness, which the traditional terminology does not do justice to. The most comprehensive discussion to date is in Lyons (1977: Ch. 9), and his terminology is followed here. All oppositions, in his technical sense, are binary, *i.e.* involving two lexemes, which are seen as being at polar extremes. Several types are recognized:

(a) Antonymy. Lyons reserves this term for those binary contrasts which are gradable, *i.e.* it is possible to identify degrees of contrast between the extremes. For example, *happy* and *sad* are antonyms, in this sense, as it is possible to compare these properties using such forms as *He is happier/very happy/as happy as ...* Lyons proposes a further classification of antonyms into three sub-types:

(i) those where the basis of comparison is explicit, *e.g. X is as happy as Y;*

(ii) those where the basis of comparison is implicit, *e.g. X is happy (i.e.* compared with some unstated norm);

(iii) those where the basis of comparison is semi-explicit, *e.g. X is very happy.*

(b) Complementarity. This term is reserved for those binary contrasts which are ungradable—they do not permit degrees of quantification, unlike antonymy. For example, *single* and *married* are complementaries, in this sense, as are *male/female, alive/dead,* and many more. It is not possible to talk (except occasionally in jest) using such forms as *He is very single/as single as/more single ...*

(c) Converseness. This term is reserved for binary contrasts which display an interdependence of meaning, such that one member of the pair presupposes the other member. This sense-relation is especially found in the definition of reciprocal social roles or spatial relationships, *e.g. buy/sell, parent/child, employer/employee, above/below.* One cannot be an employer without having employees, and vice versa. This is the essential difference with complementarity, where there is no such symmetry of dependence; these terms are also ungradable, hence there is a difference with antonymy.

(d) Others. There are several other kinds of opposition which could be identified. One such is directionality, referring to those contrasts where there is an implication of motion in one of two opposed directions with respect to a given place. Examples of directional oppositions include *up/down, to/from, come/go, arrive/depart,* and (because of the implication of consequence obtaining between them) *learn/forget.* Another relation is the "antipodal" oppositions of *north/south, left/right, black/white, summer/winter,* etc. The degree of applicability of such distinctions to the lexicon as a whole is not clear, at present; but it is intuitively obvious that there is something "different" about such sets, and it may well be that specific difficulties, in clinical terms, could be related to distinctions of this kind.

Two other observations concerning oppositions are of importance. Firstly, it should be noted that depending on the context or sense involved, many lexemes can be seen as having more than one opposite. For example, *cat* is opposed to *dog* in one context, and to *kitten* in another; *summer* may be opposed to *winter,* but *spring* seems "equally" opposed to the other three seasons (though technically one might argue that it is antipodal to *autumn*). Often, the alternatives derive from different morphological possibilities in the language, *e.g. happy* is opposed to both *sad* and *unhappy*. English has a large number of prefixes and suffixes that can form opposites in this way, *e.g. dis-, in-, -less*. Secondly, in many oppositions, one member of the pair can be said to be the more neutral of the two—"unmarked" (*cf.* p. 25). The classical test for this with opposed adjectives is using them in constructions with *How*. For example, given the antonyms *old/young*, the neutral *How* question would be to ask *How old is John?*, where the reply could cover any part of the whole age range. To ask *How young is John?*, by contrast, is odd or loaded—implying, for instance, that there is something problematic about John's age (*e.g.* a criterion for a job, perhaps). It has been argued (*cf.* H. Clark, 1973) that it is the more negative, or limiting, of the pair of antonyms which tends to be singled out, or "marked" in this way, *e.g. short* in the opposition *tall/short* (*cf. How tall is your boy now?* vs. *How short is your boy now?!*). The point has also been investigated in relation to language acquisition (*cf.* p. 181). Clinically, we might therefore expect differences in performance in relation to this distinction, as is illustrated by the following dialogue, where the marked member of the pair *near/far* was causing particular difficulty[23].

P   it's not very něar to 'Newbury/
T   'not very fàr/
P   not fàr/ yès/
        by càr it's quite fár/ yès/

Problems in the comprehension or production of oppositions are commonplace in aphasia. What is less obvious, without analysis, is whether there is any pattern in the range of difficulties displayed by P—for example, whether he is having particular difficulty with one of the above categories (see further below).

4. Non-Binary Contrasts

This label rather loosely characterizes the relationship between sets of lexemes (more than two) when there is plainly a contrast in sense, but the notion of "opposite" does not seem relevant. For example, there is a semantic relationship obtaining between *oboe* and *clarinet*, but one would not want to say that *oboe* was the "opposite" of *clarinet*, as there are several other items with which it can be put into immediate contrast, such as *flute* and *bassoon*. Sets of lexemes, where the sense of one delimits the sense of the others, are referred to under the heading of *incompatibility* by Lyons (1977: 288). Thus the lexemes *red/blue/green*, etc. are incompatible, as are the instrument terms above. Incompatibility is most clearly illustrated when there is a superordinate term to which the lexemes can be related—*woodwind*, in the above examples; and one should note in this respect the relationship between incompatibility and hyponymy:

---

[23] Experimental studies aiming to show differential ability, both in production and comprehension, have been frequent in child language acquisition, for certain areas of the vocabulary: see, for example, Eilers, Oller and Ellington (1974).

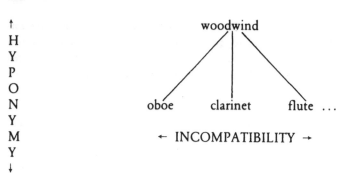

↑
H
Y
P
O
N   oboe   clarinet   flute ...
Y
M   ← INCOMPATIBILITY →
Y
↓

But there may not always be an obvious superordinate term: the term *colour*, for example, does not cover all hues in the spectrum—*black, white* and *grey* are often excluded from the category *coloured* (as on TV). What is important is that the lexemes can be seen as members of a fixed set of alternatives, sharing certain features of meaning. Lexemes such as *dog/book/car/sky* contrast in sense, but they are not incompatible terms, because they have nothing in common, and contexts where the speaker has to make a meaningful choice between them are unlikely, to say the least.

Within this general heading, some quite specific sets of incompatible items can be isolated. Lexeme sets which are *unordered* (such as colours, musical instruments) can be distinguished from those where there is a fixed internal ordering. For example, *serial* ordering is illustrated in the terms for military ranks, or scales of measurement, where there is a fixed gradation between the outermost members. In *cyclical* ordering, on the other hand, there are no outermost members, except by convention, *e.g.* days of the week, months of the year.

In many ways, incompatibility is the most problematic of all the structural semantic relations to work with clinically, in that it involves an extremely wide range of lexemes within a semantic field (*e.g.* foodstuffs, parts of the body, vehicles), and it is not immediately obvious how these should be related to each other, if at all. P may generate a set of incompatible items by loose association, producing a list of lexemes for colour, fruit, or whatever. Is there any further internal structuring that can be given to these lists? The notions of synonymy, oppositeness and hyponymy are inapplicable, so we must refer to other notions in order to analyse the similarities and the differences between the members of the list. It is here that the notion of semantic feature becomes relevant (see p. 155). But not all incompatible sets are able to be given an illuminating analysis in terms of features. Cyclical and serial sets, in particular, seem unable to be further analyzed, and have to be learned by rote: in what way is Monday different from Tuesday, for example, other than that the one precedes the other?

5. Other Paradigmatic Relations

It is unclear how many other kinds of sense-relation might be recognized on the basis of paradigmatic oppositions. It may be that there are no other categories comparable in generality to the above four logical types (sameness, oppositeness, inclusiveness and dissimilarity). But there are doubtless several relations that remain to be identified, operating in more restricted areas of the lexicon. For example, there is in English the possible marking of a lexeme for sex. This relation (male vs. female) is sometimes marked morphologically *(e.g. lion/lioness, host/hostess)*; and sometimes through the use of different lexemes *(e.g. dog/bitch)*. What is of importance is that in such pairs, one member is marked and the other unmarked in a semantic sense also: the unmarked member may be used in a wider range of contexts than the marked member, which it often subsumes, *e.g. there are lions in the safari park* allows the possibility that some of these may be female as well as male; whereas *there are lionesses in the safari park* excludes the presence of male lions. Another example of a sense-relation, which is much less restricted than this, is the distinction between parts and wholes, as in the lexemes which label parts of the body, of a car, an engine, and so on. This is distinct from hyponymy: a wheel is not a "kind of" car; it is "part of" a car. This relation is closely bound up with grammatical factors, such as the possessive construction, or the use of the verb *have* (*cf.* p. 163), but it also has a lexical structuring role, as can be seen from such hierarchical sequences as: "the page is a part of the book which is a part of the library which is part of the town . . .". Here, the sense-relation only operates if a lexeme is used with reference to a specific superordinate term in the part-whole hierarchy. To take this example a stage further, it would be strange to talk of "the page is a part of the library" or "the book is a part of the town", by omitting the intermediate steps. On the other hand, the serial chain of "second-minute-hour-day" seems more flexible in this respect. A further distinction, of potential clinical relevance, is whether the part-whole relationship is temporary or permanent: both a branch and a bird's nest may be "part of" a tree, but the former is an intrinsic feature of the identity of the tree, whereas the latter is incidental. The terms *inalienable* and *alienable* are sometimes used to identify this contrast (branches are inalienable features of trees, as are arms of bodies; nests are alienable features of trees, as are spectacles of bodies). The extent of the part-whole relationship in the lexicon is unclear: as soon as we attempt to analyze the more abstract kinds of noun, for example, we run into problems (*cf.* Lyons, 1977: 314). But the clinical importance of this category of lexical structure is considerable, as errors in identifying part-whole relationships are common.

Syntagmatic Relations

This dimension has been much less thoroughly investigated in the analysis of meaning, and the semantic literature can do little more than provide general guidelines and a few broad categories. But these can nonetheless be illuminating, in guiding clinical practice. The fundamental notion here is the linguistic constraints which lexemes have on their ability to co-occur, within a grammatical structure. The operative word is "linguistic". Some lexemes co-occur simply because the world motivates their doing so: houses have walls, hence it is not surprising that the lexeme *house* and the lexeme *wall* will co-occur fairly frequently in English sentences. Conversely, there seems little reason to expect that the lexemes *pencils* and *elephants* will co-occur (though I do not doubt that one day someone will write a children's tale called *The Elephant and the Pencil!*), that *desks* will *growl*, *sleeping* be *furious*, and so on. But apart from these cases, there are innumerable co-occurrences, of varying degrees of mutual expectancy, which cannot be explained by reference to anything in the real world. For example, a sentence such as *he was—with jealousy* will very likely have the blank filled with the lexeme *green*—though there is nothing in the colour of the individual to motivate this choice. Or again, the sentence *it was an auspicious —* will have the blank filled by a small range of lexemes, such as *occasion, event* or *omen*. Such expectancies between lexemes have been called *collocations*, and the relationship concerned is known as *collocability*[24]. They are an important part of the statement of a lexeme's total use in a language, and they thus enter into a statement of a lexeme's meaning. An oft-repeated quotation is from Firth: "you shall know a word by the company it keeps".

Collocations have not been studied very systematically, largely for practical reasons: to investigate the mutual predictability of individual lexemes would require an enormous body of informant tests, or corpora of millions of words. From an intuitive point of view, however, it is plain that there is a scale of mutual predictability, ranging from the wholly predictable to the (lexically) unpredictable. Items which are 100% predictable, or nearly so, would include: *spick (→and span), amok (run→), eke (→out)* and *rancid (→butter, bacon)*. A little less predictable would be items such as *flock (→sheep, birds, goats,* and in its verb use, *people [the people flocked . . .]), auspicious (cf.* above) and the verb *crack (→egg, joke, dawn, ice,* and a few more). Some way further down this scale would be lexemes like *table* and *letter*, which can collocate with a wide range of lexemes. What is interesting here is how these lexemes can be grouped to identify the different senses of these words, viz.:

table₁   furniture, top, legs, lamp, wine, card . . .
table₂   . figures, page, lists, column, multiplication, time, log . . .
letter₁   box, post, write, envelope, head . . .
letter₂   alphabet, spelling, law *(cf. the letter of the law)*, press, man *(sc.* of letters) . . .

At the other end of the scale would be items which have no lexical predictability at all, such as *the, to* and *is* (these items, of course, have grammatical predictability of various kinds). Somewhere above this would be such lexemes as *big, have, go, take, put,* which have extremely wide ranges of lexical occurrence. And so we could continue, throughout the lexicon. It is not possible, in our present state of knowledge, to formalize this scale, but the general idea is clear enough.

There is another way of studying lexical co-occurrence: instead of identifying mutual expectancies positively, we can talk negatively, and attempt to state the degree of unlikelihood of their co-occurrence. This includes those cases where the unli-

---

[24] See Firth (1951: 194 ff.), Halliday (1966), Robins (1971: 63—66). Sometimes the term is used for all co-occurrences between lexemes—including the *house/wall* type; nor is there as clear a boundary between these two types as the above examples might suggest—cf. Palmer (1976: 96).
In the terminology of generative theory, collocational information is partly handled under the heading of "selectional restrictions".

kelihood is motivated by our knowledge of the real world (*cf.* above): thus, *desk* and *growl* is an unlikely collocational sequence, as is *stone* and *sleep, drink* and *bacon,* and so on. But it also includes cases where there is no reason *in the world* why the items should not go together. For example, there is no reason, apart from linguistic convention in English, why *blouse* or *buxom* collocates with *girls* and not *boys,* or why *rancid* collocates with *butter/bacon* and not *eggs/cheese.* Similarly, to express the notion of "oldness", we have animate lexemes such as *elderly,* inanimate lexemes such as *antique (antique monument,* not **elderly monument)* and others which are less determinate *(ancient shop/man).*

Two other points about collocations should be made. Firstly, it should be noted that collocational expectancy is to some extent a cumulative phenomenon: you are more likely to be able to predict the lexemes occurring towards the end of a sentence than those early on. For example, *pop* has a wide range of potential lexical followers; *pop—letter* immediately reduces this range to a tiny number—probably *pillar-box,* or the like. The theoretical literature is not clear as to what the optimal grammatical range is in terms of which lexical collocations can be identified, though various suggestions have been made[25]. Secondly, it is often possible to collect a set of lexemes together, and study their potential for collocation with another set of lexemes—all the items within the one set have an identical collocation with all the items in the other set. For example, the lexemes *strong, strength, strengthen* and *strongly* all collocate with the lexemes *argue, argument, argumentative, arguable* (*cf. he argued strongly, the strength of his argument,* etc.). Such sets of lexemes are sometimes referred to as "formal scatters".

Finally, a word of warning not to confuse the notion of collocation with that of sense association: the former is a linguistic notion, the latter is a psychological one. In the study of collocations, we are dealing with those patterns which are part of the language as a whole; *i.e.* all speakers, regardless of context, would recognize the relationships between *rancid* and *butter,* and so on. Sense associations, however, have no necessary universal status; indeed, the whole point of some investigative procedures using associations (*e.g.* in psychiatry) is to obtain an individual profile of response which may yield clues as to the nature of a pathological condition. The sense associations I may have for *butter* can thus be idiosyncratic and eccentric, and these are outside the scope of linguistic investigation, and thus of semantics.

Componential Analysis

In this approach, the sense of a lexeme is analyzed into a set of sense components, or *semantic features,* some or all of which will be used as part of the analysis of other lexemes, *i.e.* they are more general in meaning. This technique, an extension of the principle of distinctive feature analysis in phonology (see p. 25), was originally devised by anthropologists as a means of describing and comparing vocabulary, but later developed into a theoretical framework which attempted to interrelate

---

[25] See, for example, the methods used by Sinclair (1966), on the basis of the approach summarised in Halliday (1966).

and explain such sense-relations as those discussed above[26]. Semantic features can be easily illustrated with reference to such lexemes as *boy, girl, man*, etc., *e.g. boy* can be seen as the "product" of *male+child*, or *male+non-adult+human*. A whole system of relationships can be established along these lines, a much-used example being:

man	woman	child
bull	cow	calf
ram	ewe	lamb
	etc.	

all of which can be analyzed in terms of the components *male* vs. *female, adult* vs. *non-adult*, and *human* vs. *bovine* vs. *ovine*. Componential analyses are usually conceived as binary opposites: one of the members is then used as a base form, the contrast being signalled through the use of plus or minus, *e.g. man=+male, +adult, +human,* or *−female, −child, −animal.* The inapplicability of a distinction can then be marked using ±, as when *soup* is held to be indeterminate with reference to the contrast *liquid/solid* (does one eat or drink it?).

Componential techniques of analysis can be valuable, in that they enable one to define more clearly some of the logical relationships that underlie sense-relations; salient contrasts can often be readily isolated, as we shall see below. But there are problems which reduce the plausibility of this approach: for instance, how do we motivate the choice of components *(e.g.* is *+male* and *−male* preferable to *+female* and *−female?)?* how do we handle lexical contrasts which are not binary (for instance, complementary and incompatible terms)? how do we restrict the applicability of the features so that they are not used unnecessarily *(e.g. male/female* is relevant only for animate things, and not for chairs, pictures, needles, etc.)? how do you decide which features are essential to define a concept, and which are irrelevant (remembering that there is an infinity of possible negative features). The various fragments of the lexicon which have been studied in these terms present occasional insights, but involve so many arbitrary assumptions that both Palmer (1976: 91) and Lyons (1977: 333) conclude that the approach does not provide a viable theoretical framework. Given this pessimism, it is perhaps surprising to see so much use being made of the notion in the literature on language acquisition; but in fact aspects of the feature methodology do have heuristic value. It is perfectly possible to analyze a lexeme into a set of features, using these to contrast the lexeme with other lexemes. The problems come when we try to establish universal principles governing the applicability of these features throughout the lexicon (or across languages) or to suggest that there is something psychologically real, either about the features themselves, or about the way they are organized.

From a clinical viewpoint, an ad hoc analysis of lexemes, within the framework of sense-relations, can be a fruitful exercise, as it can help to locate those aspects of lexical meaning with which P is having particular difficulty. This can be illustrated from any semantic field: one that turns up often in clinical sessions is the field of human movement, as categorized in terms of *run, jump, walk*, etc. It is very easy to

---

[26] See Lounsbury (1956), Katz and Fodor (1963).

underestimate the semantic complexity of even the most mundane areas of the vocabulary. Without careful preparation, T's choice of a lexeme may give rise to major and unexpected problems in P. One dictionary definition of the lexeme *walk*, for example, is as follows:

(of people and creatures with two legs) a natural and unhurried way of moving on foot in which the feet are lifted one at a time with one foot not off the ground before the other touches.

The associated verb is defined similarly: "to move (or cause to move) in this way". With all such definitions, the important thing is to note the number of features it contains, each of these providing a point of potential contrast. This definition might be broken down into five feature contrasts:

(a) of people and creatures with 2 legs   (vs. 4 legs)
(b) a natural   (vs. unnatural)
(c) and unhurried   (vs. hurried)
(d) way of moving forward on foot   (vs. not on foot backward)
(e) in which ... touches   (vs. two feet stay on the ground)

We can eliminate (a) from the present enquiry, as a consequence of (e): (a) contrasts with the definition required for creatures with 4 legs, where it is the case that two legs are always on the ground at any given time. We can however use the remaining features as a means of organizing the whole of this area of the lexicon, to see the similarities and differences of meaning between related lexemes—in other words, we can begin to work out the structure of this semantic field. A matrix presentation is a convenient way of doing this: the lexemes in question are listed vertically on the left, and the potentially relevant semantic features are listed horizontally at the top. For example:

	natural	unhurried	movement	forward	foot on ground
walk	yes	yes	yes	yes	yes
totter	no	yes	yes	yes	yes
march	no	no	yes	yes	yes

As the lexicon gets extended, so the range of potential contrasts has to be extended. For example, to add *swim* would require reference to water vs. land; to add *run* would require that the "foot on ground" criterion be split into "foot always on ground" vs. "foot regularly on ground". Here are some further examples:

a short walk for pleasure/health, etc.	stroll, jaunt, constitutional
a longer walk for pleasure/health, etc.	ramble, hike
a regular walk for professional purposes	beat, circuit, route

or again:

manner of walk (gait):	careless	slouch, shamble, shuffle, droop
	erratic	totter, stagger
	pride	mince, swagger, strut
	injury	hobble, limp

Such matrices always have to be viewed with caution; they are necessarily simplifications, omitting certain nuances. But they do suggest ways in which order might be
imposed on what would otherwise be an inventory. In this way, also, lexical *gaps* can
be identified, *i.e.* concepts for which no single lexeme exists in a language, *e.g.* in
English there is no single lexeme for the concept "hurried movement backwards
with one foot always on the ground"!

In clinical analyses, this approach can be extremely illuminating. It can identify
the reason for a particular lexical confusion, *e.g.* P may be unable to grasp the significance of a particular feature contrast, such as the distinction between hurried
and unhurried, or natural vs. unnatural. P may try to apply a particular feature to
lexemes for which it is inappropriate, either because it is already specified *(e.g. walk
with his legs)* or because it is contradictory *(e.g. he rushed slowly in)*. Perhaps P has a
special sense in mind, which he finds difficult to eliminate: there are many such
special contexts for the common lexemes in a language (indeed, it is the commonest
lexemes which raise the greatest problems in this respect); for example, *walk* has
special senses in such contexts as ghosts *(spirits walk)*, cricket *(the batsman walks)*, moving by holding *(walk his bike)*, moving an object in the manner of a walk *(walk the cup-
board)*, follow a way of life *(walk in his shoes)*, and so forth. Given this range of potential usage, it is not difficult to see why an apparently simple concept should cause
major semantic problems.

And a similar need to be aware of the complexity involved arises when we
consider remediation techniques. Providing an adequate context is obviously crucial, but this means more than simply giving a plausible occasion, or picture. It
means anticipating the reason why P should use the lexeme in the first place (why
should P *want* to identify the person in the picture as walking?), and this usually
boils down to the question of semantic contrast (what is the person in the picture
doing, as opposed to . . .?). Look how a quite different set of contrasts can be elicited,
by varying the context of a lexeme such as *walk:*

(1) That baby's just learned to walk. A month ago she couldn't walk. What was she
able to do?

(2) I was walking towards the bus-stop, but I still had a long way to go. I saw the bus
coming. What did I do?

(3) A horse was walking along the road. Its rider made it go faster. What did the
horse do?

(4) The little boy was walking beside his bicycle. Then he got on. What did he start
to do?

The responses to these questions (involving such lexemes as *crawl, run, trot/gallop,*
and *ride*) each involve the use of a sense-relation—one of the categories of oppositeness referred to above. It is these that constitute the reality of the use of *walk* in
everyday language. Such exercises contrast with the picture-showing technique
which is not only unreal (because decontextualized) but also ambiguous ("What's
the man doing?" [in the picture] can also be answered by "thinking", "breathing", or
even "nothing", given that the picture is static).

Non-Lexical Semantics

This chapter has so far concentrated on the semantic analysis of the lexicon, as this is the area where meaning is most obviously located, and where most of the research has been done. But it would be wrong to assume that meaning is restricted to the lexical level. On the contrary: it can be argued that all levels of linguistic organization contribute in some way to the meaning of an utterance—phonetic, phonological and grammatical. J. R. Firth was one who advanced the view that meaning could be seen as a "spectrum" of modes, involving all linguistic levels; but even if we do not accept his theoretical account of meaning, the insight of this approach can be given an immediate clinical interpretation. In this section, then, we look briefly at what might be involved, clinically, in phonetic and phonological meaning, with a rather more detailed look at grammatical meaning.

1. Phonetic Meaning

Here, a meaning is attributed to the sounds of a language, *i.e.* a sound-symbolism (*cf.* p. 132)—a phenomenon which is normally limited to a few cases of onomatopoeia, and to literary and rhetorical expression. It is possible to have abnormal semantic behaviour in which P attributes a meaning to sounds which they would not normally be held to possess, for example, a schizophrenic reaction in which words are avoided beginning with certain sounds, or words containing certain sounds are overused because of their connotations. An analogous reaction may be found in patients who react to the non-segmental properties of the voice in pathological ways, *e.g.* being antagonistic towards a certain voice quality, or a regional/social accent, or choosing to speak in a certain voice quality or accent, because of the imagined meaning attributed to them. To be a clinical concern, of course, such reactions need to be severe—for instance, a characteristic of neurotic or psychotic behaviour; in a mild form, attitudes to the phonetic properties of speech (*e.g.* a dislike/preference for a particular accent) are universal. A comparable example from aphasia was a patient who was able to maintain a reasonably fluent level of expression only if she used what she called her "television voice". Phonetic meaning is also clinically relevant in identifying situations where, in order to make contact or develop rapport with P, T may need to adopt a particular voice quality as a norm, *e.g.* speaking in a loud resonant voice, or with a widened pitch range. With children, it is common to find T adopting a lively exaggerated melodic style, in which the intonation patterns are widened and stressed, the aim presumably being to generate enthusiasm, interest and involvement in the teaching/therapy situation[27]—though not all children respond well to this kind of approach. To the extent that T has chosen to convey a particular personal and situational impression, or "meaning" by her choice of speech style, a factor has been introduced into clinical interaction which is certainly of semantic interest. This area does not seem to have received systematic study, however.

[27] Cf. the baby-talk prosody of parents: see the paper by Garnica, and other references in Snow and Ferguson (1977); also above, p. 93. On the social function of accents, see Trudgill (1974), Giles and Powesland (1975).

2. Phonological Meaning

In certain linguistic genres (such as poetry), patterns of phonemes in an utterance can be interpreted as conveying a meaning of sorts, for example the way in which alliteration, assonance and rhyme act to interrelate words that are spatially apart—the similarity of sound promoting a connection of sense[28]. Apart from this, phonemes have no meaning, and do not therefore provide a topic for this chapter. Non-segmental phonology, however, does permit a direct statement of meaning, in the form of the attitudes, emotions and social roles that prosodic and paralinguistic patterns signal. These points might have been discussed here, but as they have already formed part of the subject-matter of Chapter 3, a reference to the relevant section should suffice: pp. 65—66.

3. Grammatical Meaning

It has already been pointed out (Ch. 4) that the various categories and constructions of grammar can be discussed from both formal and semantic points of view. A category such as tense, or number, can be identified in terms of the formal features of syntax and morphology which mark the contrasts involved, or in terms of the meaning conveyed by these formal contrasts: for example, number in English is formally a two-term system involving an unmarked singular form and a marker of plurality (usually a form of -s); semantically, it usually conveys the difference between "one" and "more than one" (though cf. Palmer, 1971: Appendix, for a discussion of the limitations of this interpretation). A construction such as a grammatical statement can be identified formally (e.g. NP+VP, or Subject-Verb) and also semantically (e.g. Actor-Action, or Topic-Comment). It is never an easy matter to state the correspondence between formal and semantic analyses, and very little progress has been made in constructing models of the semantic side of this correspondence, but what is already evident is that there are generalizations to be made which go well beyond the terms of reference of Chapter 4 of this book, and which often provide a more illuminating analysis of a clinical condition[29]. One such makes use of the notion which different theories refer to as the "case role", "valency" or "semantic function" of an element of clause structure[30]. Without restricting the discussion to any one theoretical approach, it is evident that the main elements of sentence structure (Subject, Verb, Complement, Object, Adverbial, in the terminology of Chapter 4) can be studied, not only in terms of their syntactic form and distribution in the clause (SVO, VOA, etc.), but also in terms of the type of information that such grammatical patterns convey. An early attempt to define the semantic relations underlying these patterns was Fillmore (1968), whose notion of "case grammar" analyzed surface grammatical patterns in terms of such relations as

---

[28] Cf. Empson (1930), Firth (1951: 193—194), Leech (1969: Ch. 6).

[29] In some accounts of linguistic analysis, the patterns discussed below would in fact be handled under the heading of grammar, and not in this Chapter at all. The boundary between syntax and semantics is always somewhat arbitrarily decided.

[30] See for example Fillmore (1968), Chafe (1970).

"agentive", "instrumental" and "locative". The same instrumental "case", for example, was claimed to underlie the phrase *(with) the key* in each of the following sentences:

(i) the key opened the door

(ii) he used the key to open the door

(iii) the door was opened with the key

despite the fact that, from a surface grammatical viewpoint, the *key* is Subject in (i), Object in (ii), and Adverbial in (iii). It was argued that semantic identities of this kind are obscured by the traditional kinds of formal analysis.

Formalizing this conception of linguistic structure is however very difficult, and it is now doubtful whether a general linguistic theory based on these principles can be constructed. But the approach, and its derivatives, has proved extremely illuminating in certain areas of grammar and lexicon, and in child language studies. In clinical linguistic analysis, also, the approach can be valuable, for the analysis of Ps who seem to defy analysis in conventional grammatical terms. An approach of this kind is at present extremely primitive, as models of the semantic structure of clauses exist only in outline, and competing terms and interpretations of terms make the field controversial. Certain *semantic functions* do however seem to be widely recognized, and these will form the basis of the clinical analyses below[31]. The usual procedure is to recognize the centrality of the category of verbs, identifying the two main functions of ACTION (or DYNAMIC), *e.g. kick, run, go,* and STATIVE, *e.g. know, see, want, be*[32]. The remaining semantic functions are then specified with reference to the verb, as follows:

ACTOR (=Fillmore's AGENTIVE, Wells' AGENT): the animate being that causes an action or change of state, *e.g.* **John** *kicked the ball,* **The** *ball was kicked by* **John.**

EXPERIENCER (=Fillmore's DATIVE): the animate being that experiences an action or change of state, *e.g.* **John** *is happy,* **John** *saw a car.*

GOAL (=Fillmore's FACTITIVE, OBJECTIVE, Wells' PATIENT): the object or being which undergoes the result of an action or change of state, *e.g. John kicked* **the ball,** *John saw* **Jim.**

INSTRUMENTAL: the inanimate cause of an action or change of state, *e.g.* **The rock** *broke the window,* *He broke the window* **with a rock.**

LOCATIVE: the location of the action or state specified by the verb, or of the goal, *e.g. The car is* **in the garage, Greenland** *is cold.*

TEMPORAL (not specified in the above references): the time of the action or state specified by the verb, as expressed outside of the tense forms, *e.g.* **Later,** *he came in, We went* **at 7 o'clock.**

Several other semantic functions are illustrated in the references given below, for example BENEFACTIVE (*e.g. that is* **for Billy**), POSSESSOR (*e.g.* **John** *has a car),* COMITATIVE (*e.g. he went* **with mummy**), CONNECTIVE (*e.g.* **The boy and the girl** *came),* CLASSIFICATORY (*e.g. A tulip is* **a flower**), ATTRIBUTIVE (*e.g. The car was*

---

[31] These are based on a comparison of the functions recognised in Brown (1973), Bowerman (1973), Wells (1974), Bloom, Lightbown and Hood (1975), and Bloom and Lahey (1978), with the further references therein.

[32] Cf. the grammatical classification of Quirk, *et al.* (1972: Ch. 3).

red, *The* **red** *car...),* QUANTITATIVE *(e.g. There were* **several),** CAUSATIVE *(I went* **because...),** etc. Moreover, it is possible to recognize sub-divisions within these very general categories, *e.g.* types of instrument, or location, or time. Using just the main semantic functions, however, several observations can be made concerning the use of language by many patients.

An example is provided by the 8-year-old girl analyzed in Crystal (1979: 28-30, 110), who suffered a left CVA of unknown etiology, with a resulting (temporary) total aphasia. After six months, a spontaneous speech sample began as follows:

T wèll/ how àre you to'day/
P 'all right/
T well you've 'got a 'lot to tèll me/ as I haven't sèen you for a 'long tíme/
P I knòw/
T okày/
   'what were you 'doing for Chrìstmas/ -
P erm - erm - erm - erm - a fa -- erm - 'Christmas Dăy/ - er - 'went to - bēd/ - on 'Christmas Ĕve/ and and and -- s - erm - erm --- erm - er -- and 'lots of 'toys to plây at/ -
   òh and/ - sòme of the 'toys/ - er - a brōught/ er - Jénny's/ - er - a knóck-out/
T 'Jenny had a
P a ↑knòckout/   (name of a game)
T it's a knòckout/
   I sèe/
P yès/ er
T uhúh/
P and and - a - 'Sharon - erm cámera/
T she dìdn't/
P yés/   (laughing)
T and 'did she 'take some phŏtos/
P nó/ er -
   Gûernsey/
T Gûernsey/
P uhùh/ -
   'Guernsey on the trìp/ .
   the schòol/
T mhṁ/
P and - and er - mŷ 'presents/ Sìndy 'horse/

A conventional grammatical analysis of this data proved unilluminating. Approximately half of the sentences were of regular grammatical construction covering a wide syntactic range, and usually with little or no hesitation, *e.g.*

I knòw/   that's a pòlar 'bear/
hàlf as 'big/   'what's thát/
Mùmmy 'blow them 'up/   'Margot and 'Mary and dáddy - 'brought
'all sòrts of 'things/   sòmething/

The remainder were incomplete, problematic or deviant, often spoken with considerable hesitancy, *e.g.*

sòme of the 'toys/ - er - a brōught/ er - Jénny's/ - er - a knóckout/
a - 'Sharon - erm cámera/
mŷ 'presents/ Sìndy 'horse/
thìs 'horse/ is a 'mane - lòng/
and I 'went 'my Sìndy 'set/

A semantic functional analysis of the two types of sentence did prove helpful, however. It emerged that the majority of the deviant sentences involved P attempting to express such notions as possession, proximity, directional movement and location—especially in space, but also in time[33]. Grammatical factors do add certain complications, but basically the underlying difficulty seems to do with the expression of spatio-temporal *location*. P does have spatial and temporal concepts, but has great difficulty in relating them to objects, actions and agents. If P does not attempt to use these concepts, as in making a straightforward request or description, the sentence structure emerges with little error and hesitation.

In this example, it should be noted how the semantic notion involved "cuts across" grammatical structures. Several very different kinds of grammatical construction can be used to express the notion of location, *e.g. the car* **has** *wheels, there are wheels* **on the car,** *the car's wheels,* and so on. An analysis in terms of semantic functions seems to be the only way to demonstrate the existence of pattern in such data.

The above observations were made on the basis of an analysis in which certain semantic functions were shown not to be expressed, or, when attempted, provided P with especial difficulties. In such cases, there is usually a corresponding deficit in comprehension. The opposite kind of pattern also presents, namely P's apparent dependence on a particular semantic function, so that sentence patterns come to appear stereotyped, and a small range of lexical patterns appear overused. The following extract from a 10-year-old language-delayed boy of low-average intelligence illustrates this:

T   ... 'how long did you 'have to be a'way from schôol/
P   erm - 'Thursday at - er
      'had [brùːk]/ . er . bòok befóre/ - er
      'when I (had) . 'that wèek off/ Frìday/ .
      when . 'I (had) 'that wèek off/ a . 'all . póorly/
      I('m) 'not going óut/ . to . Mo 'Monday to Fri . Sàturday/
      yéah/ -
      erm - thēn/ . 'I come báck/ - làst wéek/
      Thùrsday I 'poorly agáın/ . 'with thát/ --
      [n] 'not 'same thíng/ .
      'then Mǒnday/ -- I 'go to dóctors/ ...
T   ... are you 'having your 'dinners at 'school todáy/

---

[33] Note the close cognitive relationship between space and time in early development, as argued by H. Clark (1973).

11*

P   yés/
     'Tuesday 'Wednesday 'Thursday 'Monday Frìday/
     ...

T   'tell me a'bout any 'dogs that you knòw/
P   erm - I 'got alsàtian nów/ -
T   you've 'got an *alsătian/
P   *bòught it/
T   you bòught it/
P   'last wèek/
T   rěally/
     in 'your *hŏuse/
P   *yéah/ -
     in 'my hòuse/ .
     (he) pòorly/ nòw/
T   it's pòorly/
P   ṁ/
T   whỳ/
P   'fighting with erm - er erm 'red sètter/ .
T   ôh/
P   'got - 'all . the [dɔɪ] - hàirs/ come òut/
T   is it a pùppy your alsátian/
P   erm yès/ .
     'last wèek/ - I bòught/
T   yès/
     but 'is it 'still a pŭppy/
P   *(2 sylls)* -- I dìd/ - er
T   'did you . yés/
P   'not my 'favourite dòg/
     I 'don't know 'what thát is/ -
T   and 'what's erm - 'where does it slêep/
P   erm - 'in hóuse/ . with . bàsket/
     (2 sylls) basket/
     'my da dád/ not màde 'kennel/ . yĕt/ . fór him/ .
     mỳ dad . 'dad 'he 'got [m] - (do) làst wéek/
     'doing . pàinting/ ànd wállpapering/
     [n n] 'not 'got 'much tìme/ do thăt/
     [leɪ] - thìs wéek/ - him . him . wòrking . mórnings/ -
     er . 'when Chrìstmas I míght/ --

This patient's focus on the expression of time relations is well illustrated by these extracts. The vast majority of his sentences involve an element whose function is to specify time of action, and this cuts across clause elements: usually adverbials are involved *(e.g. poorly now)*, but also objects *(e.g. not got much time . . .)* and complements *(e.g. when Christmas . . .)*. This focussing is also reinforced prosodically: clause elements expressing this notion are often given separate tone units, or carry the tonic syllable, often with the effect of producing an abnormal tone-unit structure for the clause, *e.g. poorly/now/, my dad/ not made kennel/ yet/ for him*. Indeed, in the above extract, apart from the incomplete clause, *all* tone units containing a temporal expression place the tonic syllable on that expression.

The contrast between a purely syntactic, as opposed to a syntactic/semantic analysis is also well illustrated by this extract. A straightforward syntactic analysis would show a wide range of clause types, ranging from sentences containing single clause elements *(e.g. in my house)* to those containing five elements *(e.g. my dad not made kennel yet for him)*. It would be difficult to see a clear grammatical pattern in, say a profile analysis of these data *(cf.* p. 101). In LARSP terms, there would be grammatical structures represented from Stages I to V, but very many gaps, and a large number of errors. Looking at the data semantically, however, produces a much clearer picture. If we divide the sentences into those containing a temporal expression and those not containing one, we find in the above data the following distribution (excluding incomplete, unintelligible, and minor sentences):

		No temporal element	Temporal element
Clause	1	4	2
elements	2	7	0
	3		6
	4		5
	5		3

In other words, the length and complexity of P's clause structure is almost entirely a consequence of his use of temporal expression. In real terms *(i.e.* in terms of Subject-Verb "core" structuring ability), P seems to be operating at the two- to three-element stage. His longer sentences may be semantically more specific, as far as time is concerned, but often this is at the expense of the more basic elements of clause structure, which he readily omits, apparently in the interests of getting to and expressing the temporal item.

There are several other semantic functional patterns evident in clinical data. A series of semantic functions may appear in an abnormal sequence, *e.g.* in a sentence a time expression may always occur first, or the agent occur last. Or again, because of poor grammatical expression, it may be unclear what semantic function a particular construction has—a particularly common problem in aphasic speech. In one exchange, T asked P to tell her about a TV programme P had seen the previous evening: P replied: *an ugly man*. The problem with such an utterance is not its syntactic form, nor the comprehension of the lexemes (there *was* an ugly man in the film), but what semantic function the phrase is supposed to have. Is the ugly man the actor of some putative sentence ("the man was doing something"), or the goal of some action ("someone did something to the man"), or is he seen as a causative factor ("something happened on account of his presence"), and so on? If P says nothing further, T must choose one interpretation from this range, in the hope of eliciting more language: she must, in other words, provide the noun phrase with a semantic function, and trust that the interpretation is compatible with P's intentions.

At an opposite extreme, P may produce long strings of grammatical elements, the majority of whose semantic function is unclear, and where there is little clear sequencing, other than a loose associative link. It is important to stress that a gram-matical analysis is often impossible with such data, as it is usually unclear where sen-tence boundaries fall. All we have to go on is the organization imposed by the prosodic structure: the data can be organized as a sequence of prosodic information units, and an analysis made in terms of recurrent semantic patterns, if any. Take the following sequence, from a 60-year-old stroke patient (the whole thing being said fairly calmly, but rapidly and jerkily):

T   did you 'do any hòuse wórk/
P   well nŏrmally/ .
     lèft it/ -
     the pàinting/ .
     the erm the erm dóors/ .
     because I 'will 'last wèek/ .
     er lôoking/ -
     some erm erm wàll páper/
     'very dèar tóo/
     cos I
     sòme of thém/ .
     but Míchael/ -
     mèasure how 'much we 'want/ -
     'work ôut/
     the 'landing and the wáll/
     and 'tell me thên/
     ăctually/
     but er -
T   you 'don't feel you could mĕasure/
P   I . well . 'probably hc còuld dó/ ...

There is often no way of sorting out such strings without external help (*e.g.* from a relative who knows what P is talking about), and in an initial assessment of such patients, it is crucial for T to use topics about which her knowledge is equal to P's (*e.g.* a television programme they have both seen). In the present case, reference to P's wife later produced the gloss that (a) P's son had come to help measure the landing and the wall for wallpaper, (b) they had looked for wallpaper, but not bought any yet—it was very expensive, (c) this visit to the shops meant that P hadn't been able to finish off painting the woodwork last week, but he hoped to next week, and (d) it also meant that he hadn't helped as usual with the housework. Given this informa-tion, it is now possible to begin the process of reconstructing P's intentions. The aim is to see whether there is any semantic pattern *either* in what P is producing, *or* in what he is omitting. Once this is known, T has guidelines for ongoing interpreta-tion, and also an indication of P's processing limits, to which she can relate her own stimuli. As things stand, T in the above dialogue was really "talking blind"—picking out, almost at random, a lexical item from P's string, and constructing a new stimu-lus using it. This technique produced a quite fluent conversation, but one whose topic structure wavered erratically. In attempting structured remediation, such an approach, with P in total control over the way the interaction went, obviously would not suffice. A semantic function labelling of the above extract produces the following:

well normally	TEMPORAL
left it	ACTION+GOAL
the painting	? ACTION
the doors	GOAL
because I will last week	CAUSE+ACTOR+TEMPORAL
looking	ACTION
some wall paper	GOAL
very dear too	ATTRIBUTE+COMMENT
cos I	CAUSE+ACTOR
some of them	QUANTITY
but Michael	CONNECTIVE+ACTOR
measure how much we want	ACTION+GOAL
work out	ACTION
the landing and the wall	GOAL
and tell me then	CONNECTIVE+ACTION+GOAL +TEMPORAL
actually	COMMENT

One stable pattern does seem to emerge: there seems to be a predictable ACTION+ GOAL sequence, though this is sometimes split prosodically. There is much less control over the ACTOR, which is sometimes omitted and sometimes left in isolation; and similarly, other semantic functions are used in an apparently random manner. On the basis of this observation, the possibility of introducing more structured interaction, using verb-object sequences, and gradually involving more sentence structure, suggests itself. It is also apparent that if P is operating at best with a two-element string, then T's stimuli ought themselves to be formally organized into sequences of a comparable order. To take a single example, presumably the stimulus "Who went to the shops to buy some paper?" would be a bad stimulus for this patient, on three counts: it contains five elements (ACTOR, ACTION, LOCATION, ACTION, GOAL), whereas P seems happy to cope with only one or two at a time; it lacks an ACTION-GOAL structure in its main clause, whereas this seems to be P's favourite pattern; and the question focusses on the ACTOR, which is one of P's weak areas. A much better stimulus, for getting P's response under control, would be "What did Michael do?", where the expected response "buy some paper" fits well with our expectations of P's response capabilities. This, at least, is the hypothesis that can be used to guide further work with P. It may be wrong, or too limiting in some way, but it is at least a start, given the lack of any structured guidelines previously.

One of the most important areas for semantic function analysis of this kind is in relation to the variety of patterns that characterize fluent aphasic speech (whether predominantly receptive, or mixed). In such patients, it is unlikely that conventional grammatical analysis will help, in carrying out an assessment, or providing guidelines for T's interaction. Unless P shows production or comprehension limitations clearly explicable in developmental terms, there is little basis for direct grammatical intervention; and in the more fluent kinds of speech, these limitations are not at all evident. On the contrary, a wide range of grammatical patterns may be apparent; and even if certain grammatical gaps do emerge (*e.g.* copula difficulties), we are left with the impression that these are not central to an explanation of the difficulties that P has, or that T has in understanding him. Under such circumstances, T has two possible lines of action, if he wishes to engage in structured therapy: he may still attempt to work grammatically, and build an alternative "dialect" to the one P uses, with the aim of motivating P to use this instead of his problematic speech; or he can try to analyze the speech patterns directly, looking for an explanation in semantic terms. It is with this latter aim that the following section is concerned.

Semantic analysis of this kind of speech will however work only if certain conditions are fulfilled:

(a) a reasonable proportion of the speech must be phonologically intelligible;
(b) T must be able to interpret P's semantic intentions, either from his own knowledge of P (or of the events that P is referring to) or by using an intermediary (as in the example above, where P's spouse provided an interpretation).

These conditions were fulfilled in the following dialogue, taken from a 66-year-old predominantly receptive aphasic man. As with the patient above, the sequence should be read quite quickly, with only the briefest of pauses at the end of each tone unit.

T   'how've you been 'getting òn/
P   yés/
     been 'going alríght/
     lóvely/
     yés/
     thánk you/
T   'had a 'game of gólf since I 'last 'saw you/
P   nó/
     (2 sylls) Sŭnday/
     on ?a Súnday/
     that's ăll/
     nó/ .
     nó/
     ànyway/ 'next Sùnday/ ànyway/
T   nèxt 'Sunday/
P   yēah/
     I (2 sýlls) .
     yés/
T   'why can't you 'play during the wèek/
P   wèll/
     it's -
     it's Mĭke/ .
     it's for the càr/ sée/ .

it's for the car
it's -
it's got 'too far awày sée/
T   oh I sèe/
so your 'son . dríves you/
P   thàt's ríght/
yéah/
T   mhm̀/
P   and the cár/ .
and the and the and the . 'whatsisname and the and . they 'give the .
    whàtsisname you sée/ .
so . other thăn/ . there's no gòod . sée/ .
T   yèah/
P   well it's nò good/ .
will a bús/ get me . clúbs/ and all thát/
(   ) dòn't it/ rĕally/
T   *oh you 'can't get on a bùs/*
do you 'not know any ôther 'people who 'play 'golf/ who could 'play in the
    wèek/
P   nò/
I'm afraid .
I'm afràid not/ rèally not/ -
not 'nobody over 'there with er - with the pĕople/ rĕally/
ôtherwise/ I I'd lìke to/ rĕally/ - ?to gò there/ rĕally/ cos it's it's sēe/
    alrìght/ sée/
T   rathĕr/
P   you knōw/ but er . I mèan/ er . Míke/ and . Éddy/ .
he's at Néwbury/
he 'likes down thére/
and er . that's ìt/ sée/ -
so they 'just got . real .
what's thàt/ .
the 'only thing ìs/ *(3 sylls)* whatsisname *(2 sylls)* whatsisname *(1 syll)* whàtsis-
    name/ - *(2 sylls)*
ōtherwise/ it's 'only for one - Sŭnday/
and they only .
it it
I mean there 'really ìs sée/

This sample satisfies the conditions above: most of the data is intelligible—there are
just a few short stretches of jargon; and T was later able to make a reasonable interpretation of what P was attempting to say, because of her familiarity with P's family
background and habits. It emerged that Mike and Eddy, P's sons, now live at Newbury, and are thus unable to give P a weekly lift to the golf course, which is some way
from where P lives; a bus ride is awkward so P has little chance to play; however, the
next Sunday, the possibility has arisen of Eddy being available to give P a lift.

How, then, can we use this information in order to demonstrate a semantic pattern underlying P's speech. The first thing that must be done is to delete or put on one side those features of the sample which are performance inadequacies almost certainly irrelevant to the analysis, and those which are impossible to analyze, under any circumstances. The aim is to reduce the sample to its nucleus of apparently coherent information. For Ts who have been used to focussing primarily on the jargon, automatic phrasing, and so on of aphasic speech, this may seem to be a radical change of emphasis, but it is an essential one, if progress is to be made in understanding P's semantic system. From the semantic point of view, the automatic speech, etc. is least important.

To arrive at an information nucleus, several decisions must be made:
(1) delete all tone-units containing unintelligible speech, along with any tone-units that seem to depend grammatically upon them;
(2) delete all non-fluencies, *e.g. er*, repetitions of words or word-partials, and incomplete tone-units;
(3) delete all comment clauses, *e.g. you know, I mean*, semantically empty and stereotyped (automatic) speech;
(4) conflate any structural expansions in immediate sequence, retaining the most developed, *e.g. cat—a cat—a big cat came in→a big cat came in;*
(5) mark candidates for sentence status in the residue; this is the "information nucleus" referred to above;
(6) put ambiguous sentences on one side; expand the remainder, using contextual information, so that all unstated semantic functions are made explicit;
(7) analyze (a) the semantic functions expressed, (b) the semantic functions provided by reference to context.

This heuristic can be seen to operate, by taking the final sequence from the above extract, and applying the steps in the order given:

Step (1)

you knōw/ but er . I mèan/ er . Míke/ and . Éddy/ .
he's at Néwbury/
he 'likes down thére/
and er . that's ìt/ sée/ -
so they 'just got . real .
what's thàt/ .
ōtherwise/ it's 'only for one - Sŭnday/
and they only .
it it
I mean there 'really ìs sée/

Step (2)

you knōw/ . I mèan/ . Míke/ and . Éddy/ .
he's at Néwbury/
he 'likes down thére/
and . that's ìt/ sée/ -

what's thàt/ .
ōtherwise/ it's 'only for one - Sŭnday/
I mean there 'really ìs sée/

Step (3)

Míke/ and . Éddy/ .
he's at Néwbury/
he 'likes down thére/
ōtherwise/ it's 'only for one - Sŭnday/

Step (4) does not apply; there are no ambiguous sentences nor are any expansions
needed (Step [6]); and putative sentences (Step [5]) have already been identified by
the transcription (separate lines). We may therefore proceed to an analysis of the
clause structure directly (*PRO* stands for a "pro-form", such as a pronoun):

Míke/ and Éddy/	ACTOR
he's at Néwbury/	PRO-ACTOR+LOCATIVE
he 'likes down thére/	PRO-ACTOR+STATIVE+PRO-LOCATIVE
it's 'only for one Sŭnday/	?PRO+TEMPORAL

The pattern that stands out is that in each sentence there is really only one major
semantic function expressed. The first sentence expresses a specific ACTOR; the
second expresses a specific LOCATION, with the agent being referred to by a pro-
form; the third sentence expresses a specific STATIVE, with both agent and location now covered by pro-forms; and the last sentence expresses a specific TEMPO-
RALITY, with the subject slot unclear semantically, but probably referring to the
action of going to the golf course, and thus a pro-form. P seems limited to a single
specific semantic notion per sentence. To conflate the first three sentences into, say,
Mike and Eddy like living at Newbury, is presumably quite beyond him. A great deal
has been omitted, semantically, between the third and the fourth sentences, and it is
unclear, just from this example, whether this was a random jump, or whether it is
indicative of a specific semantic weakness; but the fourth sentence, like the others,
is restricted to a single specific semantic function.

How far does this hypothesis about P's processing limitations apply to the rest
of the data? Here are the relevant sentences, taken from the above dialogue, using
the above heuristic:

on a Súnday/	it's nò good/
that's ăll/	will a bús/ get me . clúbs/ and all thát/
'next Sùnday/	I'm afràid not/
it's Mĭke/	not 'nobody over 'there with the pĕople/
it's for the càr/	I'd lìke to/ gò there/ cos it's alrĭght/
it's got 'too far awày/	
and the cár/	
there's no gòod/	

The single-unit hypothesis certainly seems supported by this sample. Note how on
the only occasion when he attempts more than one unit (the *bus-clubs* sentence), the
grammatical structure breaks down, and the prosodic structure is abnormal.

What are the implications of this way of proceeding for subsequent remedial work with P? One important point is to note the mismatch, in the above extract, between the level of semantic complexity found in T's stimuli, and P's restricted processing ability, as measured by his ability to express semantic functions using specific lexical items. In terms of the admittedly crude measure of number of semantic functions expressed, it is plain that there are considerable differences. Here are T's stimuli (excluding her opening, phatic question, and minor sentences):

1 had a game of golf since I last saw you	STATIVE+GOAL+TEMPORAL: AGENT+ACTION+TEMPORAL+ GOAL
2 next Sunday	TEMPORAL
3 why can't you play during the week	CAUSE+ACTOR+ACTION+ TEMPORAL
4 so your son drives you	CONNECTIVE+ACTOR+ACTION+ GOAL
5 do you not know any other people who play golf who could play in the week	ACTOR+STATIVE+GOAL: ACTION+GOAL: ACTION+ TEMPORAL

Over and above the various grammatical constructions used (question forms, tenses, pronominals, etc.), T's stimuli regularly involve five or six semantic functions—a pattern which continues throughout the conversational part of the data. Regardless of P's comprehension ability, if he is expected to respond to such stimuli, and if he is, in effect, limited to single semantic functions in order to do so, it is likely that the complexity of such stimuli will itself be a source of the confusion. The extract above provides some support for this view. In the table below, we see, first, the stimulus complexity of each sentence, in terms of number of semantic functions T uses; then the number of processing units in P's response, measured in terms of the number of whole or incomplete tone units (but ignoring any obvious non-fluency); and then the number of "empty" whole or partial tone-units, as identified by the above procedure:

		T's semantic functions	P's tone-units or incompletes	P's "empty" tone-units
	1	8	9	4
	2	1	3	2
	3	4	8	5
Stimulus	4	2	2	0
no.	5	0	5	3 (plus non-
	6	0	6	3 fluency)
	7	7	13	8
	8	0	17	12

The correlation is suggestive (though, without much more data analysis, not yet convincing): the worst P responses are those where T produces stimuli of greatest semantic complexity, or where no semantically specific stimulus at all is provided. The best example above is where T gives a stimulus just one unit more complex than the level at which P seems to be functioning (*cf.* Stimulus no. 4).

This is only the beginning of a semantic analysis of P's output: it is based solely on a length index, and as we have seen, length by itself is of only limited value. It could indeed at times be positively misleading, *e.g.* Wells (1974: 263) shows that in acquisition, clauses which appear relatively early often contain more elements than those appearing later, *e.g.* directional locative clauses with agent expressed (such as "X put Y on Z") turn up quite early in his data, whereas agent function clauses (such as "X sang") turn up quite late—but the former tend to have four semantic units, whereas the latter may have only two. In other words, analysis should now proceed to take into account the semantic *type* of units which P prefers to respond to, or tends to omit, *e.g.* whether he has more problems with units expressing actions, goals, times, or whatever. "Deeper" semantic analyses, less obviously related to the surface syntactic structure of the clause, might be made. But some illustration of these issues has already been given. Before remediation could proceed in a fully systematic way, moreover, some kind of acquisitional framework would need to be provided—a possibility which we must now consider.

Semantic Acquisition

Having outlined the main theoretical and descriptive conclusions of structural semantics, and illustrated their application, we may now move on to the question of how this information should be graded, in order to provide the basis for an assessment and remediation procedure. It is here that the research clinician faces considerable difficulties, given that semantic studies of language acquisition have been ongoing for little more than a decade, and that the focus of attention has been on constructing theoretical models of acquisition and not on the descriptive application of these models. There is a marked shortage of facts, compared with the other levels of linguistic description. Nor is the situation likely to improve in the immediate future. Semantics, unlike grammar and phonology, is a subject about which descriptive generalizations are difficult to make. There are, after all, only 40 or so phonemes in English, and a reasonably small sample will provide the basis for an analysis which will have considerable generality. The several hundred grammatical constructions that make up English can also be discussed generally, with reference to fairly small samples of data. But the language's lexicon is so large (approaching a million lexemes, according to recent dictionaries) that it becomes much more difficult to see general patterns of organization and acquisition, and very large samples will be required before the general applicability of a research finding can be demonstrated. For example, we may take a corner of the lexicon, such as Andersen (1975) did in her study of the way children acquire the distinction between *cups* and *glasses,* and draw certain general conclusions about the kinds of semantic discrimination being gradually introduced by the children. One conclusion, for example, was that the primary perceptual properties of size, shape and material formed an important stage in acquiring the distinction, with reference to such features as handle, stem, glass, paper and breakability. But whether these properties, or features, are equally relevant for other areas of the lexicon at similar ages, remains to be shown. Would a study of children's discriminations in furniture show similar patterns? or in cutlery? or in other containers? The descriptive task is enormous, and it is for this reason that semantic scales of any detail have not been constructed.

What does this mean, in real clinical terms? It means that we are unlikely to see a semantic assessment or remedial procedure developed in the immediate future. Lack of descriptive detail means that two of the cardinal criteria for developing such procedures would not be met: they would lack comprehensiveness, and they would lack discrimination. Even if all the descriptive information in the child language literature were brought together and graded along the lines of, say, LARSP, there would be insufficient material to make a discerning and fruitful assessment. There would be no guarantee that the lexemes and lexemic structures referenced on the semantic chart would be those in use by the patient population, and, more seriously, there would be no way of guaranteeing that the lexicon referenced would relate to those semantic areas which cause greatest difficulty for the patient, in his learning (or relearning) of the semantic system. A great deal of the cogency of procedures like LARSP is the way they draw a clear dividing-line between those structures which are felt to be clinically important, as far as differential diagnosis is concerned, and those which are not (grouped in LARSP under the heading of "Other"). It would be very difficult to motivate a distinction between clinically important lexicon and "other lexicon", in the present state of knowledge.

Does this mean, then, that there is nothing that can be said, developmentally, about the semantics of a language? By no means. Several important trends in semantic acquisition have been quite thoroughly investigated, and while the findings may lack the descriptive generality referred to above, the theoretical implications for clinical work are considerable. At least if we are aware of the *kind* of thing that is going on, semantically, at a given age range, or at a certain point in linguistic development, it can provide a guideline for looking generally at P's vocabulary, and can sensitize us to the range of difficulties likely to be encountered in remedial work. What general pointers of this kind have been established?

There are two main research paradigms in semantic acquisition, reflecting the theoretical distinction between lexical and grammatical meaning.

Lexical Patterns

Lexical acquisition studies aim to establish the developing patterns in the size, type and structure of a child's vocabulary. Several typological steps have been proposed by different authors[34], and while there are many differences in method of analysis

---

[34] See Nelson (1973, 1974), Clark (1973), Bloom (1973), Anglin (1977), Bloom and Lahey (1978: Ch. 4). Summaries may be found in Clark and Clark (1977: Ch. 13) and Fletcher and Garman (1979: Chs. 8, 9).

and terminology, it is possible to see important parallels. It is these which are here summarized, beginning with the lexicon typical of the earliest period.

(1) Social lexemes: lexemes that are learned as part of social routines, and which have no semantic productivity outside of those routines, *e.g. hi, bye, ta, night-night.* Other labels for these items include "personal-social" and "expressive".

(2) Relational lexemes: lexemes which identify the relation of an object to itself or to other objects of the same class ("reflexive" lexemes), *e.g. more, gone, there, again.* From the viewpoint of the child's "here and now", the main factors are the object's existence, appearance, disappearance, reappearance, recurrence, and other such states. The role of perceptual change of state and movement at this stage is held to be of particular importance in the cognitive development of the child; and lexemes associated with such development thus constitute a large proportion of the early lexicon. They can be grouped into several basic classes, relatable to the growth in the child's cognitive awareness. Bloom, for example, suggests a developmental sequence for four major semantic classes: (a) existence of an object in the child's context (also referred to as nomination [Brown, 1973]), *e.g. that, this, there;* (b) non-existence, or non-occurrence of an object which the child expects to be present in the context, *e.g. no, gone,* or a high rising tone on a specific lexeme, *e.g.* ↑*dáda;* (c) disappearance of an object from the context, or cessation of some activity, *e.g. all-gone, bye, no;* (d) recurrence (either reappearance, or other instances of the same object), *e.g. more, again.* It should be noted that a lexeme may be assigned to different classes, depending on the context and behaviour of the child: as Bloom (1973) has pointed out, a lexeme such as *no* may have several interpretations. And while it is sometimes extremely difficult to be sure from context and behaviour which interpretation is the correct one (often impossible), there are a sufficient number of clear cases documented to demonstrate the important role that context has in the development of early lexical meaning. From a clinical point of view, this stage is a significant one, as it marks a stage of context-dependence, which many patients find difficult to leave. Items such as *there, this* and *more* are "easy" lexemes, in the sense that they avoid P having to use semantically more specific lexemes: examples are given on p. 121.

(3) Specific lexemes: lexemes which have a direct labelling or categorizing function with reference to the objects, events, states of affairs, etc., in the external or mental world, *e.g. boy, car, black, run, know.* It is here that the open-endedness of the lexicon is apparent; social and relational lexemes are relatively few in number. Several semantic types of lexemes have been distinguished within this enormous field: (a) Everyone recognizes the importance of a major class of *substantive* (also called *referential* or *object*) lexemes, in which objects in the external world (or their conceptual representations) are identified and gradually distinguished from each other. While in theory it is possible to establish this semantic class independently of grammar, in practice grammatical criteria invariably influence decisions—hence, the members of this class will be nouns, certain noun phrases *(e.g. puss in boots),* and noun-like items *(e.g. the rich, the Chinese).* The class also includes higher-order lexemes, such as *animal, vehicle* and abstractions relatable to object properties, such as *beauty, time, history.* The notion of "object" is thus viewed as a point of departure, and not as a limitation to physical entities only.

(b) *Activity* lexemes constitute a second major class. In the first instance, these refer to the observable events and actions of the external world, *e.g. run, move, go,* and the term *dynamic* is sometimes used to characterize the sub-class. But the class also covers activities where there is no immediate external action observable, *e.g. know, hear, be,* and here the term *static* is often used for the sub-class[35]. Grammatical influence is apparent here too, in that activity lexemes will be seen as verbs and verb-like items *(e.g. be born).*

(c) *Attribute* lexemes constitute a third major class. The tradition here is to restrict this class to the properties of substantives, *e.g. big, white, clean, expensive.* Not only adjectives are involved, however: many attributes are expressed using prepositional phrases, such as *a house of brick, man in a suit.* It would also be possible, in theory, to extend the class to include properties of activities, but for present purposes these are covered separately below.

(d) *Scope* lexemes are here recognized as a major class, though this is not normal practice in the semantic acquisition literature. The term relates primarily to two semantic notions that *are* widely recognized in this literature, however: lexemes used as part of the expression of *location* and *time*—sometimes summarized in the single phrase, *spatio-temporal location.* From a grammatical point of view, it is the class of adverbials that is primarily involved, and we are thus dealing with properties of activities, *e.g. something happened in the garden, yesterday.* There is sometimes ambiguity in deciding whether a lexeme is a property of an activity or a substantive (*cf.* [c] above), as when a phrase could equally well be assigned to some preceding noun or verb, *e.g. the boy went to bed hungry;* but on the whole there is no difficulty. The class must also be extended, though, to include the whole range of semantic functions carried by adverbials, such as manner, *e.g. quickly, in a hurry.*

(e) *Proper names,* often included under the substantive heading, are here classified separately, on the grounds that they are basically ostensive items, incapable of generalization, and lacking the kind of structural relationships typical of the rest of the lexicon, such as class membership, *e.g. London, Jim Smith, Mummy* have referential identities, but are not members of classes.

This classification is admittedly crude, and would be of limited value if it were applied to the study of the normal adult vocabulary; but in clinical contexts, where we are dealing with a limited lexicon, broad divisions of this kind can be very useful, as part of a semantic screening procedure. It must be recognized, however, that there will always be a large category of "problems" in carrying out such analyses, especially when the lack of grammatical or clear non-linguistic context makes it impossible to say whether a lexeme is being used as a substantive, activity or property. For instance, the lexeme *sore* referring to a picture of a boy with a wounded knee could be substantive or attribute—or even (in the mind of the child) activity or scope. The less developed the patient's language, the more difficult it will be to make decisions of this kind. But simply calling the linguistic situation indeterminate does not eliminate the problem for the clinician: therapy has to proceed and

---

[35] Some lexemes may of course be used in both a static and a dynamic interpretation. *Cf.* Quirk *et al.* (1972: Ch. 3), though their purpose is to identify the grammatical constraints operating upon verbs, and not to provide a semantic classification in its own right.

interpretations have to be made; analyses have to be assigned to the lexemes, given the available evidence and the expectations of the clinician. And while the clinician can often never know whether the correct interpretation has been made, at least by providing plausible interpretations from her point of view, she is giving P targets which in due course may influence his developing skills. But the clinician must always be aware, just as much as the language acquisition scholar, of the dangers of reading in normal adult values to the emerging or re-emerging lexicon of the patient.

Semantic Field Emergence

How far is it possible to plot the emergence of semantic fields in children? The difficulty here is that children's social situations vary so much, from family to family, and from one time (of day/year) to another, that generalizations are impossible without enormous samples—and these have not been made. Studies of the vocabulary of even the first 50 or 100 lexemes of children show quite marked differences. However, with more samples coming to be analyzed[36], the importance of certain fields is becoming clearer. Chief amongst these are food and drink, body-parts (facial terms earliest), clothing, animals, vehicles, living routines, body functions, household items, and people. Factors which seem to promote the learning of lexemes within these fields include the importance of the immediate environment of the child (the so-called "here and now"); his awareness of movement (of people, other animates, and of entities that move), of actions and the results of actions; and his awareness of location, recipients, and instruments (*i.e.* objects which facilitate the performance of an action).

How do children learn semantic fields? The point has received little attention, but it seems likely that they are the result of a mixture of constraints, some cognitive (the developing perceptual abilities of the child), some social (the repetitive nature of activity in the home), and some personal (individual characteristics of the child and his family). Parents are extremely selective in their use of lexemes to their children, but they are not random. Using only one of the basic "felicity conditions" for conversation (see p. 201), that utterances address a single theme (unless the speaker indicates to the contrary), all the child need assume is that the sequence of lexemes his parent produces on a specific occasion are all related in some way. Not all the lexemes in the sequence will belong to the same semantic field, of course, but a fair number will be, as the following monologue illustrates. The mother is washing dishes, just after the father has left for work; her 18-month-old child is playing on the floor, and says *dada gone;* mother replies: (with fairly long pauses between each sentence) "yes, daddy's gone; he's gone to work; he'll be back later; see him at tea-time; he's gone in his car, hasn't he; you like going in cars, don't you ..." It would not take much exposure to this kind of input to enable the child to build up quite an

---

[36] See Nelson (1973), Chambers and Tavuchis (1976), Cruse (1977), Andersen (1978), Clark (1979), Rescorla (1981), and, for an early review, Nice (1915).

extensive comprehension lexicon for the "routine" of home and work. But exactly what strategies parents use is unclear. An important aspect of this question would be to discover how parents introduce the different levels of categorization within a taxonomy, *e.g.* referring to a range of entities as "types of animal" or "types of drink". Do they opt for a particular "generic" level of categorization, as has been suggested[37]? For example, the entity sleeping in front of the fire could be labelled "animal", "dog", "labrador", or given an attribute, such as "big dog". How does the parent introduce these taxonomic levels, and interrelate them? To a child, the term "dog" would be the most appropriate one to use, in a picture naming task; to an adult, this could be too "obvious", and the likelihood would be that a more specific term would be used. If there are norms, they could be extremely useful, in remedial work.

From the clinical point of view, given the selectivity of the acquisition studies, and their concentration on the earliest months of lexical emergence, any attempt at applying the notion of semantic fields has to take into account criteria of a logical kind (*cf.* the logical classifications of the lexicon referred to on p. 144). It is not possible to construct a framework for lexical organization on purely developmental lines. Semantic profiles have to be primarily constrained by adult cognitive distinctions, but there is no reason why they should not be influenced by our expectations about cognitive development in children, and by what is known so far about lexical development. As an exercise, such frameworks are certainly worth constructing, despite their tentativeness: they have the merit of bringing out into the open the kinds of assumptions we have about vocabulary, and the arbitrary divisions we tend to work with[38]. Only by doing this kind of thing do we come to realize that, for example, there is little point in postulating a semantic field of "toys" for the young child (as is often done): cognitively there may be, in the sense of "things to play with"—but as almost anything can be played with, the range of lexemes that could be classed as "toys" (including *wool, spoons, dirt*) becomes impossibly large. Likewise at an older age, we may think, entering a toy shop, that it contains items whose lexemes constitute a semantic field; but in fact the lexemes in question are *soldiers, cars, bricks,* and the like, which belong to their own semantic fields, and where the function as toys is derivative.

Semantic Mismatch

The lexemes referred to so far have been discussed in terms of their normal adult semantic values; but the process of acquiring these values is not a simple one. There are several kinds and degrees of approximation to the adult norm, or target, as lexical items come to be used[39]. Three processes in particular have been identified:

(a) *underextension,* in which the child's use of a lexeme is to a narrower range of referents than the corresponding adult use, *e.g. bus* being used for red buses only.

---

[37] See Berlin, Breedlove and Raven (1973); also Anglin (1977), Clark (1979).

[38] One such framework is illustrated in Crystal (1982).

[39] See Bloom and Lahey (1978: 116 ff.), Clark (1974), Anglin (1977), Reich (1976).

From the point of view of comprehension, such narrowings are fairly easy to observe: given a red bus and some other bus, for instance, and asked to identify a bus, only the red one will be selected. From the point of view of production, however, underextension is difficult to observe, as the child's use of the term *bus* for the red bus is of course correct. It is always a problem deciding whether a child's lack of use of a lexeme is because of his lack of knowledge of the lexeme's application, or a lack of initiative or incentive to use it.

(b) *overextension*, in which the child's use of a lexeme is to a wider range of referents than the corresponding adult use, *e.g. bus* being used for cars, buses and trains. This category, unlike (a) above, is easy to spot in productive language use: obviously, to label a train a *bus* will be immediately apparent. It is more of a problem deciding whether a similar process of overextension affects the child's comprehension ability[40]. Two main types of growth in overextension patterns have been noted. Firstly, there are the so-called "chain" associations, in which a lexeme comes to be used in a succession of situations, each pair of situations being linked by a common (but semantically unsystematic) feature, *e.g. drink* might be used first for milk, then for milk-bottles, then for a milkman, then for his milkfloat, and then for cars in general. Secondly, there are semantically more principled associations (sometimes called "holistic" associations) in which the lexeme is applied to new situations on the basis of some perceived similarity in form or in function between the situations (see below), *e.g.* the *bus* example above, or the use of *dog* for other types of animal.

(c) *no overlap*, in which the child's use of a lexeme bears no relationship at all to the adult's use, *e.g. car* being used for a toothbrush. Insofar as the context of use is clear, such a mislabelling will be immediately noticed; but often in connected speech, it will not, *e.g.* a child sitting near a window and mislabelling his shoe as *car* will almost certainly be misinterpreted by his mother as having seen a car outside. (Such cases might of course be seen as cases of overextension, in which the "natural history" has been unobserved.)

It is not clear how much of the young child's vocabulary varies in its extension in the above ways: certain lexemes (*e.g.* vehicles, letters) seem to overextend more readily than others, for example (see Rescorla, 1980). Also, while it is fairly obvious why children should start to vary the extension of lexemes (a process of trial and error as they apply lexemes to an increasingly varied range of situations, learning which extensions will be acceptable and which will not), it is not so obvious when or how they come to stop extending lexemes in this way. To some extent, of course, this trial and error strategy is always with us: many new lexemes which adults learn involve decisions about extension similar to those a young child must use (*e.g.* we might use the term *beetle* to apply to all horrid wriggly things until we are told off by a coleopterist for doing so). It is the scope and frequency of the extensional changes in vocabulary between the ages of about $1\frac{1}{2}$ and 3 which is so striking, and which has attracted analysts' attention. The processes involved are evidently extremely important as aids to lexical learning, and must be taken as indices of development,

---

[40] See the discussion in Thomson and Chapman (1977), Fremgen and Fay (1980).

12*

rather than simply as "errors". From a clinical point of view, accordingly, the development of over-extension patterns (especially of the holistic kind) can be seen as a positive sign, on which it will be possible to build; the continuance of underextension or no overlap patterns will likewise be an important aspect of assessment. The study of no overlap patterns is particularly important in working with aphasics, where the search for system in the misidentifications patients make is a primary analytic goal (see below).

Semantic Features

The use of the semantic feature model as an explanatory principle in lexical acquisition has led to some illuminating observations. Two main categories of features have been recognized: the physical attributes of objects, and the functions of objects[41]. Under the first heading, the importance of shape to the young child as a means of grouping and distinguishing objects has been stressed, but other properties have also been identified as performing important roles in lexical development, especially texture, size, sound and taste. Not all properties seem to be important early on, *e.g.* smell and colour are little used as a basis of differentiation. Under the second heading, the importance of movement is crucial, as children come to identify how and where things move, who is affected by movement, and what limitations there are on the movements of objects (what can be rolled, thrown, picked up, etc.)[42]. Other functional differences can be illustrated by contrasting *dog* and *cow:* over and above their physical differences, there are such functional notions as where they live, whether one plays with them, whether one obtains food from them, etc. Both formal and functional notions are part of the full definition of a lexeme: the classical definitional form "An X is a Y that does/has Z" illustrates the complementarity of the two, *e.g.* "A chair is a piece of furniture with legs (etc.) that you sit on (etc.)"[43].

In language acquisition studies, semantic features have been useful in the way they can explain the process of holistic overextension—the child focussing on a certain feature and using that as the main test of whether a lexeme should be used (*e.g.* for one child it may be the four-legs-ness of the dog that motivates its application to cat and horse; in another case it might be size alone, in which case there might be an extension to cat, but not to horse; in a third case it might be texture; and so on). The possibility that there might be a developmental ordering of features, so that certain types of formal or functional feature might be developmentally prior, has been a major theme of research. According to the "Semantic Feature Hypothesis" (E. Clark, 1973), children learn the adult meanings of lexemes by acquiring the semantic features of the lexemes in a fixed order, starting with the more general features and

---

[41] See E. Clark (1973), Nelson (1974).

[42] See Bloom, Lightbown and Hood (1975), Bloom and Lahey (1978: 134).

[43] The acquisition of definitional form and function is discussed by Litowitz (1977) and Wehren, De Lisi and Arnold (1981).

later learning the more specific. Lexemes which share semantic features are acquired in order depending on the number and type of features needed to define them. Several small semantic fields have been investigated from this point of view, and orders of emergence postulated (*e.g.* for dimensional terms, such as *big, small,* and for kinship terms, such as *father, brother, cousin*)[44]. Certain tendencies have been observed, but because of the methodological difficulties of carrying out this research, and the limited lexical range to which these notions have been applied, results are of limited generalisability. It would not be possible, in the present state of knowledge, to propose a general ordering of semantic features which could be directly applied to clinical analysis. All we can reasonably do is take some of the experimental observations as guidelines along which to work (rather than as a framework within which to work). If we happen to be working on size adjectives, or kinship terms for example, it would be worthwhile bearing in mind the developmental trends observed. Similarly, some of the theoretical notions propounded have considerable relevance, *e.g.* the notion of marked vs. unmarked terms (*cf.* p. 151), where it has been argued that children will first learn the linguistically unmarked term, the marked term being initially interpreted as if it had the meaning of the unmarked term (*e.g. long* will be learned first, and *short* will, in its early use, be interpreted as having the meaning "long"). The hypothesis is a controversial one, as far as language acquisition is concerned, but it is at least agreed that it is worth investigating. Likewise, in clinical language studies, which also suffer from a dearth of hypotheses to search for organization in the lexicon, the idea could be illuminating. At the very least, there is a great deal to be gained by keeping the feature model in mind, as we look at patient data: it is usually possible to notice if a particular feature is facilitating for a patient, or of particular difficulty, in his acquisition of vocabulary; and idiosyncratic classifications of lexemes also occur, on the basis of an unexpected or eccentric component of meaning.

Semantic Fuzziness

One reason for the limited applicability of the semantic feature approach is that there are several areas of the lexicon where it is not possible to identify clear-cut components of meaning, or to group them into binary contrasts. Alternative models to handle this kind of indeterminancy have been slow to develop. One important notion which emerged in the 1970s is that of "prototypical" meaning[45]. An instance of a specific class—say, a particular car—is said to be identified as such in terms of how close it is to an internalized representation of "car-ness" in our memory. This internal representation has developed (it is argued) as the result of our assimilating many examples of cars and car-like entities, from which we have

---

[44] For the former, see Eilers, Oller and Ellington (1974), Bartlett (1976); for the latter, Haviland and Clark (1974), Chambers and Tavuchis (1976).

[45] See Rosch (1973), Rosch and Lloyd (1978), Anglin (1977). For the relevant cognitive psychological support, see, *e.g.* Posner (1973), Reed (1972).

refined a "core" meaning, and an inventory of criterial distinctive features. Any new instance of a car-like entity can then be evaluated against this prototype of car, and judged to be a clear case or a marginal case, in terms of how many features it shares with the prototype. How this takes place, from an acquisitional point of view, is quite unclear, but there is certainly some evidence that children learn first to identify instances which adults would consider to be central rather than marginal instances of a class. And the clinical relevance of the notion is evident: in assessing comprehension, for example, we would want to present patients with instances which were the best possible exemplars of their class, if we hope to elicit the lexemes, and be aware of the increasing difficulty which would come as less central instances were presented. Clinical interaction is full of examples of the way marginal instances turn up and interfere with therapy. Asked to point to a shop, in a high street picture, one P pointed to a pub, to which T replied "well, yes, but it's not *really* a shop, is it? it's a *sort of* shop, but it's not the kind of place where you'd usually do your shopping, is it? show me a shop like the ones you usually go to". P then pointed to a building that looked suspiciously like a betting-shop! The example illustrates the way in which T's prototype of shop—at least for the purposes of the session—was "place for making domestic purchases". P might have agreed; but it is also possible that he was working with a different prototype of shop, *e.g.* "place where you can buy something", or "building in the centre of a town". The importance of lexemes such as *very, quite, sort of, kind of,* and the like has been much underestimated in T-P interaction, and has only recently begun to be looked at in acquisitional or normal adult terms[46].

There are many other ways in which semantic analysis becomes fuzzy. One obvious way is if there is no lexeme commonly available in the language for an entity, activity or attribute. We tend to underestimate, in fact, how many things in the world we are *unable* to talk about using single lexemes, and have to resort to circumlocutions, vague modifiers (*cf.* above) and empty fillers (such as "sort of thing",

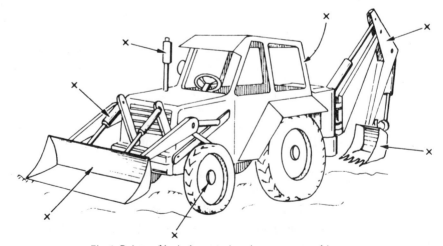

Fig. 1. Points of lexical uncertainty in a common object

46 See, for example, Berndt and Caramazza (1978), Crystal and Davy (1975).

"whatsit"). Picking up any simple (sic) toy in a clinic will illustrate the difficulty. What does one reply when P asks "What's that called?", pointing to the points marked X on the bulldozer in Fig. 1? There may be technical terms for these notions, but (a) we will probably not know them, and (b) if we did, we would jib at introducing them to P. To provide an approximation, using some lexeme that seems vaguely appropriate, is what usually happens—but an ad hoc answer of this kind may be confusing (especially if P, later, obtains a different ad hoc answer from someone else).

Lexeme Relations

Developmental norms dealing with the learning of the various categories of lexemic relation described earlier in this Chapter (p. 147) are almost totally lacking. Hyponymy has sometimes been discussed with reference to the general problem of cognitive categorization, but not usually distinguished clearly from it. Certain types of opposite have been used as part of the investigation of the semantic feature hypothesis, but only for limited semantic fields. There are obviously major research initiatives needed here, as well as with reference to synonymy and incompatibility, in order to provide a developmental perspective for handling this problem clinically. In the absence of such a perspective, we have to apply sense relations in an ad hoc way, as soon as P's lexical inventory is large enough to suggest that an analysis on the basis of primitive semantic fields would be fruitful. Having an inventory of the various possibilities is useful, in carrying out an assessment; but the lack of a developmental dimension makes the exercise of limited value.

A similar point applies to syntagmatic lexical relations. Here, various general observations can be made, but they are too general to be of much help in individual analyses. For example, there is evidence to show that early on in lexical development, children use items of very low collocational predictability, *e.g. see, get, make, put, do, go* are among the first verbs to be frequently used, whereas *hit, jump, run, eat* are later. Apart from any cognitive considerations, the former verbs are semantically extremely non-specific—almost anything can be "seen", "got", "done", "put", etc. The latter verbs are much more specific: there is a limited range of lexemes that can eat or be eaten, jump or be jumped over, etc. Often, we may express the same meaning using either the specific verb or a circumlocution involving an empty verb, *e.g. make go* for *start*, and this is an avoidance strategy which many patients use, as the p. 124 example illustrates. Later, more restricted collocational sequences emerge, and children begin to produce metaphorical and other patterns[47]. But in all of this there is a total lack of the detailed descriptive data which is prerequisite for assessment or remedial work. Here, too, therefore, all that can be done is to bear in mind the logical possibilities presented by the theory, and investigate apparent difficulties in an ad hoc way.

---

[47] See Winner (1979), Gardner (1974), Gardner, Kircher, Winner and Perkins (1975).

Sentential Functions

Attempts to identify an order of emergence for the semantic functions operating within sentence structure (*cf.* p. 161) have been a major focus of attention in the 1970s[48]. The findings are not easy to summarize, unfortunately, because of several differences in terminology and analytical criteria; also, with samples still relatively small, individual differences loom large. But certain notions recur. After an initially unstructured stage, in which lexemes come to be juxtaposed within prosodic contours (*cf.* p. 69), it is suggested that abstract semantic functions develop, to which individual lexemes are assigned. An early pattern is to use a specific lexeme along with a relational lexeme, which may be a simple demonstrative or other deictic, *e.g. that mummy, more drink.* Activity relations are the first major class to emerge, in the form of action+actor (*e.g. daddy go*) and action+goal (*e.g. push daddy*) combinations. There is evidence to suggest that dynamic precedes static, within the activity category (*e.g. fall, go,* etc. before *want, see,* etc.). Locative relations are the next major class to emerge, being used along with both actors and goals (*e.g. daddy there, ball there*) and actions (*e.g. jump there*). There is some evidence to suggest that dynamic locatives precede static locatives (*e.g. go in box* before *see in box*). An actor+goal relationship is also found (*e.g. man ball,* for the man kicking a ball), as is the experiencer+goal (*e.g. daddy happy*) and experiencer+action (*e.g. daddy see*) relationships. Several attributive relationships also emerge during this period, though their sequence of emergence is unclear (*e.g. big house, daddy beard, my car*). Much later, a further set of relationships appear, including benefactive (*e.g. give daddy*) and instrumental (*e.g. write pencil*). By this time, more complex 3-element combinations of functions have begun to appear, *e.g.* actor+action+goal (*daddy kick ball*), actor+action+location (*daddy go garden*), actor+action+benefactive (*daddy give man*). In each case, the elements in question may appear in grammatically "fuller" forms, *e.g. daddy is kicking the ball,* according to the language's norms for grammatical development. Lastly, the canonical four-element clause structure develops, in such structures as actor+action+goal+location (*e.g. daddy kicked the ball into the bushes*), actor+action+goal+benefactive (*e.g. daddy gave a letter to the man*). The whole process takes about a year to become established, from around 18 months until 2½, on average.

Other semantic generalizations have been made about this period. For example, Wells suggests that the earlier two-element structures encode relations about the outside world, whereas the later structures encode relations concerning inner states and perception. Bloom makes much of the way in which dynamic relations precede static ones. Some have tried to trace the antecedents of the above relations in the single element stage of speech production, relying on non-verbal information in the context to support their interpretations (*e.g.* Greenfield and Smith, 1976). There have also been attempts to take the semantic approach a stage further, to incorporate the patterns of clause sequencing which emerge late in the second

---

[48] See Brown (1973), Bowerman (1973), Wells (1974), Bloom, Lightbown and Hood (1975), Greenfield and Smith (1976), Bloom and Lahey (1978: Ch. 4), Macrae (1979). For a critique, see Howe (1976) and the further discussion in *Journal of Child Language*, 8. 2. (1981).

year, beginning with the unspecified coordinating role of *and*, and continuing with more specific functions (such as temporal and causal), using *and* and other conjunctions (especially *because, when, what* and *so*)[49]. And certain general semantic strategies have been repeatedly noticed, such as the way in which acquisition is facilitated if order-of-mention is preserved *(i.e.* the order of events taking place in the world is paralleled by the sequence of linguistic units referring to them, *e.g. the cat bit the dog*, as opposed to *the dog was bitten by the cat*, or *after he knocked, he went in* vs. *he went in after he knocked)*[50].

Given the limited empirical findings, it would be difficult to draw up a scale of semantic development which would show patterns of delay or deviance in the emergence of semantic functions. The provision of such a scale should certainly be an aim of future research. But evidence is plain that there is little point in studying lexical emergence in the early years without some reference being made to these functions. To know that a child has used the word *man*, for example, is to know very little; what is more important is to see the semantic role he attaches to this lexeme— whether he is using the lexeme as actor, goal, recipient, or whatever. The developmental studies seem to show that there is no automatic use of a lexeme in all possible semantic functions in the clause; on the contrary, there is no guarantee that just because a lexeme has been used in, say, actor function, that it will emerge as confidently in, say, goal or locative function. Even without the descriptive details, this principle is an important guideline for clinical practice. In teaching a lexeme, there is more to be done than to teach the meaning of the lexeme, as defined in terms of its reference, sense relations, features, etc.: we must also teach its semantic function in clause structure. A patient who has been taught to use such sentences as *the horse kicked the man* may be unable to use sentences such as *the man kicked the horse*, even though he apparently knows the meaning of each individual lexeme in the sentence. But to establish the way in which such limitations operate in language acquisition will require an understanding of the interface between grammatical and semantic structure that at present theoretical linguistics has been unable to elucidate[51].

Types of Semantic Disability

It would certainly be premature to attempt to discuss this topic in terms of semantic "symptoms" or "diagnosis". All that has been done above is to suggest a set of methods which can identify semantic difficulties or abnormalities encountered in clinical situations. Several different kinds of pattern seem to emerge, but it is by no means clear how applicable all the linguistic distinctions are, how exhaustive a classification could be established on the basis of these examples, or how easy it will be

---

[49] See Bloom, Lahey, Hood, Lifter and Fiess (1980).
[50] See Clark (1971), Hatch (1971), French and Brown (1977), Coker (1978).
[51] For an example of the interaction between grammatical and semantic variables in an area of considerable clinical importance, we may refer to the development of question forms, p. 103.

to relate the linguistic symptomatology to medical conditions. The following classification is, accordingly, proposed in the spirit of exploration rather than of presenting a solution.

Two broad types of semantic disability are suggested: *lexical* and *sentential.*
Within each category, the standard distinctions between delay and deviance, and
comprehension and production, are recognized.

Lexical Delay

In the present state of knowledge, only gross patterns of delay can be isolated:
(i) patients whose vocabulary is largely or wholly composed of social/relational/
stereotyped lexemes, or who lack specific lexemes; (ii) patients who, within the area
of specific lexemes, show inability to use the later semantic fields; (iii) patients who
continue to under-extend or over-extend vocabulary beyond the developmental
peak period; (iv) patients who are unable to use the more advanced semantic feature
contrasts to develop and extend their vocabulary; (v) patients who fail to develop
sense relations, *e.g.* hyponymy, opposites; (vi) patients who fail to develop the expected range of collocational relations. The clearest cases of semantic delay would
be children whose lexicon, in terms of number of lexemes, lexeme meaning and
interrelationship, was a replica of their juniors. As usual with the notion of delay,
however, such clear cases may not exist; instead, we more regularly encounter
"unbalanced" delays, in which these variables are used to different levels of
maturity, and where deviant patterns intervene. The possibility of different delay
patterns in comprehension and production must also be recognized[52].

Lexical Deviance

Given the lack of developmental detail, it is often very difficult to be sure whether
an abnormal lexical use in a patient is an instance of lexical delay or something
which would be outside the path of normal lexical development. For example, any
of the paradigmatic sense relations could "go wrong", in that pairs of lexemes could
be interrelated in unacceptable ways, *e.g.* lexemes taken as synonyms when in fact
they are not; assigning a lexeme to the wrong superordinate term; treating two
lexemes as antonyms, when in fact they are not. On first encounter with such problems, they inevitably strike one as deviant usages, but it may be that systematic
observation will show that they are features of normal development. For example,

---

[52] See Goldin-Meadow, Seligman and Gelman (1976), Benedict (1979). Average number of (different) lexemes in production are: 10 by 1:2, 50 by 1:6, 100 by 1:7, 200 by 1:9, and 300 by 2:0. However, in the
early period, the ratio of number of lexemes comprehended to number produced is about 5:1, with often a gap of several months between comprehension and production. On average, comprehension development moves at the rate of just over 20 new lexemes per month; production just under 10 per
month. The distinction becomes much less important after age 2.

using a circumlocution instead of a synonym, in response to a "What's another name for...?" question may be a quite normal response, for certain areas of the lexicon. Or again, "What's the opposite of ...?" may produce unexpected, but not necessarily deviant responses: one patient produced *fat* as the opposite of *pretty, baby* as the opposite of *big*. The same point applies to syntagmatic responses. Redundant collocations, such as *lick with my tongue, kick with my legs* may be common in normal children, or they may not. To observe an aphasic responding to a simile completion task *(e.g. the house was as big as --)* with "as big as big" might strike one immediately as deviant; but reference to, say, Gardner *et al.* (1975) would suggest that this would be quite expected for a pre-schooler. Even word-finding problems have their counterparts in the non-fluencies of the young child. One 2½-year-old, for example, would be able to name objects in a book in rapid sequence, but quite often, especially at bedtime, he would pause at (well-known and often-named) objects, and be unable to produce their names until prompted by the parent. There would even be phonological perseveration, as when a petrol pump was referred to as a *pet shop* (from earlier in the book).

However, it is by no means clear how widespread such phenomena are, and they by no means invalidate the delay/deviance distinction. Certainly, the anomalous responses to collocational patterns *(cf.* Lesser, 1978: 34) and the general problem of word-finding, as encountered in aphasia, in their extreme forms present problems which seem to have no counterpart in normal child development, and require separate study. But before proceeding with this issue, there is a much-needed clarification: the traditional term "word-finding" would, in the sense of this chapter, be better referred to as "lexeme-finding". This seems to be the usual meaning, *i.e.* a lexeme is unavailable to the speaker, *whatever grammtical context he is provided with.* For instance, lacking the lexeme *walk* would mean that P would be unable to complete any of the following contexts: *We - to town; I'm going for a -; He's - down the street; He's a fast -.* On the other hand, if a patient lacked only the verb use of *walk,* and retained his ability to use the lexeme in other grammatical contexts, then we would not want to say he had a lexeme-finding problem—for he *can* "find" the lexeme under certain grammatical conditions. Rather, we would here say, in the sense of this chapter (*cf.* p. 138) that he has a *word-finding* problem—*i.e.* a problem of retrieving a lexeme in a specific grammatical form. As the latter category are less common, it may be as well to provide an example of the kind of problem which arises:

T	'show me the bìg one/	(indicating two boxes)
P	thàt's the bíg one/	(correct)
T	'very gòod/	
	now 'look at thìs/	(adding third size)
	'which one's bìggest/	
P	thàt one/	(correct)
	thàt's the bíggest/	
T	yès/	
	now tèll me/ of thèse 'two/ 'which one's bìgger/	
P	'that one's --	(pointing to the correct box)
	'that one's --	

T   ˈgo ón/
     thát one's/
P   ˈnot bǐg/
     bìggest/
     nò/ --
     that's làrger than thát one/   (proudly, and correct)
     it's ˈbig -- ˈbig
T   bìgger/
P   bìg/
     yès/
T   bìgger/
P   bìgger/

Whatever is happening to this patient, it is not consistent to refer to his difficulty as a word-finding problem, in the same sense as someone who is unable to retrieve a lexeme under any grammatical circumstances. In what follows, it will be assumed that only genuine lexeme-finding difficulties are involved.

The main problem for the analyst is to determine whether there is evidence of pattern underlying the lexeme-finding behaviour of the patient, and whether this pattern is governed by linguistic (specifically semantic) factors. There are several logical possibilities which need to be systematically considered, before a decision can be arrived at.

(1) the lexeme seems totally unavailable, *i.e.* for all modalities (auditory, speech, reading and writing) and for all tasks (comprehension, production, imitation)[53].

(2) the lexeme is sometimes available (*i.e.* in some modalities, in some tasks), and when it is used, it is compatible with T's use of the lexeme.

(3) the lexeme is available (in some modalities and tasks), but is not compatible with T's use, *i.e.* P has a different semantic system, at least for the field to which the lexeme belongs. The distinction between (2) and (3) is summarized, from a different point of view, by Lesser (1978: 96): "It may be that the aphasic patient's problem is not so much one of difficulty in retrieval from an intact store of words [*sc.* lexemes] which have maintained their integrity, but is one of changes in the pattern of inter-relationships amongst word meanings ..."

(4) the lexemes may be used inconsistently, sometimes as (2), sometimes as (3).

There are 12 possible states that need to be taken into account, as shown in Fig. 2. The search for pattern is in fact a double task: we may investigate whether there is pattern in the correct use of lexemes, and also in the incorrect use. In both cases, the range of factors outlined earlier in this chapter will be relevant. For example, a patient might have no difficulty in using lexemes from one sub-set of semantic fields, but have difficulty with those from another; within a field, he might or might not have difficulty in using a particular sense-relation, such as hyponymy. From the linguistic point of view, what the analyst will try to establish is whether there is any sign of systematicness in the patient's use, and will operationalize this with refer-

---

    53 *Cf.* Aram and Nation (1975), and fn. 16 in Ch. 4.

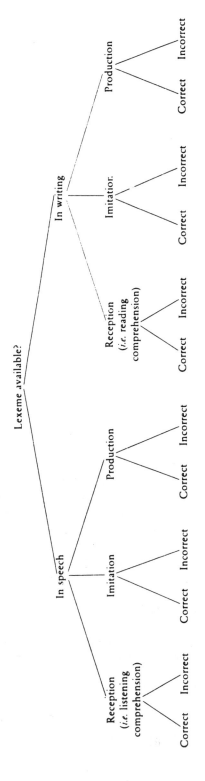

Fig. 2. Availability of lexemes in language modalities

ence to the notion of semantic structure used above. Thus, if the relationship between target lexeme and produced lexeme does *not* demonstrate synonymy, oppositeness, hyponymy, incompatibility (whether defined logically, or in terms of
semantic features), is not an expected collocation, does not belong to the same
semantic field, and cannot be explained by grammatical or phonological interference, then by definition it will be said to be unrelated. We may summarize this
view in the following way:

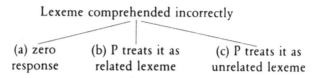

For example, asked to point to the door, P under (a) looks uncertain and does nothing; under (b) he may point to the window; under (c) he may point to a tree.

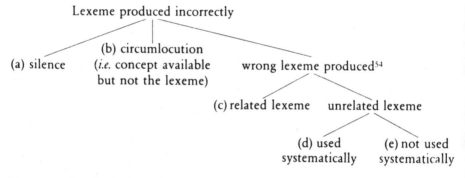

For example, asked what is happening in a picture clearly showing a man running,
under (a) P might say *man is* followed by silence; under (b) he might say *man is going
fast;* under (c) he might say *man is dashing* or *man is walking—no;* under (d) he might say
man is angry, and does so whenever presented with this picture; and under (e) he
might say *man is angry,* and then at a later showing say *man is regular,* or whatever[55].

Sentential Delay

In the present state of knowledge, only gross patterns of delay can be isolated:
(i) patients whose sentential semantic expression is incomplete, being dependent
on context to make the meaning clear (or non-verbal behaviour, *e.g.* gesture);
(ii) patients whose sentences seem restricted to a single, early-emerging semantic

---

[54] It is obviously important for T to know the target item, before a decision about relatedness can
be made; similarly, a lot depends on the unambiguity of the stimulus.

[55] These strictly intra-linguistic observations of course constitute only a part of a theory of lexical
retrieval—but they are an important part. For broader, psycholinguistic accounts, within which structural semantic notions might be incorporated, see Forster (1978), Morton (1979).

function, *e.g.* reflexive meaning only, activity only, locative only; (iii) patients with a restricted range of two- or three-element semantic function sentences; (iv) patients unable to connect sentences semantically, or who seem restricted to a certain strategy, *e.g.* order-of-mention. The comments made above concerning lexical delay (p. 186) are equally applicable.

Sentential Deviance

Assuming that research does not show the following patterns to be a feature of normal development (*cf.* p. 186), then the range of abnormal conditions under this heading includes:
(i) inability to express a specific semantic function (or set of functions), unrelated to any developmental order of emergence; (ii) ability to use only a single semantic function, unrelated to developmental order; or to develop semantic functions in an unexpected developmental order; (iii) ability to use a semantic function, whether developmentally early or not, but in an abnormal way, *e.g.* restricting locative expressions to the semantic field of vehicles; (iv) the unnecessary use of a semantic function either because it is repeated, or because it is redundant in context, or because it is simply irrelevant to the context. In relation to grammatical ability, several other possibilities emerge, such as a mismatch between the order of grammatical elements and the semantic values attributed to them (*e.g.* subject-verb-object being interpreted as goal-action-actor), or the introduction of grammatical deviance because of the attempted use of a certain semantic function, or sequence of functions. In all such cases, the disentangling of semantic and grammatical factors is not easy, and analytical problems abound. For example, in the sentence *I put on the wall,* is the error a grammatical problem arising out of poor control of clause structure, or is it a semantic problem due to a locative relationship being applied to both the activity and the goal? In the sentence *My dog was for a walk,* is the problem of the wrong choice of verb due to grammatical or semantic reasons? Are a patient's difficulties in disambiguating or defining due to grammatical or semantic reasons, or both, or of course to non-linguistic reasons (such as unfamiliarity with the task)? Faced with such puzzles, it will be evident that the study of sentential disability is in its infancy.

6 Diagnosis and Management

Linguistic Diagnosis

It will be plain, from the very large number of "don't knows" encountered in Chapters 2 to 5, that clinical linguistics is still at a primitive stage of development. There is a great deal of hard work that needs to be done before the generalizations envisaged in Chapter 1 can be achieved. Chapters 2 to 5 represent a first step in the direction of a theory and praxis of language disability, but the information they contain needs to be supplemented in two main ways. First, there are several important gaps that need to be filled by empirical research and theoretical model-building. Secondly, there needs to be a synthesis of the information obtained from each of the levels, so that an integrated view of a patient can emerge. It is always valuable to work with an analytical model, which allows us to examine in detail the parts of a phenomenon, in order to add to our understanding of the whole. But there has to be a corresponding synthesis, especially in a field like language disability, where patients often (perhaps even usually) present with symptoms which we can analyze on several linguistic levels at once. We can see this by looking at some of the commonly recognized conditions in linguistic pathology, and interpreting them in relation to the model of language used in this book.

Voice disorders. The traditional focus on the non-segmental phonetic character of voice disorders is undoubtedly correct, but more detailed and comprehensive models of the non-segmental variables involved need to be constructed, and the relationship between the phonetic and the phonological features of speech in these patients needs to be more fully explored. Specifically, most voice profiles I have seen might profitably be supplemented with reference to the following kinds of information:

(i) a more precise account of the laryngeal and associated sub- and supra-laryngeal settings involved in dysphonia[1];

---

[1] See Laver (1968) (1980). Laver's approach in fact makes use of several other variables: supralaryngeal settings, defined both longitudinally (*e.g.* raised and lowered larynx) and latitudinally (labial, lingual, faucal and mandibular settings), velopharyngeal settings (types of nasalisation), and laryngeal (*i.e.* phonatory) settings.

(ii) a comparably detailed account of the phonetic variables other than those contributing to dysphonia (*cf.* p. 60);

(iii) the multiple role of pitch should be recognized, with particular attention paid to the distinction between pitch direction and range, and between syllabic and polysyllabic ranges of application (*cf.* p. 62);

(iv) the syllabic vs. polysyllabic distinction also needs to be fully considered with reference to the loudness and timbre dimensions, in order to supplement such notions as "intermittent" phonation already in use;

(v) the synchronic vs. diachronic distinction should be more systematically used, so that the concept of change in voice quality over time can be more precisely identified: all of the phonetic variables can, in principle, change in the short and long term, and a profile chart needs to allow for this;

(vi) separate account should be given to those aspects of phonation and resonance which overlap with other areas of linguistic structure: chief among these is articulation (needed in order to make sense of the notions of vocal "attack" and "termination", and also of "nasal" and "denasal", whose values vary depending on the kind and distribution of segments involved in the utterance); but the possible relevance of semantic and grammatical factors also needs to be considered (*e.g.* the effect on comprehension of abnormal breaks in the grammar of laryngectomee speech);

(vii) above all, the interaction between non-segmental phonetic and phonological variables needs to be anticipated (*cf.* p. 74)[2].

Cleft palate. The multiple character of the linguistic disability associated with cleft palate syndrome is well-known. From the linguistic point of view, the following variables would seem to be particularly important:

(i) The analysis of the speech in phonological terms, to determine the extent to which an adequate phonological system is being obscured by purely phonetic deviance, or whether there is in addition an underlying disturbance of a phonological type; if the latter, whether it is something unique to the cleft palate condition, or a manifestation of some general pattern of delay (*cf.* p. 45);

(ii) the phonological, as well as the phonetic statement, must be interpreted in perceptual as well as production terms; the known association of the condition with hearing-loss will lead to one set of predictions, but the possibility of a more abstract problem of perceptual organization must not be discounted;

(iii) particularly in cleft palate speech, the analysis of the voice component of the problem must take into account the distribution of segments within the utterance: it is not possible to be consistent in rating degree of severity of nasal resonance, for example, on a unidimensional scale, without allowing for the "interference" of nasal consonants, and the differing degrees of nasal perceptibility on the range of vowel qualities;

---

[2] There are, in addition, other factors of a more general methodological kind which would need to be incorporated into a voice profile chart, especially a more motivated way for indicating frequency of a problem than is often found. There are several possibilities (linear scales, *e.g.* estimating frequency in percentages, or impressionistic categories [*e.g.* intermittent, mild, severe]; numerical categories [*e.g.* utterance length marked in seconds, etc.], some of which may be more efficient than others with reference to the categorization of a voice parameter.

(iv) the non-segmental structuring of the child's speech needs to be considered, in the light of problems arising out of inadequate breathing or voicing control, and associated difficulties in fluency (see below);

(v) in view of the recognized association of the condition with language delay, precise statement of the grammatical and semantic level of achievement of the child seems essential.

Fluency. The comprehensive analysis of the notion of "transition smoothness" in Dalton and Hardcastle (1977) clearly relates to the range of factors reviewed in the present book:

(i) at the segmental phonetic level, the combinatorial effects of prolongations, blocks, repetitions and abnormalities in muscular tension will be to produce a range of phonological difficulties which will need analysis in terms of the constructs of Chapter 2: chief amongst these will be the distribution of non-fluent segments within the word, but attention also needs to be paid to the way in which feature contrasts can be affected (due to such variables as length and tension no longer falling within normal perceptual limits);

(ii) transition smoothness at the prosodic level is evidently of great importance, special reference being made to pause, tempo, intonation and rhythm; once again, the phonological, as well as the phonetic consequences of disturbances in this area need to be systematically considered;

(iii) the distribution of non-fluency with reference to grammatical structure in the adult, and emerging grammatical structure in the child, need to be more systematically incorporated into fluency profiles (*cf.* p. 115);

(iv) the full range of semantic problems promoted by the non-fluency (*e.g.* avoidance of certain lexical items, circumlocutions) needs to be taken into account;

(v) in due course, we would hope to obtain from sociolinguistics a more systematic account of the nature of the social and psychological variables affecting interaction, as part of the statement of the severity of a dysfluent condition.

Aphasia. Repeated reference to this condition having been made throughout this book, the main points involved in linguistic analysis may perhaps be reviewed briefly. Lesser (1978) provides a comprehensive review of the relevant literature.

(i) For those patients whose grammatical production is plainly affected, the importance of a properly qualitative account of their difficulties is strongly stressed;

(ii) for those patients whose semantic organization is plainly affected, the importance of a properly qualitative account of their difficulties is strongly stressed— as a long-term goal, at any rate, given the limitations in our current state of knowledge;

(iii) the importance of the non-segmental organization of language, for the adequate handling of both the comprehension and the production of speech, suggests the need for a more systematic and detailed statement of this variable than is usually carried out in aphasia studies; distinguishing phonological from phonetic information under this heading is particularly important;

(iv) the multiple analysis of phonological problems, using the notions of segment, feature and process, is fruitful, with particular attention being paid to the distribution of the phonological difficulty in grammatical and semantic terms (*e.g.* to determine the possible systematicity of perseverative tendencies);

(v) there is a potentially important role for sociolinguistic and psycholinguistic analysis of the interaction and task settings in which aphasia remediation takes place; variable performance by patients is well-known, and a more systematic account of the range of factors involved in linguistic interaction could be helpful in bringing this variability more under control.

Dyspraxia. This condition is one which offers most scope for linguistic investigation, given the limited analysis it has received within traditional paradigms of enquiry. In particular, the extent of the systemicness of the data referred to as dyspraxic needs to be established:

(i) the most fruitful hypothesis would seem to be to see dyspraxia in terms of phonological realization, requiring multiple analysis in terms of segments, features, and especially processes (of the phonotactic type, in particular: *cf.* p. 30);

(ii) in more severe cases, disturbances in non-segmental phonology need to be systematically analyzed;

(iii) the limitations of the patient's expressive grammatical ability need to be established, especially in developmental conditions (where the possibility of semantic factors ought not to be discounted).

Dysarthria. This disability is most fruitfully seen as a phonetic problem, in the first instance, but depending on the degree of severity of the condition, several higher-order problems may emerge:

(i) the breakdown of transitions between phonological segments may lead to an attempted reorganization of phonological resources, especially in children; these will require separate analysis, especially in feature terms;

(ii) unclear boundary markers between grammatical and lexical units may lead to associated problems of expression or listener comprehension;

(iii) the extent to which non-segmental organization is disturbed needs careful investigation, and here too the distinction between phonetic and phonological properties of speech turns out to be critical.

Deafness. This is plainly an area where the whole range of linguistic variables is of relevance, the extent of their involvement however being less predictable, as so many different kinds and degrees of deafness exist. In principle, at least, we may expect the following:

(i) segmental phonological problems, which will need definition in terms of Chapter 2; there should not, however, be an over-reliance on analysis in terms of segments, which often omits the existence of important characteristics of deaf speech;

(ii) non-segmental phonological organization, and the underlying phonetic abilities involved, need careful study—a point which has received particular attention in recent years, in relation to advances in instrumentation[3];

(iii) the whole range of grammatical structure provides an essential (though traditionally neglected) dimension of analysis;

(iv) the whole range of semantic structure provides an essential dimension of analysis (avoiding the traditional focus on quantitative measures of vocabulary: *cf.* p. 140);

(v) sociolinguistic interaction studies are again important, as a means of defining the functional demands made on the deaf person by his environment;

---

[3] See for example Fourcin and Abberton (1971).

(vi) the continued study of the linguistic organization of both natural and contrived signing behaviour is important, but it should not be divorced from the study of oral expression and speech comprehension in the deaf, in view of the many possible ways in which linguistic information can be simultaneously transmitted and perceived (*e.g.* grammatical base with phonological cueing, semantic base with occasional grammatical structuring, etc.)[4].

These examples should indicate the range of applicability of the linguistic notions discussed in this book, and should also make very plain the need for future research. Already, however, it is possible to draw some general conclusions about the nature of linguistic disability, particularly with reference to the way in which it has been studied in the past. Two points in particular have been repeatedly referred to in this book. First, it no longer seems profitable to attempt to operate with the distinction between disorders of *speech* and disorders of *language*. The notion of "spoken language", used throughout Chapter 1, illustrates the nature of the confusion, but the reasons for rejecting the distinction are several:

(a) it gives exclusive emphasis to sound as a medium of communication, as opposed to the visual or tactile media—an understandable emphasis (*cf.* p. 12), but a theoretically restricting one, for anyone wishing to deal with writing or signing disability;

(b) it apparently gives priority to motor disorders of communication, as opposed to the sensory ones. Why is not *hearing* mentioned, as being a category of disability comparable in generality to *speech,* and a classification of "hearing" vs. "language" disorders maintained?

(c) there is a confusion because of the everyday meaning of the term "speech" to mean "spoken language", in which, inevitably, meaning and grammatical structure is involved[5].

(d) above all, there are the problems posed by the recognition of a phonological level of language organization. Phonology is often seen as falling "mid-way" between phonetics and other levels of linguistic organization[6]. Because it constitutes the sound system of language, it is thus intimately connected with the transmission of meaning. In segmental phonology, meaning is involved as a consequence of the oppositions which distinguish lexical items. In non-segmental phonology, the relation between sound system and meaning may be even more direct (as in the emotional function of intonation, for example). On the other hand, phonology is also intimately connected with phonetics—that is, with the physical realization of sound through the use of the vocal organs. So how should disorders of phonology (whether segmental or non-segmental) be classified, in traditional terms? As disorders of speech or of language? The impossibility of giving a satisfactory answer to this question suggests that the question is an unreal one. Phonological disabilities form a unique class: they should not be identified with the meaning-generating

---

[4] See further Schlesinger and Namir (1978), Siple (1978).

[5] Some textbooks on disability in fact use the term in this general sense, and thus constitute a different tradition from the classical "speech vs. language" one, *e.g.* Berry and Eisenson (1956), who include chapters on aphasia, language delay and hearing. This of course is one reason for the terminological dissatisfaction with the notion of "speech" clinician: see Crystal (1980: Ch 1).

[6] It is called an "interlevel" by Halliday, McIntosh and Strevens (1964), for example.

levels of language, nor should they be identified with the phonetic manifestations of language. A more satisfactory model of disability would be as in Fig. 3[7].

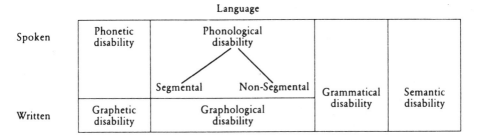

Fig. 3. Main categories of linguistic pathology

    The second notion which needs to be viewed with considerable caution is that of *deviance* vs. *delay*. As an initial orientation to disability typology, it has a certain value, but as soon as we try to apply it in any serious, discriminating way, the distinction becomes less useful. I have attempted to use it throughout this book, but usually on close examination the disability, whether phonological, grammatical or semantic, turns out to involve factors of both kinds, or factors whose status in terms of the distinction is unclear. This may to some extent be a temporary problem: in the absence of clear models of delay (*e.g.* in phonology and semantics) the distinction will inevitably appear muddled. But the difficulty is more serious than this, for it proves difficult to work with the distinction even in those areas where reasonably clear developmental guidelines exist. There is certainly no such thing as a "pure" category of delay, in which a patient's language is a replica of his juniors. Quantitative and qualitative differences are invariably present, and thus the notion of deviance is involved. We may, at best, salvage the notion by talking about "predominantly delayed" language patterns, if we wish; but we would do better to concentrate on refining the notion of deviance, which seems so pervasive. This at any rate has been the intention behind the examination of individual cases throughout this book[8].

Linguistic Management

The above suggestions are the result of trying to use a model of linguistic behaviour as a supplement to, and sometimes as a replacement for the traditional medical model of clinical investigation. The primary aim is to demonstrate that there is system in the behaviour of a patient, with reference to his production and comprehension/perception of language, but that this system is limited, by comparison with child and adult norms. In due course, it is anticipated that the detailed study of

---

    [7] This model is discussed further in Crystal (1980).
    [8] For a fuller discussion of deviance, see Crystal, Fletcher and Garman (1976: 28 ff.), Crystal (1979a: 27 ff.), in relation to grammar; see also Leonard (1972).

individual patients will be supplemented by an analysis of the linguistic characteristics of groups of patients matched in medical, psychological and other terms. At this point, a real contribution to differential diagnosis might be forthcoming. Looking still further ahead, it is possible to see how such correlations will raise fundamental theoretical questions of the kind addressed by Whitaker (see p. 6). The outcome might be a viable theory of language pathology.

But in the meantime, clinicians have to get on with the job, and this means developing a viable theory of linguistic management—not an easy task, obviously, in the absence of a general theory of disability within which to work. To what extent, then, can linguistics be of assistance in this direction? Our main expectations here must derive from the way theoretical linguistics has in recent years taken increasing cognisance of the importance of social and psychological context as determinants of linguistic behaviour. This movement has been noted at several points in the above chapters. In segmental phonology, we had to consider the environmental factors which might influence the development of perception ability. In non-segmental phonology, the role of tonicity in linguistic stimuli proved to be influential. In grammar, the relationship between grammatical stimulus and patient's response was stressed at several places. And in semantics, the role of the clinician and the parent in developing and maintaining the meaning patterns and expectations of the individual was a central theme. We may summarize this by stressing the significance of the study of linguistic *interaction* to our understanding of disability, and the need for this to proceed in a properly scientific way.

The most relevant subjects would seem to be sociolinguistics and psycholinguistics (see p. 20), especially the former. In a putative "clinical sociolinguistics", there would be three main themes, corresponding to the triadic organization of earlier chapters: an account of interaction in theoretical terms (partly social, social psychological, and linguistic)[9]; a descriptive framework within which the relevant linguistic variables could be identified and classified; and a characterization of the range of linguistic interactional disabilities encountered in the clinical population. In the present state of knowledge, it is not possible to say a great deal about the last two themes (which is why this topic does not rank as a separate chapter in this book), but it is possible to illustrate the type of information involved.

An important characteristic of remedial interaction is that it is typically a three-way process—this contrasting with the two-way interactions found in most normal adult conversations. A normal conversation proceeds in a series of overlapping dyads: A speaks to B, and B replies, but in the course of replying produces a stimulus to which A in turn will reply; A's reply then acts as a further stimulus to B; and so on. Any clearly definable sequence involving a change of speaker is known as a conversational "turn", and the rules governing turn-taking have been a particular focus of attention in recent years[10]. The analysis turns out to be more complex than might appear at first sight because of the way real conversations operate in practice—full of interruptions, re-phrasings and parallel speech (the various "attention signals", such as *mhm, yeah* and *I see,* as well as the non-verbal features which we use while

---

    [9] For an account of sociolinguistic theory, see Labov (1972), Hymes (1964), Trudgill (1974).

    [10] See Sacks, Schegloff and Jefferson (1974), Gumperz and Hymes (1972).

someone else is speaking). But the notion of a two-way turn, consisting of stimulus and response, seems valid enough, and indeed rather obvious. What is less obvious is the way in which speakers depart from this norm to achieve certain communicative or social effects, and here the distinctiveness of remedial conversation is a primary example. The three-way nature of the conversational turn is best illustrated by such sequences as:

T   'where's the càr/
P   in the gàrage/
T   in the gàrage/ 'good bòy/

What we have here is a clinical stimulus, a patient response, and then a clinical *reaction* to the response. Providing such paraphrases and reactions of praise to our interlocutors in adult speech would be extremely odd, to say the least!

A profile of clinical linguistic interaction thus has to take into account three variables, not two. A comprehensive typology of such interactions does not seem to have been made, but at least the following exist:

Example

1. T   stimulus   T   do you lìke fóotball/
   P   zero response   P   ---
   T   new/rephrased stimulus   T   you were 'playing 'football with the
                                           bòys/
                                      P   ---
                                      T   'that 'book's all abòut fóotball/
                                           ìsn't it/
                                      P   ---

2. T   stimulus   T   'what's thàt 'called/
   P   response   P   a bàll/
   T   reaction   T   'good bòy/ -
       new stimulus   and 'what's thàt 'called/

3. T   stimulus   T   'what 'colour's thìs 'man's 'shirt/
   P   response   P   yèllow/
   T   new stimulus   T   'what 'colour's thìs/
   P   response   P   blùe/

4. T   stimulus   T   and will he 'not come bàck to sée
                                           her/
   P   response   P   not ex'pect he wìll/
   T   reaction+new stimulus   T   you 'don't ex'pect he wìll/
       (in same sentence)   P   m̀/

5. P   stimulus   P   'I have X̀mas 'toy/
   T   response   T   you've 'got a 'new tòy/
       new stimulus   'what ìs it/
   P   response   P   càr/

6. P	stimulus		P	'now 'what abóut/ er - nèxt 'week/ you 'going to erm - 'give me a lètter/
T	response		T	'that's rìght/
P	new stimulus		P	'where is it/
T	response		T	it's thère/
7. P	stimulus		P	some 'people 'see in wìndow/
T	response+new stimulus (in same sentence)		T	'what are they dòing/
P	response		P	lòoking/
8. T	stimulus		T	'I've 'got a 'blue càr/
P	new stimulus		P	'I got 'red hòrse/
T	new stimulus		T	'I've 'got a 'black tràin/
			P	'I got 'green còw/

We can group these into certain more general types:

T-initiations

A. *Failure*—type 1 above.
B. *Primitive*—types 2 and 3. In the first of these, the elementary pattern of stimulus→response is reinforced by the addition of a reaction. In the second, this has been dropped, and the interaction is thus somewhat more advanced in the direction of normal conversation. But in its regularity it is still very primitive.
C. *Advanced*—types 4 and 8. Type 8 is a somewhat exceptional interaction, only found in the context of a turn-taking game (in the above example, taking things out of a bag). It is type 4 which is closest to the conversational norm found in non-clinical settings.

P-initiations

A. *Single*—type 5. P initiates a conversational turn, but T then takes the initiative, and P falls into a response pattern above.
B. *Recurrent*—type 6. P takes the initiative on repeated occasions, but T's responses are very limited.
C. *Normal*—type 7. P takes the initiative, and T responds to him as he would to anyone else, providing a response and a new stimulus, to which P then responds.

There are several differences here with adult conversational norms. Even in the P-initiated interactions, it is T who has the initiative: the "conversational ball" does not pass so readily backwards and forwards as it does in normal settings. There is an absence of P reactions: P does not usually use *mhm* (etc.) while T is speaking—unless it is to over-use it (as with much aphasic speech). The clinical interactions are far too symmetrical to be normal: in normal conversations, blocks of sentences alternate, as the conversational initiative changes; conversations where the speakers say equivalent amounts in rotation are unusual (except in prepared arguments). There are few interpolations or interruptions in clinical interaction. And generally, there is a lack of concern on P's part to maintain the "felicity conditions" necessary to promote a coherent conversation[11].

An interaction typology of this kind does not take us very far, however: it needs to be followed up immediately by a more detailed analysis of the stimulus types used by T, and of the types of response and reaction which follow. It is at this level that factors will emerge indicating in what respects P's interaction performance is being facilitated or hindered by T's interventions. Unfortunately there are several theoretical problems in the way of devising adequate descriptive frameworks at this level. Stimuli can be classified not only in grammatical or semantic terms, but also in terms of their *pragmatic* function. "Pragmatics" is a loosely-used term in contemporary linguistics which refers to the study of language from the point of view of the user, especially of the choices he makes and the constraints he encounters in using language in social interaction, and the effects his use of language has on other participants in an act of communication. It is in trying to make such notions as "choices", "constraints" and "effects" precise that difficulties arise. It is not easy to make an exhaustive list of all the factors which have to be taken into account in order to understand the social intent behind a sentence. If someone says "I'm cold", for example, it might be a simple statement of fact, a statement made in order to keep conversation going, an implied request for someone else's coat, a suggestion that a window be shut, and so on. Moreover, whatever the intended meaning in the mind of the speaker, there is always the possibility that what he says may be misinterpreted by the hearer, and a different effect produced from the one intended. All these variables constitute the focus of *speech-act* theory—the "act of speaking" being defined with reference to the speaker's intentions (the so-called "illocutionary" force of his utterance) and the effects he achieves on the listener (the "perlocutionary" effect)[12]. Examples of speech-acts that have been much discussed in the literature on language acquisition include *directives* (the speaker tries to get the listener to do something, *e.g.* requesting, commanding), *commissives* (the speaker commits himself to a future course of action, *e.g.* promising), *expressives* (the speaker expresses his feelings, *e.g.* apologizes, welcomes), and many more[13]. As soon as we attempt a list such as this, though, the theoretical problem is immediately apparent: how do we know when a list is exhaustive? how do we distinguish one type of "social force" from another (*e.g.* how clear is the difference between "requesting", "inviting", "soliciting", "begging", "accosting" . . .?)? how do we correlate these intangibles with the formal features of language? Faced with such a mass of imponderables, it is not surprising that the theoretical debate in this field is making slow progress.

---

[11] "Felicity conditions" refer to the criteria which must be satisfied if a speech act (see below) is to achieve its purpose, *e.g.* "preparatory conditions" relate to whether the person performing a speech act has the authority to do so (*e.g.* not everyone is qualified to say "I baptise/arrest/marry . . ."). An utterance which does not satisfy these conditions cannot function as a valid instance of the type of speech act to which they apply, *e.g. will you drive?* is inappropriate as a request, if the speaker knows that his hearer has not learned to drive. See Lyons (1977: Ch. 16).

[12] See Austin (1962), Searle (1969), and the discussion in Lyons (1977: Ch. 16).

[13] Some relevant child language studies are: Keenan (1974), Bruner (1975), Garvey (1975), Bates (1976), and the papers in Snow and Ferguson (1977) and Ochs and Schieffelin (1979).

In remedial settings, the theoretical problems are fortunately not as serious as they might be, because of the much more circumscribed nature of these settings, and the much more limited types of speech-act normally encountered there. Even so, an inventory of types can become quite complicated, as the following attempt suggests (the list is restricted to P-directed stimuli, and excludes the utterances T uses to others, *e.g.* parents, kin, phone-callers). Only the main grammatical categories are used.

A. *Minor sentences*[14]

organization, *e.g.* rìght/, nòw/ (*i.e.* let's move on to something new)

vocative, *e.g.* Jòhnny/, Mr Smìth/ (many functions, depending on the intonation, such as attention-seeking, warning)

continuity, *e.g.* mhm̀/, yés/ (*i.e.* carry on, I'm listening)

formulae, *e.g.* 'up the réds/ (said by T as P came in wearing a football scarf)

exclamation, *e.g.* gòsh/, òoh/

B. *Major sentences*

Statements (*i.e.* statement in form, but not necessarily functioning as a statement of fact):

neutral, *e.g.* descriptive narrative about a picture, event, etc.

identification (following P's zero response), *e.g.* it's a càr/, he's rùnning/

correction (following P's wrong response), *e.g.*   P   it's a càr/
                                                       T   it's a vǎn/

checking (a repeat of P's utterance, but with a high rising tone), *e.g.* it's ↑cár/

supplementary information, *e.g.*   T   it's a vàn/
                                             it's 'not got any wìndows/

commentary on action, *e.g.* we'll 'have to 'do that agàin/

prompt, *e.g.* it's ↑ā - (intonation being crucial here)

tag (used as question, though not a question in form), *e.g.* he's 'eating his dìnner I sup'pose/

command, *e.g.* it 'goes thère/, I'm wǎtching/

Questions (*i.e.* question in form, but not necessarily in function):

general—wholly deictic (*cf.* p. 121), *e.g.* 'what's thàt/

       using empty verb (*cf.* p. 124), *e.g.* 'what's thàt 'called/, 'what's he dóing/

specific—lexical item provided, *e.g.* 'what's he èating/

forced alternative, *e.g.* is he éating or drìnking/

clarification, *e.g.* 'more whàt/

checking (incorporates P's utterance, or part of it), *e.g.* 'did you 'say réd/

rephrase by T, *e.g.* is he rǔnning/
                      is the 'man rǔnning/

rhetorical (no expectation of a response), *e.g.* you're tìred/ àren't you/

instruction, *e.g.* will 'you 'sit stìll/

---

[14] For the minor vs. major distinction in grammar, see Crystal, Fletcher and Garman (1976: Ch. 3). Essentially, minor sentences are unproductive, *i.e.* they have a sentence structure which has no potential for development using the normal grammatical rules of the language.

Commands

general, *e.g.* 'go ón/, lòok/, dòn't/

specific, *e.g.* 'put the 'pig in the bòx/, 'let's 'find a còw/, 'say blúe/

Exclamatory

general, *e.g.* hów clèver/

specific, *e.g.* 'what a 'big càr/

The differential effect the selection of one rather than another of these stimuli may have on P's response ability is much in need of study. Aspects of the problem have been referred to earlier in this book (*e.g.* p. 125) and elsewhere, but only in an illustrative way[15].

A classification of T's reaction patterns would also be an important feature of an interaction profile, and an initial attempt at this has been made in Crystal (1979 a: 55 ff.). Several of the categories referred to above may of course turn up as reactions as well as stimuli (*e.g.* checking). A particularly important factor here seems to be the extent T provides P with formal guidance in his responses as to how P should proceed. At one extreme, T may provide no formal guidance at all, but simply a general positive or negative reinforcement (*e.g.* yès/, 'good bòy/, it's nòt/). At the other extreme he may provide P with an explicit correction, consciously drawing P's attention to the existence of an error (*e.g.* 'say it lòuder/, 'finish it òff/). In between, there are several reaction strategies that can be used, some of which have been noted as being of importance in language acquisition, *e.g.* the parental techniques of structural expansion and semantic amplification[16]:

P   'there càr/
T   'there's a càr/ (structural expansion)
     your dàddy's 'got a 'car like thát/ (amplification)

Lastly, we would need to provide a categorization of P's responses, not this time in terms of the phonological, grammatical or semantic acceptability of his sentences, as formally constructed entities, but in terms of their appropriateness to the ongoing situation. It is this range of possibilities which introduces the idea of interactional disability, referred to on p. 20. Several types of problem have been noted in the clinical literature. In addition to the patients whose language output falls *below* what is socially normal (the majority of language-disordered, by definition), there are also groups of patients whose language output rises to well *above* what is socially acceptable. Meaning may be present (*e.g.* in the outpourings of some schizophrenic patients) or it may be largely absent (as in "fluent" dysphasic speech, or the "cocktail party" speech of hydrocephalic children)[17]. A third possibility is that language may be normal in quantity, but moving "in parallel" with T, and not genuinely interacting with his utterances. A good example is the language habits of

---

[15] For example, in Crystal, Fletcher and Garman (1976: Ch. 6), concerning the use of different question forms. See also Schachter, Fosha, Stemp, Brotman and Ganger (1976).

[16] See further, Brown and Bellugi (1965), Nelson, Carskaddon and Bonvillian (1973), Bushnell and Aslin (1977).

[17] See Schwartz (1974), Swisher and Pinsker (1971), Bloom and Lahey (1978: 295–296).

the child of 3;3 analyzed by Blank, Gessner and Esposito (1979), from which the following extract is taken:

Father	John
That's Pat's house. What's everyone doing at Pat's house?	
	Knock, knock, knock. *(Knocking on door in book)*
Come in!	
	Nobody's home.
Nobody's home? Well, isn't Pat home? *(Pat is evident in the picture)*	
	Come back later.
O.K., let's go to Pat's new house.	
	Pat's old house. *(Looking at book)*

The general feel of conversations such as this is of the adult doing a great deal of work to no effect. The child's utterances sometimes make contact with lexicon from the adult, but not in any coherent manner, and without any willingness to move the conversation in a given direction. It is as if a basic felicity condition has been broken: the adult is interested in having a conversation about a topic, but the child is not—though he nonetheless produces a great deal of speech, and if the adult withdraws from the exchange, he immediately becomes upset. Similar patterns have been observed in the language of young schizophrenic and autistic children, and they are probably common in adult psychopathological conditions also, though the point has been little investigated[18].

It is my hope that clinical sociolinguistics will develop as a major field of inter-disciplinary enquiry—though whether it will be called this, as opposed to "clinical pragmatics", "clinical discourse analysis", or several other possible titles remains to be seen! Similarly, the clinical application of psycholinguistics provides a further important interdisciplinary field, over and above the contribution that has come from language acquisition studies in their various forms. The study of language ability (as opposed to learning) in relation to such factors as memory, perception and attention is at the centre of much clinical language practice. All have been referred to at various points in this book, along with the emphasis on individual differences and the role of task variation in mediating linguistic response. From a remedial point of view, this perspective is essential in order to develop and make sense of the notion of a "structured" language situation, and of teaching "at the right level" for a patient. The linguistic factors in these notions can be identified and described using the techniques of this book; but they cannot be implemented without a systematic awareness of the interaction between these factors and the psychological ones. For

---

[18] See Kanner (1973). Other abnormal interaction patterns also exist, *e.g.* the various kinds of echolalia. For adults, see Rochester and Martin (1979), Shapiro (1979), whose title ("clinical psycho-linguistics") refers to the interaction between linguistics and clinical psychology, and is thus a more restricted sense than the one used earlier in this book.

example, there may be excellent grounds for using forced alternative questions to a patient, to enable him to focus on a relevant lexical or grammatical feature (see Crystal, Fletcher and Garman, 1976: 120 ff.), but if this strategy exceeds P's memory span, it will not achieve its aims. And a similar point might be made in relation to any area of linguistic intervention. But the foundations of a clinical psycholinguistics, in this sense, are to be found not only in linguistics, but also in psychology. They are therefore not given systematic treatment in this book[19].

The goal of a theory of linguistic management is thus one to which linguistics can make an important contribution, but it is a limited one. It is limited by the need for the clinician to be aware of the whole range of psychological, social and of course medical factors which affect the well-being of his patient. There is thus no need for the concern which was once expressed to me by a speech therapist at a conference on the role of clinical linguistics a few years ago, that with developments in this subject, one day there would be nothing left for her to do! To look after the patient, was the only proper answer, with all that that involves. Clinical linguistics may be one of the foundation-stones of speech pathology, but it is no more than that. The aim of this book has been to show that it is no less than that, either.

---

[19] See further, Dato (1975), Allen and Cortazzo (1974), and on specific issues, Moore (1973), Corrigan (1978) and Tyler and Marslen-Wilson (1978).

References

Alajouanine, T. (1956): Verbal realization in aphasia. Brain 79, 1–28.

Allen, G. D., Hawkins, S. (1978): The Development of Phonological Rhythm. In: Syllables and Segments (Bell, A., Hooper, J. B., eds.), pp. 173–185. Amsterdam: North-Holland.

Allen, R. M., Cortazzo, A. D. (eds.) (1974): Psycholinguistic Development in Children: Implications for Children with Developmental Disabilities. Coral Gables: University of Miami Press.

Andersen, E. S. (1975): Cups and glasses: learning that boundaries are vague. J. Child Lang. 2, 79–103.

Andersen, E. S. (1978): Lexical Universals of Body-Part Terminology. In: Universals of Language (Greenberg, J. H., ed.), Vol. 3, pp. 335–368. Stanford: Stanford University Press.

Anderson, J. (1969): Syllabic or non-syllabic phonology. J. Ling. 5, 136–142.

Anglin, J. (1977): Word, Object and Conceptual Development. New York: Norton.

Antinucci, F., Miller, R. (1976): How children talk about what happened. J. Child Lang. 3, 167–190.

Aram, D. M., Nation, J. E. (1975): Patterns of language behavior in children with developmental language disorders. J. Sp Hear. Res. 18, 229–241.

Ardery, G. (1980): On coordination in child language. J. Child Lang. 7, 305–320.

Atkinson-King, K. (1973): Children's Acquisition of Phonological Stress Contrasts. UCLA Working Papers in Phonetics 25.

Austin, J. L. (1962): How to Do Things with Words. Oxford: Clarendon.

Ayer, A. J. (1936): Language, Truth and Logic. London: Gollancz.

Baldie, B. J. (1976): The acquisition of the passive voice. J. Child Lang. 3, 331–348.

Bartlett, E. J. (1976): Sizing things up: the acquisition of the meaning of dimensional adjectives. J. Child Lang. 3, 205–219.

Bates, E. (1976): Language and Context: the Acquisition of Pragmatics. New York: Academic Press.

Benedict, H. (1979): Early lexical development: comprehension and production. J. Child Lang. 6, 183 to 200.

Beresford, R. (1971): Some Comparative Descriptions of Children's Language. In: Applications of Linguistics (Perren, G., Trim, J., eds.), pp. 121–131. Cambridge: C.U.P.

Beresford, R. (1972): Deviant Language Acquisition: The Phonological Aspect. In: The Child with Delayed Speech (Martin, J. A., Rutter, M., eds.), pp. 161–167. London: Heinemann.

Beresford, R., Grady, P. A. E. (1968): Some aspects of assessment. B. J. Dis. Comm. 3, 28–35.

Berlin, B., Breedlove, D. E., Raven, P. H. (1973): General principles of classification and nomenclature in folk biology. Am. Anth. 75, 214–242.

Berndt, R. S., Caramazza, A. (1978): The development of vague modifiers in the language of preschool children. J. Child Lang. 5, 279–294.

Berry, M. F., Eisenson, J. (1956): Speech Disorders: Principles and Practice of Therapy. New York: Appleton-Century-Crofts.

Blank, M., Gessner, M., Esposito, A. (1979): Language without communication: a case study. J. Child Lang. *6*, 329—352.

Bloom, L. (1973): One Word at a Time: the Use of Single-word Utterances before Syntax. The Hague: Mouton.

Bloom, L., Hood, L., Lightbown, P. (1974): Imitation in language development: if, when and why. Cogn. Psychol. *6*, 380—420.

Bloom, L., Lahey, M. (1978): Language Development and Language Disorders. New York: Wiley.

Bloom, L., Lahey, M., Hood, L., Lifter, K., Fiess, K. (1980): Complex sentences: acquisition of syntactic connectives and the semantic relations they encode. J. Child Lang. *7*, 235—261.

Bloom, L., Lightbown, P., Hood, L. (1975): Structure and Variation in Child Language. Monogr. Soc. Res. Child Dev. *40* (Serial No. 160).

Bloomfield, L. (1933): Language. New York: Holt, Rinehart, Winston.

Blount, B. G., Padgug, E. J. (1977): Prosodic, paralinguistic, and interactional features in parent-child speech: English and Spanish. J. Child Lang. *4*, 67—86.

Blumstein, S., Cooper, W. E. (1974): Hemispheric processing of intonation contours. Cortex *10*, 146 to 158.

Blumstein, S., Goodglass, H. (1972): The perception of stress as a semantic cue in aphasia. J. Sp. Hear. Res. *15*, 800—806.

Bolinger, D. L. (1961): Syntactic blends and other matters. Lang. *37*, 366—381.

Bolinger, D. L. (1964): Intonation as a universal. In: Proc. IX Int. Cong. Ling. pp. 833—844. The Hague: Mouton.

Bolinger, D. L. (1972): Accent is predictable (if you're a mind-reader). Lang. *48*, 633—644.

Bonvillian, J. D., Raeburn, V. P., Horan, E. A. (1979): Talking to children: the effects of rate, intonation and length on children's sentence imitation. J. Child Lang. *6*, 459—467.

Boomer, D. S., Laver, J. (1968): Slips of the tongue. B. J. Dis. Comm. *3*, 2—12.

Bosma, J. F. (1975): Anatomic and Physiologic Development of the Speech Apparatus. In: Human Communication and Its Disorders (Tower, D. B., ed.), Vol. 3. New York: Raven Press.

Bowerman, M. (1973): Early Syntactic Development: a Cross-linguistic Study with Special Reference to Finnish. Cambridge: C.U.P.

Bresnan, J. W. (1971): Sentence stress and syntactic transformation. Lang. *47*, 257—281.

Bridges, A. (1979): Directing two-year-olds' attention: some clues to understanding. J. Child Lang. *6*, 211—226.

Bridges, A. (1980): SVO comprehension strategies reconsidered: the evidence of individual patterns of response. J. Child Lang. *7*, 89—104.

Brown, J. W. (1977): Mind, Brain and Consciousness. New York: Academic Press.

Brown, R. (1968): The development of wh-questions in child speech. JVLVB. *7*, 279—290.

Brown, R. (1973): A First Language: the Early Stages. Cambridge, Mass.: Harvard University Press.

Brown, R., Bellugi, U. (1965): Three Processes in the Child's Acquisition of Syntax. In: New Directions in the Study of Language (Lenneberg, E. H., ed.), pp. 131—161. Cambridge, Mass.: M.I.T. Press.

Bruner, J. S. (1975): The ontogenesis of speech acts. J. Child Lang. *2*, 1—19.

Bushnell, E. W., Aslin, R. N. (1977): Inappropriate expansion: a demonstration of a methodology for child language research. J. Child Lang. *4*, 115—122.

Cairns, H. S., Hsu, J. R. (1978): Who, why, when and how: a development study. J. Child Lang. *5*, 477 to 488.

Carlson, P., Anisfeld, M. (1969): Some observations on the linguistic competence of a two-year-old. Child Dev. *40*, 569—575.

Catford, J. C. (1977): Fundamental Problems in Phonetics. Edinburgh: Edinburgh University Press.

Chafe, W. L. (1970): Meaning and the Structure of Language. Chicago: University of Chicago Press.

Chambers, J. C., Tavuchis, N. (1976): Kids and kin: children's understanding of American kin terms. J. Child Lang. *3*, 63—80.

Chao, Y. R. (1943): The Non-Uniqueness of Phonemic Solutions of Phonetic Systems. Repr. in: Readings in Linguistics (Joos, M., ed.), Vol. 1, pp. 38—54. Chicago: University of Chicago Press 1957.

Charney, R. (1979): The comprehension of "here" and "there". J. Child Lang. *6*, 69—80.

Chomsky, C. S. (1969): The Acquisition of Syntax in Children from 5 to 10. Cambridge, Mass.: M.I.T. Press.

Chomsky, N. (1957): Syntactic Structures. The Hague: Mouton.

Chomsky, N. (1964): Current Issues in Linguistic Theory. The Hague: Mouton.

Chomsky, N. (1965): Aspects of the Theory of Syntax. Cambridge, Mass.: M.I.T. Press.

Chomsky, N. (1966): Cartesian Linguistics. New York: Harper & Row.

Chomsky, N. (1967): Discussion Comment. In: Brain Mechanisms Underlying Speech (Millikan, C. H., Darley, F. L., eds.). New York: Grune & Stratton.

Chomsky, N. (1970): Deep Structure, Surface Structure and Semantic Interpretation. In: Studies in General and Oriental Linguistics (Jacobson, R., Kawamoto, S., eds.), pp. 52—91. Tokyo: TEC Corp.

Chomsky, N. (1975): Reflections on Language. Glasgow: Collins.

Chomsky, N., Halle, M. (1968): The Sound Pattern of English. New York: Harper & Row.

Clark, E. V. (1971): On the acquisition of the meaning of "before" and "after". JVLVB. *10*, 266—275.

Clark, E. V. (1973): What's in a Word? On the Child's Acquisition of Semantics in His First Language. In: Cognitive Development and the Acquisition of Language (Moore, T., ed.), pp. 65—110. New York: Academic Press.

Clark, E. V. (1978): From Gesture to Word: on the Natural History of Deixis in Language Acquisition. In: Human Growth and Development (Bruner, J. S., Garton, A., eds.). London: O.U.P.

Clark, E. V. (1979): Building a Vocabulary: Words for Objects, Actions and Relations. In: Language Acquisition (Fletcher, P., Garman, M., eds.), pp. 149—160. Cambridge: C.U.P.

Clark, E. V., Garnica, O. K. (1974): Is he coming or going? On the acquisition of deictic verbs. JVLVB. *13*, 559—572.

Clark, E. V., Sengul, C. J. (1978): Strategies in the acquisition of deixis. J. Child Lang. *5*, 457—475.

Clark, H. H. (1973): Space, Time, Semantics and the Child. In: Cognitive Development and the Acquisition of Language (Moore, T., ed.), pp. 28—64. New York: Academic Press.

Clark, H. H., Clark, E. V. (1977): Psychology and Language: an Introduction to Psycholinguistics. New York: Harcourt, Brace, Jovanovich.

Clark, R. (1974): Performing without competence. J. Child Lang. *1*, 1—10.

Clark, R. (1977): What's the use of imitation? J. Child Lang. *4*, 341—358.

Clark, R., Hutcheson, S., Van Buren, P. (1974): Comprehension and production in language acquisition. J. Ling. *10*, 39—54.

Coker, P. L. (1978): Syntactic and semantic factors in the acquisition of "before" and "after". J. Child Lang. *5*, 261—277.

Collinson, R. L. (1981): A History of Foreign-language Dictionaries. London: Deutsch.

Compton, A. (1970): Generative studies of children's phonological disorders. J. Sp. Hear. Dis. *35*, 315 to 339.

Connor, P., Stork, F. C. (1972): Linguistics and speech therapy—a case study. B. J. Dis. Comm. *7*, 44—48.

Corrigan, R. (1975): A scalogram analysis of the development of the use and comprehension of "because" in children. Child Dev. *46*, 195—201.

Corrigan, R. (1978): Language development as related to stage 6 object permanence development. J. Child Lang. *5*, 173—189.

Critchley, M. (1970): Aphasiology and Other Aspects of Language. London: Edward Arnold.

Crosby, F. (1976): Early discourse agreement. J. Child Lang. *3*, 125—126.

Cross, T. G. (1977). Mother's Speech Adjustment: The Contribution of Selected Child Listener Variables. In: Talking to Children: Language Input and Acquisition (Snow, C. E., Ferguson, C. A., eds.), pp. 151—188. Cambridge: C.U.P.

Cruse, D. A. (1977): A note on the learning of colour names. J. Child Lang. *4*, 305—311.

Cruttenden, A. (1972): Phonological procedures for child language. B. J. Dis. Comm. *7*, 30—37.

Cruttenden, A. (1974): An experiment involving comprehension of intonation in children from 7 to 10. J. Child Lang. *1*, 221—231.

Cruttenden, A. (1979): Language in Infancy and Childhood. Manchester: Manchester University Press.

Crystal, D. (1969): Prosodic Systems and Intonation in English. Cambridge: C.U.P.

Crystal, D. (1971): Linguistics. Harmondsworth: Penguin.

Crystal, D. (1975): The English Tone of Voice. London: Edward Arnold.

Crystal, D. (1976): Child Language, Learning and Linguistics. London: Edward Arnold.

Crystal, D. (1978): The Analysis of Intonation in Young Children. In: Communicative and Cognitive Abilities—Early Behavioral Assessment (Minifie, F. D., Lloyd, L. L., eds.), pp. 257—271. Baltimore: University Park Press.

Crystal, D. (1979 a): Working with LARSP. London: Edward Arnold.
Crystal, D. (1979 b): Prosodic Development. In: Language Acquisition (Fletcher, P., Garman, M., eds.), pp. 33—48. Cambridge: C.U.P.
Crystal, D. (1980): An Introduction to Language Pathology. London: Edward Arnold.
Crystal, D. (1981): Directions in Applied Linguistics. London: Academic Press.
Crystal, D. (1982): Profiling Linguistic Disability. London: Edward Arnold.
Crystal, D., Davy, D. (1975): Advanced Conversational English. London: Longman.
Crystal, D., Fletcher, P. (1978): Profile Analysis of Language Disability. In: Individual Differences in Language Ability and Language Behaviour (Fillmore, C., Wang, W., eds.), pp. 167—188. New York: Academic Press.
Crystal, D., Fletcher, P., Garman, M. (1976): The Grammatical Analysis of Language Disability. London: Edward Arnold.
Cutler, A. (1976): Phoneme-monitoring reaction time as a function of preceding intonation contour. Percept. Psychophys. 20, 55—60.
Dale, P. S. (1976): Language Development: Structure and Function, 2nd ed. New York: Holt, Rinehart, Winston.
Dalton, P., Hardcastle, W. J. (1977). Disorders of Fluency. London: Edward Arnold.
Dato, D. P. (ed.) (1975): Developmental Psycholinguistics. Washington: Georgetown University Press.
Dever, R. B. (1972). TALK (Teaching the American Language to Kids). Experimental Materials, Final Report 27.3. Bloomington: Indiana University, Center for Innovation in Teaching the Handicapped.
Dinneen, F. P. (1967): An Introduction to General Linguistics. New York: Holt, Rinehart, Winston.
Donaldson, M. (1978): Children's Minds. London: Fontana.
Dore, J. (1975): Holophrases, speech acts and language universals. J. Child Lang. 2, 21—40.
Dore, J., Franklin, M. B., Miller, R. T., Ramer, A. L. H. (1976): Transitional phenomena in early language development. J. Child Lang. 3, 13—28.
Edwards, M. L. (1974): Perception and production in child phonology: the testing of four hypotheses. J. Child Lang. 1, 205—219.
Edwards, R. P. A., Gibbon, V. (1973): Words Your Children Use, 2nd ed. London — Toronto: Burke Books.
Eilers, R. E. (1975): Suprasegmental and grammatical control over telegraphic speech in young children. J. Psycholing. Res. 4, 227—239.
Eilers, R. E., Oller, D. K. (1976): The role of speech discrimination in developmental sound substitutions. J. Child Lang. 3, 319—329.
Eilers, R. E., Oller, D. K., Ellington, J. (1974): The acquisition of word-meaning for dimensional adjectives: the long and short of it. J. Child Lang. 1, 195—204.
Eilers, R. E., Wilson, W. R., Moore, J. M. (1979): Speech discrimination in the language-innocent and the language-wise: a study in the perception of voice onset time. J. Child Lang. 6, 1—18.
Emerson, H. F. (1979): Children's comprehension of "because" in reversible and non-reversible sentences. J. Child Lang. 6, 279—300.
Emerson, H. F. (1980). Children's judgements of correct and reversed sentences with "if". J. Child Lang. 7, 137—155.
Empson, W. (1930). Seven Types of Ambiguity. London: Chatto & Windus.
Erreich, A., Valian, V., Winzemer, J. (1980): Aspects of a theory of language acquisition. J. Child Lang. 7, 157—179.
Ervin-Tripp, S. (1970): Discourse Agreement: How Children Answer Questions. In: Cognition and the Development of Language (Hayes, J., ed.), pp. 79—107. New York: Wiley.
Ferguson, C. A. (1977): Baby Talk As a Simplified Register. In: Talking to Children: Language Input and Acquisition (Snow, C. E., Ferguson, C. A., eds.), pp. 219—236. Cambridge: C.U.P.
Ferguson, C. A., Farwell, C. B. (1975): Words and sounds in early language acquisition. Lang. 51, 419 to 439.
Ferguson, C. A., Peizer, D., Weeks, T. (1973): Model-and-replica phonological grammar of a child's first words. Lingua 31, 35—65.
Fillmore, C. J. (1968): The Case for Case. In: Universals in Linguistic Theory (Bach, E., Harms, R., eds.), pp. 1—88. New York: Holt, Rinehart, Winston.

Fillmore, C. J. (1971): Santa Cruz Lectures on Deixis. Bloomington: Indiana University Linguistics Club.

Fillmore, C. J., Langendoen, D. T. (eds.) (1971): Studies in Linguistic Semantics. New York: Holt, Rinehart, Winston.

Firth, J. R. (1948): Sounds and prosodies. Trans. Phil. Soc. 127—152.

Firth, J. R. (1951): Modes of meaning. Essays Stud. 118—149. Repr. in: Papers in Linguistics 1934 to 1951, 190—215.

Fletcher, P. (1979): The Development of the Verb Phrase. In: Language Acquisition (Fletcher, P., Garman M., eds.), pp. 261—284. Cambridge: C.U.P.

Fletcher, P., Garman, M. (eds.) (1979): Language Acquisition: Studies in First Language Development. Cambridge: C.U.P.

Flores D'Arcais, G. B., Levelt, W. J. M. (eds.) (1970): Advances in Psycholinguistics. Amsterdam: Elsevier.

Folger, J. P., Chapman, R. S. (1978): A pragmatic analysis of spontaneous imitations. J. Child Lang. 5, 25—38.

Forster, K. I. (1978): Accessing the Mental Lexicon. In: Explorations in the Biology of Language (Walker, E., ed.), pp. 139—174. Hassocks: Harvester Press.

Fourcin, A., Abberton, E. (1971): First applications of a new laryngograph. Med. Biol. Illus. 21, 172 to 182.

Fraser, C., Bellugi, U., Brown, R. (1963): Control of grammar in imitation, comprehension and production. JVLVB. 2, 121—135.

Fremgen, A., Fay, D. (1980): Overextensions in production and comprehension: a methodological clarification. J. Child Lang. 7, 205—211.

French, L. A., Brown, A. L. (1977): Comprehension of "before" and "after" in logical and arbitrary sequences. J. Child Lang. 4, 247—256.

Fries, C. C. (1952): The Structure of English. London: Longman.

Fries, C. C. (1964): On the intonation of "yes—no" questions in English. In: In Honour of Daniel Jones (Abercrombie, D., et al., eds.), pp. 242—254. London: Longman.

Fromkin, V. (1973): Speech Errors as Linguistic Evidence. The Hague: Mouton.

Fry, D. B. (1947): The frequency of occurrence of speech sounds in Southern English. Arch. Néerl. de Phon. Exp. 20, 103—106.

Fry, D. B. (1977): Homo Loquens: Man as a Talking Animal. Cambridge: C.U.P.

Fudge, E. C. (1969): Syllables. J. Ling. 5, 253—286.

Fudge, E. C. (ed.) (1973): Phonology. Harmondsworth: Penguin.

Furrow, D., Nelson, K., Benedict, H. (1979): Mothers' speech to children and syntactic development: some simple relationships. J. Child Lang. 6, 423—442.

Gardner, H. (1974): The naming of objects and symbols by children and aphasic patients. J. Psycholing. Res. 3, 133—149.

Gardner, H., Kircher, M., Winner, E., Perkins, D. (1975): Children's metaphoric productions and preferences. J. Child Lang. 2, 125—141.

Garnica, O. (1973): The Development of Phonemic Speech Perception. In: Cognitive Development and the Acquisition of Language (Moore, T., ed.), pp. 215—222. New York: Academic Press.

Garnica, O. (1977): Some Prosodic and Paralinguistic Features of Speech to Young Children. In: Talking to Children (Snow, C. E., Ferguson, C. A., eds.), pp. 63—88. Cambridge: C.U.P.

Garvey, C. (1975): Requests and responses in children's speech. J. Child Lang. 2, 41—63.

Geschwind, N. (1964): The development of the brain and the evolution of language. Georgetown Monogr. Ser. Lang. Ling. 17, 155—169.

Gilbert, J. H. V. (1977): A voice onset time analysis of apical stop production in 3-year-olds. J. Child Lang. 4, 103—110.

Gilbert, J. H. V., Purves, B. A. (1977): Temporal constraints on consonant clusters in child speech production. J. Child Lang. 4, 417—432.

Giles, H., Powesland, P. F. (1975): Speech Style and Social Evaluation. London: Academic Press.

Gimson, A. C. (1980): An Introduction to the Pronunciation of English, 3rd ed. London: Edward Arnold.

Gleason, H. A. (1965): Linguistics and English Grammar. New York: Holt, Rinehart, Winston.

Glucksberg, S., Danks, J. H. (1975): Experimental Psycholinguistics: an Introduction. Hillsdale: Erlbaum.

Goldin-Meadow, S., Seligman, M. E. P., Gelman, R. (1976): Language in the two-year-old. Cognition *4*, 189—202.

Goodglass, H. (1968): Studies on the Grammar of Aphasics. In: Developments in Applied Linguistic Research (Rosenberg, S., Koplin, J. H., eds.), pp. 177—208. New York: Macmillan.

Goodglass, H., Fodor, I. G., Schulhoff, C. (1967): Prosodic factors in grammar: evidence from aphasia. J. Sp. Hear. Res. *10*, 5—20.

Greenberg, J. H. (1966): Synchronic and diachronic universals in phonology. Lang. *42*, 508—517.

Greene, M. C. L. (1964): The Voice and its Disorders, 2nd ed. London: Pitman.

Greenfield, P., Smith, J. H. (1976): The Structure of Communication in Early Language Development. New York: Academic Press.

Grunwell, P. (1975): The phonological analysis of articulation disorders. B. J. Dis. Comm. *10*, 31—42.

Grunwell, P. (1977): The Analysis of Phonological Disability in Children, 2 Vols. PhD Thesis, University of Reading. Published as: The Nature of Phonological Disability in Children. London: Academic Press 1981.

Gumperz, J. J., Hymes, D. (1972): Directions in Sociolinguistics: the Ethnography of Communication. New York: Holt, Rinehart, Winston.

Haas, W. (1963). Phonological analysis of a case of dyslalia. J. Sp. Hear. Dis. *28*, 239—246.

Haas, W. (1968): Functional phonetics and speech therapy. B. J. Dis. Comm. *3*, 20—27.

Hall, R. A. (1960): Linguistics and Your Language. New York: Doubleday.

Halliday, M. A. K. (1966): Lexis as a Linguistic Level. In: In Memory of J. R. Firth (Bazell, C. E., Catford, J. C., Halliday, M. A. K., Robins, R. H., eds.), pp. 148—162. London: Longman.

Halliday, M. A. K. (1967—1968): Notes on transitivity and theme in English. J. Ling. *3*, 37—81, 199 to 244; *4*, 179—215.

Halliday, M. A. K. (1975): Learning How to Mean. London: Edward Arnold.

Halliday, M. A. K., McIntosh, A., Strevens, P. D. (1964): The Linguistic Sciences and Language Teaching. London: Longman.

Hardcastle, W., Roach, P. J. (1981): The Experimental Study of Speech Production. London: Academic Press.

Hartley, L. M. (1966): Analysis of the Linguistic Data of Dyslalia. In: Signs, Signals and Symbols (Mason, S., ed.), pp. 152—158. London: Methuen.

Hatch, E. (1971): The young child's comprehension of time connectives. Child Dev. *42*, 2111—2113.

Haviland, S. E., Clark, E. V. (1974): "This man's father is my father's son": a study of the acquisition of English kin terms. J. Child Lang. *1*, 23—47.

Head, H. (1926): Aphasia and Kindred Disorders of Speech. Cambridge: C.U.P.

Henderson, E. J. A. (ed.) (1971): The Indispensable Foundation. London: O.U.P.

Higgs, J. A. W. (1970): The articulation test as a linguistic technique. Lang. Speech *13*, 262—270.

H.M.S.O. (1972): Speech Therapy Services. London.

H.M.S.O. (1975): A Language for Life. London.

H.M.S.O. (1978): Special Educational Needs. London.

Hockett, C. F. (1958): A Course in Modern Linguistics. New York: Macmillan.

Hockett, C. F., Altmann, S. (1968): A Note on Design Features. In: Animal Communication (Sebeok, T. A., ed.), pp. 61—72. Bloomington: Indiana University Press.

Hooper, J. B. (1972). The syllable in phonological theory. Lang. *48*, 525—540.

Horgan, D. (1978 a): The development of the full passive. J. Child Lang. *5*, 65—80.

Horgan, D. (1978 b): How to answer questions when you've nothing to say. J. Child Lang. *5*, 159—165.

Howe, C. J. (1976): The meanings of two-word utterances in the speech of young children. J. Child Lang. *3*, 29—47.

Hsieh, H.-I. (1972): Lexical diffusion: evidence from child language acquisition. Glossa *6*, 89—104.

Huddleston, R. (1976): An Introduction to English Transformational Syntax. London: Longman.

Hyman, L. M. (1975): Phonology: Theory and Analysis. New York: Holt, Rinehart, Winston.

Hyman, L., Schuh, R. (1974): Universals of tone rules: evidence from West Africa. Ling. Inqu. *5*, 81 to 115.

Hymes, D. (ed.) (1964): Language in Culture and Society. New York: Harper & Row.

Ingram, D. (1974 a): Phonological rules in young children. J. Child Lang. *1*, 49—64.

Ingram, D. (1974 b): Fronting in child phonology. J. Child Lang. *1*, 233—241.

Ingram, D. (1976): Phonological Disability in Children. London: Edward Arnold.

Ingram, D. (1979): Phonological Patterns in the Speech of Young Children. In: Language Acquisition (Fletcher, P., Garman, M., eds.), pp. 133—148. Cambridge: C.U.P.

Irwin, O. C., Chen, H. P. (1943): Speech sound elements during the first years of life: a review of the literature. J. Sp. Dis. *8*, 109—121.

Jakobson, R. (1941): Kindersprache, Aphasie und allgemeine Lautgesetze. Uppsala: Almqvist & Wiksell. Trans. by Keiler, A. R. (1968): Child Language, Aphasia and Phonological Universals. The Hague: Mouton.

Jakobson, R. (1955): Aphasia as a Linguistic Topic. Clarke University Monographs on Psychology and Related Disciplines, Worcester. Repr. in Selected Writings, Vol. 2 (1971), pp. 229—238. The Hague: Mouton.

Jakobson, R. (1964): Towards a Linguistic Typology of Aphasic Impairments. In: Disorders of Language (De Reuck, A. V. S., O'Connor, M., eds.), pp. 21—42. London: Churchill.

Jakobson, R., Halle, M. (1956): Fundamentals of Language. The Hague: Mouton.

Jespersen, O. (1909—1949): A Modern English Grammar on Historical Principles, Vols. 1—7. London: Allen & Unwin.

Jespersen, O. (1926): Lehrbuch der Phonetik. Leipzig.

Johnson, S., Somers, H. (1978): Spontaneous and imitated responses in articulation testing. B. J. Dis. Comm. *13*, 107—116.

Jones, D. (1950): The Phoneme. Cambridge: Heffer.

Kail, M., Segui, J. (1978): Developmental production of utterances from a series of lexemes. J. Child Lang. *5*, 251—260.

Kanner, L. (1973): Childhood Psychosis: Initial Studies and New Insights. New York: Wiley.

Kaplan, E. L. (1970): Intonation and language acquisition. Stanford Papers and Reports on Child Language Development *1*, 1—21.

Karmiloff-Smith, A. (1979): Language Development After Five. In: Language Acquisition (Fletcher, P., Garman, M., eds.), pp. 307—323. Cambridge: C.U.P.

Katz, J.J. (1964): Mentalism in linguistics. Lang. *40*, 124—137.

Katz, J.J., Fodor, J. A. (1963): The structure of a semantic theory. Lang. *39*, 170—210.

Keenan, E. L. (ed.) (1975): Formal Semantics of Natural Language. Cambridge: C.U.P.

Keenan, E. O. (1974): Conversational competence in children. J. Child Lang. *1*, 163—183.

Kohler, K. (1966): Towards a phonological theory. Lingua *16*, 337—351.

Konopczynski, G. (1975): Etude expérimentale de quelques structures prosodiques employées par les enfants français entre 7 et 22 mois. Travaux de l'Institut de Phonétique de Strasbourg *7*, 171—205.

Kornfeld, J. (1971): Theoretical issues in child phonology. Papers from the Chicago Linguistics Society, 7th Regional Meeting, pp. 454—468.

Kuhn, D., Phelps, H. (1976): The development of children's comprehension of causal direction. Child Dev. *47*, 248—251.

Labov, W. (1972): Sociolinguistic Patterns. Philadelphia: University of Pennsylvania Press.

Ladefoged, P. (1975): A Course in Phonetics. New York: Harcourt, Brace, Jovanovich.

Lamb, S. M. (1966): Outline of Stratificational Grammar. Washington: Georgetown University Press.

Lasky, E. Z., Weidner, W. E., Johnson, J. P. (1976): Influence of linguistic complexity, rate of presentation, and interphase pause time on auditory-verbal comprehension of adult aphasic patients. Brain Lang. *3*, 386—395.

Lass, N. J. (ed.) (1976): Contemporary Issues in Experimental Phonetics. New York: Academic Press.

Laver, J. (1968): Voice quality and indexical information. B. J. Dis. Comm. *3*, 43—54.

Laver, J. (1970): The Production of Speech. In: New Horizons in Linguistics (Lyons, J., ed.), pp. 53—75. Harmondsworth: Penguin.

Laver, J. (1980): The Phonetic Description of Voice Quality. Cambridge: C.U.P.

Lee, L. L. (1974): Developmental Sentence Analysis: a Grammatical Assessment Procedure for Speech and Language Disorders. Evanston: Northwestern University Press.

Leech, G. N. (1969): A Linguistic Guide to English Poetry. London: Longman.

Leech, G. N. (1974): Semantics. Harmondsworth: Penguin.

Lenneberg, E. H. (1967): Biological Foundations of Language. New York: Wiley.

Lenneberg, E. H. (1976): The Concept of Language Differentiation. In: Foundations of Language Development (Lenneberg, E. H., Lenneberg, E., eds.), Vol. 1., pp. 17—33. New York: Academic Press.

Leonard, L. B. (1972): What is deviant language? J. Sp. Hear. Dis. *37*, 427—446.

Leonard, L. B. (1973): The role of intonation in recall of various linguistic stimuli. Lang. Speech *16*, 327 to 335.

Leonard, L. B., Schwartz, R. G., Folger, M. K., Wilcox, M. J. (1978): Some aspects of child phonology in imitative and spontaneous speech. J. Child Lang. *5*, 403—415.

Lepschy, G. C. (1970): A Survey of Structural Linguistics. London: Faber & Faber.

Lesser, R. (1978): Linguistic Investigations of Aphasia. London: Edward Arnold.

Levelt, W. J. M. (1975): What Became of LAD? In: Contributions to an Understanding of Linguistics (Ut Videam). Lisse: Peter de Ridder Press.

Lewis, M. M. (1951): Infant Speech: a Study of the Beginnings of Language, 2nd ed. London: Routledge & Kegan Paul.

Li, C. N., Thompson, S. A. (1977): The acquisition of tone in Mandarin-speaking children. J. Child Lang. *4*, 185—199.

Lieberman, P. (1967): Intonation, Perception and Language. Cambridge, Mass.: M.I.T. Press.

Limber, J. (1976): Unravelling competence, performance and pragmatics in the speech of young children. J. Child Lang. *3*, 309—318.

Lingua (1967): Word Classes. Reprint of Lingua *17*, 1—261. Amsterdam: North-Holland.

Litowitz, B. (1977): Learning to make definitions. J. Child Lang. *4*, 289—304.

Lounsbury, F. G. (1956): A semantic analysis of the Pawnee kinship system. Lang. *32*, 158—194.

Lund, N. L., Duchan, J. F. (1978): Phonological analysis: a multifaceted approach. B. J. Dis. Comm. *13*, 119—126.

Luria, A. R. (1964): Factors and Forms of Aphasia. In: Disorders of Language (De Reuck, A. V. S., O'Connor, M., eds.), pp. 143—161. London: Churchill.

Lust, B. (1977): Conjunction reduction in child language. J. Child Lang. *4*, 257—287.

Lust, B., Mervis, C. A. (1980): Development of coordination in the natural speech of young children. J. Child Lang. *7*, 279—304.

Lyons, J. (1968): Introduction to Theoretical Linguistics. Cambridge: C.U.P.

Lyons, J. (1972): Human Language. In: Non-verbal Communication (Hinde, R. A., ed.), pp. 49—85. Cambridge: C.U.P.

Lyons, J. (1975): Deixis as a Source of Reference. In: Formal Semantics and Natural Language (Keenan, E., ed.), pp. 61—83. Cambridge: C.U.P.

Lyons, J. (1977): Semantics, Vols. 1, 2. Cambridge: C.U.P.

McCarthy, D. (1954): Language Development in Children. In: Manual of Child Psychology (Carmichael, L., ed.), pp. 429—630. New York: Wiley.

Macken, M. A., Barton, D. (1980): The acquisition of the voicing contrast in English: a study of voice onset time in word-initial stop consonants. J. Child Lang. *7*, 41—74.

Macrae, A. (1976): Movement and location in the acquisition of deictic verbs. J. Child Lang. *3*, 191 to 204.

Macrae, A. (1979): Combining Meanings in Early Language. In: Language Acquisition (Fletcher, P., Garman, M., eds.), pp. 161—176. Cambridge: C.U.P.

McReynolds, L. V., Huston, K. (1971): A distinctive feature analysis of children's misarticulations. J. Sp. Hear. Dis. *36*, 155—166.

Maratsos, M. P. (1973): The effects of stress on the understanding of pronominal co-reference in children. J. Psycholing. Res. *2*, 1—8.

Maratsos, M. P. (1976): The Use of Definite and Indefinite Reference in Young Children. Cambridge: C.U.P.

Marckworth, M. L. (1976): Effect of temporal expansion of speech on aphasic comprehension. Can. J. Ling. *21*, 79—94.

Martinet, A. (1949): Phonology as Functional Phonetics. Oxford: Philological Society.

Matthews, P. H. (1974): Morphology: an Introduction to the Theory of Word-structure. Cambridge: C.U.P.

Matthews, P. H. (1979): Generative Grammar and Linguistic Competence. London: Allen & Unwin.

Matthews, P. H. (1981): Syntax. Cambridge: C.U.P.

Menn, L. (1971): Phonotactic rules in beginning speech. Lingua *26*, 225—251.

Menn, L. (1976): Pattern, Control and Contrast in Beginning Speech. PhD Thesis, University of Illinois at Urbana-Champaign. Univ. Micro. *76—24*, 139.

Menyuk, P. (1969): Sentences Children Use. Cambridge, Mass.: M.I.T. Press.

Menyuk, P., Bernholtz, N. (1969): Prosodic features and children's language production. M.I.T. Quart. Progr. Rep. *93*, 216—219.

Menyuk, P., Klatt, M. (1975): Voice onset time in consonant cluster production by children and adults. J. Child Lang. *2*, 223—231.

Menyuk, P., Menn, L. (1979): Early Strategies for the Perception and Production of Words and Sounds. In: Language Acquisition (Fletcher, P., Garman, M., eds.), pp. 49—70. Cambridge: C.U.P.

Miller, G. A., Nicely, P. E. (1955): An analysis of perceptual confusions among some English consonants. J. Acoust. Soc. Amer. *27*, 338—352.

Minifie, F., Darley, F., Sherman, D. (1963): Temporal reliability of seven language measures. J. Sp. Hear. Res. *6*, 139—148.

Minifie, F., Lloyd, L. L. (eds.) (1978): Communicative and Cognitive Abilities: Early Behavioral Assessment. Baltimore: University Park Press.

Mittins, W. H. (1962): A Grammar of Modern English. London: Methuen.

Monrad-Krohn, G. H. (1947): Dysprosody or altered melody of language. Brain *70*, 405—415.

Moore, T. (ed.) (1973): Cognitive Development and the Acquisition of Language. New York: Academic Press.

Morehead, D. M., Ingram, D. (1973): The development of base syntax in normal and linguistically deviant children. J. Sp. Hear. Dis. *16*, 330—352.

Morse, P. (1974): Infant Speech Perception: A Preliminary Model and Review of the Literature. In: Language Perspectives: Acquisition, Retardation and Intervention (Schiefelbusch, R. L., Lloyd, L. L., eds.), pp. 19—53. Baltimore: University Park Press.

Morton, J. (1979): Word Recognition. In: Structures and Processes (Morton, J., Marshall, J. C., eds.), pp. 107—156. London: Elek.

Moskowitz, A. (1970): The two-year-old stage in the acquisition of English phonology. Lang. *46*, 426 to 441.

Nation, J. E., Aram, D. A. (1977): Diagnosis of Speech and Language Disorders. St. Louis: Mosby.

Nelson, K. (1973): Structure and Strategy in Learning to Talk. Monogr. Soc. Res. Child Dev. *38* (Serial no. 149).

Nelson, K. (1974): Concept, word and sentence: interrelations in acquisition and development. Psychol. Rev. *81*, 269—285.

Nelson, K. E., Carskaddon, G., Bonvillian, J. D. (1973): Syntax acquisition: impact of experimental variation in adult verbal interaction with the child. Child Dev. *44*, 497—504.

Nesfield, J. C. (1898): English Grammar: Past and Present. London: Macmillan.

Nice, M. M. (1915): The development of a child's vocabulary in relation to environment. Ped. Sem. *22*, 35—64.

Ochs, E., Schieffelin, B. B. (eds.) (1979): Developmental Pragmatics. New York: Academic Press.

O'Connor, J. D. (1973): Phonetics. Harmondsworth: Penguin.

O'Connor, J. D., Trim, J. L. M. (1953): Vowel, consonant and syllable: a phonological definition. Word *9*, 103—122.

Ogden, C. K., Richards, I. A. (1923): The Meaning of Meaning. London: Routledge & Kegan Paul.

Oller, D. K. (1973): Regularities in abnormal child phonology. J. Sp. Hear. Dis. *38*, 36—47.

Oller, D. K., Wieman, L. A., Doyle, W. J., Ross, C. (1976): Infant babbling and speech. J. Child Lang. *3*, 1—11.

Olmsted, D. L. (1971): Out of the Mouth of Babes. The Hague: Mouton.

Olney, R. L., Scholnick, E. K. (1976): Adult judgement of age and linguistic differences in infant vocalization. J. Child Lang. *3*, 145—155.

Osgood, C. E. (1953): Method and Theory in Experimental Psychology. London: O.U.P.

Osgood, C. E., Suci, G. J., Tannenbaum, P. H. (1957): The Measurement of Meaning. Urbana: University of Illinois Press.

Palmer, F. R. (ed.) (1970): Prosodic Analysis. London: O.U.P.

Palmer, F. R. (1971): Grammar. Harmondsworth: Penguin.

Palmer, F. R. (1974): The English Verb. London: Longman.

Palmer, F. R. (1976): Semantics: a New Outline. Cambridge: C.U.P. (2nd ed. 1981.)

Panagos, J. M. (1974): Persistence of the open syllable reinterpreted as a symptom of language disorder. J. Sp. Hear. Dis. *39*, 23—31.

Piaget, J. (1926): The Language and Thought of the Child. London: Routledge & Kegan Paul.

Pollack, E., Rees, N. (1972): Disorders of articulation: some clinical applications of distinctive feature theory. J. Sp. Hear. Dis. *37*, 451–461.

Posner, M. (1973): Cognition: an Introduction. Glenview: Scott Foresman.

Postman, L., Kleppel, G. (1970): Norms of Word Association. London–New York: Academic Press.

Powers, M. H. (1957): Functional Disorders of Articulation–Symptomatology and Etiology. In: Handbook of Speech Pathology (Travis, L. E., ed.), pp. 707–768. New York: Appleton-Century-Crofts.

du Preez, P. (1974): Units of information in the acquisition of language. Lang. Speech *17*, 369–376.

Priestley, T. M. S. (1977): One idiosyncratic strategy in the acquisition of phonology. J. Child Lang. *4*, 45–66.

Priestley, T. M. S. (1980): Homonymy in child phonology. J. Child Lang. *7*, 413–427.

Procter, P. (ed.) (1978): Longman Dictionary of Contemporary English. London: Longman.

Quirk, R. (1968): The Use of English, 2nd ed. London: Longman.

Quirk, R., Greenbaum, S., Leech, G. N., Svartvik, J. (1972): A Grammar of Contemporary English. London: Longman.

Ramer, A. L. H. (1976): Syntactic styles in emerging language. J. Child Lang. *3*, 49–62.

Reed, S. (1972): Pattern recognition and categorization. Cog. Psych. *3*, 382–407.

Rees, N. S. (1971): Bases of decision in language training. J. Sp. Hear. Dis. *36*, 283–304.

Reich, P. A. (1976): The early acquisition of word meaning. J. Child Lang. *3*, 117–123.

Rescorla, L. A. (1980): Overextension in early language development. J. Child Lang. *7*, 321–335.

Rescorla, L. A. (1981): Category development in early language. J. Child Lang. *8*, 2.

Richards, M. M. (1979): Adjective ordering in the language of young children: an experimental investigation. J. Child Lang. *6*, 253–277.

Roberts, P. (1956): Patterns of English. New York: Harcourt, Brace, World.

Robins, R. H. (1967): A Short History of Linguistics. London: Longman.

Robins, R. H. (1971): General Linguistics: an Introductory Survey, 2nd ed. London: Longman. (3rd ed. 1980.)

Robinson, G. M. (1977): Rhythmic organization in speech processing. J. Exp. Psychol. Hum. Percept. P. *3*, 83–91.

Rochester, S., Martin, J. R. (1979): Crazy Talk: a Study of the Discourse of Schizophrenic Speakers. New York: Plenum.

Rodgon, M. M., Jankowski, W., Alenskas, L. (1977): A multi-functional approach to single-word usage. J. Child Lang. *4*, 23–43.

Rosch, E. (1973): On the Internal Structure of Perceptual and Semantic Categories. In: Cognitive Development and the Acquisition of Language (Moore, T., ed.), pp. 111–144. New York: Academic Press.

Rosch, E., Lloyd, B. (eds.) (1978): Cognition and Categorization. Hillsdale: Erlbaum.

Sachs, J., Devin, J. (1976): Young children's use of age-appropriate speech styles in social interaction and role-playing. J. Child Lang. *3*, 81–98.

Sachs, J., Truswell, L. (1978): Comprehension of two-word instructions by children in the one-word stage. J. Child Lang. *5*, 17–24.

Sacks, H., Schegloff, E., Jefferson, G. (1974): A simplest systematics for the analysis of turn-taking in conversation. Lang. *50*, 696–735.

Salus, P. H., Salus, M. W. (1974): Developmental neurophysiology and phonological acquisition order. Lang. *50*, 151–160.

Sander, E. K. (1961): When are speech sounds learned? J. Sp. Hear. Dis. *37*, 55–63.

de Saussure, F. (1916): Cours de Linguistique Generale. Paris: Payot. Trans. by Baskin, W. (1959): Course in General Linguistics. New York: Philosophical Library.

Savić, S. (1975): Aspects of adult-child communication: the problem of question acquisition. J. Child Lang. *2*, 251–260.

Schachter, F. F., Fosha, D., Stemp, S., Brotman, N., Ganger, S. (1976): Everyday caretaker talk to toddlers vs. threes and fours. J. Child Lang. *3*, 221–245.

Schane, S. A. (1973): Generative Phonology. Englewood Cliffs, N. J.: Prentice-Hall.

Schlesinger, I. M. (1977): Production and Comprehension of Utterances. Hillsdale: Erlbaum.

Schlesinger, I. M. (1979): Cognitive structure and semantic deep structures: the case of the instrumental. J. Ling. *15*, 307–324.

Schlesinger, I. M., Namir, L. (eds.) (1978): Sign Language of the Deaf: Psychological, Linguistic and Sociological Perspectives. New York: Academic Press.

Schwartz, E. (1974): Characteristics of speech and language development in the child with myelomingocele and hydrocephalus. J. Sp. Hear. Dis. *39*, 465–468.

Schwartz, R. G., Leonard, L. B., Wilcox, M. J., Folger, M. K. (1980): Again and again: reduplication in child phonology. J. Child Lang. *7*, 75–87.

Searle, J. R. (1969): Speech Acts. Cambridge: C.U.P.

Sebeok, T. A., Hayes, A. S., Bateson, M. C. (eds.) (1964): Approaches to Semiotics. The Hague: Mouton.

Shapiro, T. (1979): Clinical Psycholinguistics. New York: Plenum.

Shatz, M. (1978): Children's comprehension of their mother's question-directives. J. Child Lang. *5*, 39–46.

Shibamoto, J. S., Olmsted, D. L. (1978): Lexical and syllabic patterns in phonological acquisition. J. Child Lang. *5*, 417–456.

Shvachkin, N. (1973): The Development of Phonemic Speech Perception in Early Childhood. In: Studies of Child Language Development (Ferguson, C. A., Slobin, D. I., eds.), pp. 91–127. New York: Holt, Rinehart, Winston.

Sinclair, J. McH. (1966): Beginning the Study of Lexis. In: In Memory of J. R. Firth (Bazell, C. E., Catford, J. C., Halliday, M. A. K., Robins, R. H., eds.), pp. 410–430. London: Longman.

Siple, P. (ed.) (1978): Understanding Language Through Sign Language Research. New York: Academic Press.

Slobin, D. I. (1973): Cognitive Prerequisites for the Acquisition of Grammar. In: Studies of Child Language Development (Ferguson, C. A., Slobin, D. I., eds.). New York: Holt, Rinehart, Winston.

Slobin, D. I., Welsh, C. A. (1971): Elicited Imitation As a Research Tool in Developmental Psycholinguistics. In: Language Training in Early Childhood Education (Lauatelli, C. S., ed.), pp. 170–185. Carbondale: University of Illinois Press.

Smith, C. (1980): The acquisition of time talk: relations between child and adult grammar. J. Child Lang. *7*, 263–278.

Smith, M. (1933): The influence of age, sex and situation on the frequency, form and function of questions asked by preschool children. Child Dev. *4*, 201–213.

Smith, N. V. (1973): The Acquisition of Phonology: a Case Study. Cambridge: C.U.P.

Smith, N. V. (1974): The acquisition of phonological skills in children. B. J. Dis. Comm. *9*, 17–23.

Smith, N. V. (1975): Universal Tendencies in the Child's Acquisition of Phonology. In: Language, Cognitive Deficits and Retardation (O'Connor, N., ed.), pp. 47–65. London: Butterworth.

Snow, C. E. (1977): The development of conversation between mothers and babies. J. Child Lang. *4*, 1–22.

Snow, C. E., Ferguson, C. A. (eds.) (1977): Talking to Children: Language Input and Acquisition. Cambridge: C.U.P.

Sparks, R. W., Holland, A. L. (1976): Melodic intonation therapy for aphasia. J. Sp. Hear. Dis. *41*, 287 to 297.

Stampe, D. (1969): The acquisition of phonetic representation. Papers from the Chicago Linguistic Society, 5th Regional Meeting, pp. 443–454.

Stankiewicz, E. (1964): Problems of Emotive Language. In: Approaches to Semiotics (Sebeok, T., Hayes, A., Bateson, M., eds.), pp. 239–264. The Hague: Mouton.

Stark, R. E., Poppen, R., May, M. Z. (1967): Effects of alterations of prosodic features on the sequencing performance of aphasic children. J. Sp. Hear. Res. *10*, 844–884.

Stark, R. E., Rose, S. N., McLagen, M. (1975): Features of infant sounds: the first eight weeks of life. J. Child Lang. *2*, 205–221.

Steinberg, D. D., Jakobovitz, L. A. (eds.) (1971). Semantics. Cambridge: C.U.P.

Strang, B. M. H. (1968): Modern English Structure, 2nd ed. London: Edward Arnold.

Strawson, P. F. (1971): Logico-linguistic Papers. London: Methuen.

Svartvik, J. (ed.) (1973): Errata: Papers in Error Analysis. Lund: Gleerup.

Swisher, L. P., Pinsker, E. J. (1971): The language characteristics of hyperverbal hydrocephalic children. Dev. Med. Child Neurol. *13*, 746–755.

Templin, M. (1957): Certain Language Skills in Children: Their Development and Interrelationships. Institute for Child Welfare Monograph *26*. Minneapolis: University of Minnesota Press.

Thomson, J., Chapman, R. (1977): Who is "daddy" revisited: the status of two-year-olds' over-extended words in use and comprehension. J. Child Lang. *4*, 359—376.

Thorndike, E. L., Lorge, I. (1944): The Teachers' Word-book of 30,000 Words. New York: Columbia University.

Timm, L. A. (1977): A child's acquisition of Russian phonology. J. Child Lang. *4*, 329—339.

Travis, L. E. (ed.) (1957): Handbook of Speech Pathology. New York: Appleton-Century-Crofts.

Trier, J. (1934): Das sprachliche Feld. Eine Auseinandersetzung. Neue Jahrbücher für Wissenschaft und Jugendbildung *10*, 428—449.

Trubetzkoy, N. S. (1939): Grundzüge der Phonologie. Trans. by Baltaxe, C.A.M. (1969): Principles of Phonology. Berkeley-Los Angeles: University of California Press.

Trudgill, P. (1974): Sociolinguistics: an Introduction. Harmondsworth: Penguin.

Tse, J. K.-P. (1978): Tone acquisition in Cantonese: a longitudinal case study. J. Child Lang. *5*, 191 to 204.

Tulving, E. (1972): Episodic and Semantic Memory. In: Organization in Memory (Tulving, E., Donaldson, W., eds.), pp. 382—403. New York: Academic Press.

Twaddell, W. F. (1960): The English Verb Auxiliaries. Providence: Brown University Press.

Tyack, D., Ingram, D. (1977): Children's production and comprehension of questions. J. Child Lang. *4*, 211—224.

Tyler, L. K., Marslen-Wilson, W. (1978): Some developmental aspects of sentence processing and memory. J. Child Lang. *5*, 113—129.

Ullmann, S. (1973): Meaning and Style. Oxford: Blackwell.

Van Lancker, D. (1975): Heterogeneity in Language and Speech: Neurolinguistic Studies. UCLA Working Papers in Phonetics *29*.

Van Lancker, D., Fromkin, V. W. (1973): Hemispheric specialization for pitch and "tone": evidence from Thai. J. Phonet. *1*, 101—109.

Van Uden, A. (1970): A World of Language for Deaf Children, Part I. Basic Principles. Rotterdam: Rotterdam University Press.

Vihman, M. M. (1978): Consonant Harmony: Its Scope and Function in Child Language. In: Universals of Human Language: Phonology (Greenberg, J. H., ed.), Vol. 2. Stanford: Stanford University Press.

de Villiers, J. G., de Villiers, P. A. (1973): The development of the use of word order in comprehension. J. Psycholing. Res. *2*, 331—341.

de Villiers, J. G., de Villiers, P. A. (1978): Language Acquisition. Cambridge, Mass.: Harvard University Press.

Wales, R. (1979): Deixis. In: Language Acquisition (Fletcher, P., Garman, M., eds.), pp. 241—260. Cambridge: C.U.P.

Walsh, H. (1974): On certain practical inadequacies of distinctive feature systems. J. Sp. Hear. Dis. *39*, 32—43.

Warden, D. (1976): The influence of context on children's use of identifying expressions and references. B. J. Psychol. *67*, 101—112.

Waterson, N. (1971): Child phonology: a prosodic view. J. Ling. *7*, 179—221.

Webb, P. A., Abramson, A. (1976): Stages of egocentrism in children's use of "this" and "that": a different point of view. J. Child Lang. *3*, 349—367.

Wehren, A., De Lisi, R., Arnold, M. (1981): The development of noun definition. J. Child Lang. *8*, 165 to 175.

Weigl, E., Bierwisch, M. (1970): Neuropsychology and linguistics: topics of common research. Found. Lang. *6*, 1—18.

Weir, R. (1962): Language in the Crib. The Hague: Mouton.

Wells, G. (1974): Learning to code experience through language. J. Child Lang. *1*, 243—269.

Wepman, J. M., Jones, L. V. (1961): Language Modalities Test for Aphasia. Chicago: Education Industry Service.

Wheldall, K., Swann, W. (1976): The effect of intonational emphasis on sentence comprehension in severely subnormal and normal children. Lang. Speech *19*, 87—99.

Whitaker, H. A. (1971 a): On the Representation of Language in the Human Brain. Edmonton: Linguistic Research Inc.

Whitaker, H. A. (1971 b): Neurolinguistics. In: A Survey of Linguistic Science (Dingwall, W. O., ed.). College Park: University of Maryland.

Winner, E. (1979): New names for old things: the emergence of metaphoric language. J. Child Lang. 6, 469–491.

Wittgenstein, L. (1953): Philosophical Investigations. Oxford: Blackwell.

Wode, H. (1980): Grammatical Intonation in Child Language. In: The Melody of Language: Intonation and Prosody (Waugh, L. R., van Schooneveld, C. H., eds.), pp. 331–345. New York: Academic Press.

Wolff, P. H. (1969): The Natural History of Crying and Other Vocalizations in Early Infancy. In: Determinants of Infant Behaviour (Foss, B., ed.), Vol. 4, pp. 81–109. London: Tavistock.

Zurif, E. B., Mendelsohn, M. (1972): Hemispheric specialization for the perception of speech sounds: the influences of intonation and structure. Percept. Psychophys. 11, 329–332.

Additional References

For the paperback edition of this book, I have added a number of relevant references which appeared during the period from 1981 to 1986, and indicated in brackets the page and footnote of *Clinical Linguistics* to which these references relate. Readers should also note the appearance of the journal *Clinical Linguistics & Phonetics*, which commenced publication in 1987 (publisher: Taylor & Francis), and of *Child Language Teaching and Therapy*, which commenced publication in 1985 (publisher: Edward Arnold).

Andrick, G. R., Tager-Flusberg, H. (1986): The acquisition of colour terms. J. Child Lang. 13, 119–34. (p. 177, fn. 34)

Bernstein, M. E. (1983): Formation of internal structure in a lexical category. J. Child Lang. 10, 381–99. (p. 174, fn. 34)

Borden, G. J., Harris, K. S. (1980): Speech Science Primer. Baltimore: Williams & Wilkins. (p. 2, fn. 3)

Boysson-Bardies, B., Bacri, N., Sagart, L., Poizat, M. (1981): Timing in late babbling. J. Child Lang. 8, 525–39. (p. 34, fn. 14)

Chomsky, N. 1986: Knowledge of Language: its Nature, Origin and Use. New York: Praeger. (p. 96, fn. 6)

Code, C., Ball, M. (eds.) (1984): Experimental Clinical Phonetics. Beckenham: Croom Helm. (p. 2, fn. 3)

Connolly, J. H. (1984): A commentary on the LARSP procedure. B. J. Dis. Comm. 19, 63–71. (p. 108, fn. 29)

Cruttenden, A. (1985): Intonation comprehension in ten-year-olds. J. Child Lang. 12, 643–61. (p. 73, fn. 18)

Crystal, D. (1984a): Linguistic Encounters with Language Handicap. Oxford: Blackwell. (p. 196, fn. 5)

Crystal, D. (1984b): Language input variables in aphasia. In: Advances in Neurology (Rose, F.C., ed.), pp. 145–58. New York: Raven Press. (p. 65, fn. 6)

Crystal, D. (1985a): Linguistics, 2nd edn. Harmondsworth: Penguin. (p. 3, fn. 4)

Crystal, D. (1985b): Who Cares About English Usage? Harmondsworth: Penguin. (p. 95, fn. 2)

Crystal, D. (1986): Listen to your Child. Harmondsworth: Penguin. (p. 20, fn. 27)

Fletcher, P. (1985): A Child's Learning of English. Oxford: Blackwell. (p. 102, fn. 16)

Fletcher, P., Garman, M. (eds.) (1986): Language Acquisition, 2nd edn. Cambridge: C.U.P. (p. 34, fn. 14)

French, L. A., Nelson, K. (1985): Young Children's Knowledge of Relational Terms: some *ifs*, *ors*, and *buts*. New York: Springer. (p. 102, fn. 16)

Garnham, A. (1985): Psycholinguistics: Central Topics. London: Methuen. (p. 20, fn. 27)

Gleitman, L., Newport, E. L., Gleitman, H. 1984): The current status of the motherese hypothesis. J. Child Lang. 11, 43–79. (p. 201, fn. 13)

Gopnik, A. (1984): The acquisition of *gone* and the development of the object concept. J. Child Lang. 11, 273–92. (p. 174, fn. 34)

Greene, M.C.L. (1980): The Voice and its Disorders, 4th edn. Tunbridge Wells: Pitman. (p. 59, fn. 2, p. 74, fn. 20)

Grunwell, P. (1982): Clinical Phonology. Beckenham: Croom Helm. (p. 23, fn. 1, p. 34, fn. 15)

Grunwell, P. (1985): PACS: Phonological Assessment of Child Speech. Windsor: NFER-Nelson. (p. 32, fn. 10)

Harris, J., Cottam, P. (1985): Phonetic features and phonological features in speech assessment. B.J.Dis.Comm. 20, 61–74. (p. 45, fn. 34)

Hawkins, P. (1984): Introducing Phonology. London: Hutchinson. (p. 23, fn. 1)

Hewlett, N. (1985): Phonological versus phonetic disorders: some suggested modifications to the current use of the distinction. B.J.Dis.Comm. 20, 155–64. (p. 45, fn. 34)

Hurford, J.R., Heasley, B. (1983): Semantics: a Coursebook. Cambridge: C.U.P. (p. 131, fn. 1)

Ilson, R. (1986): Lexicography: an Emerging International Profession. Manchester: Manchester University Press. (p. 133, fn. 8)

Ingram, D. (1986): Explanation and phonological remediation. Child Language Teaching and Therapy 2, 1–19. (p. 45, fn. 34)

Kent, R.D., Bauer, H.R. (1985): Vocalizations of one-year-olds. J. Child Lang. 12, 491–526. (p. 34, fn. 14)

Klein, H.B. (1984): Learning to stress: a case study. J. Child Lang. 11, 375–90. (p. 92, fn. 34)

Kuczaj, S.A., Barratt, M.D. (eds.) (1986): The Development of Word Meaning: Progress in Cognitive Development Research. New York: Springer. (p. 174, fn. 34)

Kyle, J.G., Woll, B. (1985): Sign Language: the Study of Deaf People and their Language. Cambridge: C.U.P. (p. 12, fn. 12)

Ladefoged, P. (1982): A Course in Phonetics, 2nd edn. New York: Harcourt, Brace, Jovanovich. (p. 2, fn. 3)

Lass, R. (1984): Phonology. Cambridge: C.U.P. (p. 23, fn. 1)

Leech, G.N. (1981): Semantics, 2nd edn. Harmondsworth: Penguin. (p. 131, fn. 1)

Leech, G.N. (1983): Pragmatics. London: Longman. (p. 201, fn. 11)

Lepschy, G.C. (1983): A Survey of Structural Linguistics, 2nd edn. Oxford: Blackwell. (p. 96, fn. 6)

Letts, C. (1985): Linguistic interaction in the clinic: how do therapists do therapy? Child Language Teaching & Therapy 1, 321–31. (p. 203, fn. 15)

Levinson, S. (1983): Pragmatics. Cambridge: C.U.P. (p. 201, fn. 11)

Lyons, J. (1981): Language and Linguistics. Cambridge: C.U.P. (p. 3, fn. 4)

Mack, M., Lieberman, P. (1985): Acoustic analysis of words produced by a child from 46 to 149 weeks. J. Child Lang. 12, 527–50. (p. 34, fn. 14)

Matthews, P.H. (1981): Syntax. Cambridge: C.U.P. (p. 99, fn. 11)

McCabe, A., Petersson, C. (1985): A naturalistic study of the production of causal connectives by children. J. Child Lang. 12, 145–59. (p. 106, fn. 24)

McTear, M.F. (1985a): Pragmatic disorders: a question of direction. B.J.Dis.Comm. 20, 119–27. (p. 210, fn. 15)

McTear, M. (1985b): Children's Conversation. Oxford: Blackwell. (p. 201, fn. 13)

Palmer, F.R. (1981): Semantics, 2nd edn. Cambridge: C.U.P. (p. 131, fn. 1)

Palmer, F.R. (1984): Grammar, 2nd edn. Harmondsworth: Penguin. (p. 95, fn. 2)

Penn, C., Gaunt, C. (1986): Towards a classification scheme for aphasic syntax. B.J.Dis.Comm. 21, 21–38. (p. 108, fn. 29)

Quirk, R., Greenbaum, S., Leech, G., Svartvik, J. (1985): A Comprehensive Grammar of the English Language. London: Longman. (p. 96, fn. 4)

Radford, A. (1981): Transformational Syntax. Cambridge: C.U.P. (p. 17, fn. 19)

Schiefelbusch, R.L., Pickar, J. (eds.) (1984): The Acquisition of Communicative Competence. Baltimore: University Park Press. (p. 201, fn. 13)

Scott, C.M. (1984): Adverbial connectivity in conversations of children 6 to 12. J. Child Lang. 11, 423–52. (p. 102, fn. 18)

Stern, D.N., Spieker, S., Barnett, R.K., MacKain, K. (1983): The prosody of maternal speech: infant age and context-related changes. J. Child Lang. 10, 1–15. (p. 65, fn. 6)

Stoel-Gammon, C., Cooper, J.A. (1984): Patterns of early lexical and phonological development. J. Child Lang. 11, 247–71. (p. 42, fn. 29)

Stubbs, M. (1983): Discourse Analysis. Oxford: Blackwell. (p. 201, fn. 13)

Trudgill, P. (1983): Sociolinguistics, 2nd edn. Harmondsworth: Penguin. (p. 20, fn. 26, p. 24, fn. 3)

Wagner, K.R. (1985): How much do children say in a day? J. Child Lang. *12*, 475–87. (p. 140, fn. 18, p. 186, fn. 52)

Wren, C.T. (ed.) (1983): Language Learning Disabilities: Diagnosis and Remediation. Rockville, Md.: Aspen Systems. (p. 7ff)

Author Index

Subject Index

Cole & Whurr Journals of related interest

THE BRITISH JOURNAL OF DISORDERS OF COMMUNICATION

The British Journal of Disorders of Communication is an academically rigorous and intellectually challenging journal which presents the latest clinical and theoretical research and is a principal forum for the discussion of the entire range of communication disorders. The journal contains a representative and balanced selection of articles, with contributions from North America, Australasia and Continental Europe, as well as the UK. Among the leading articles published in recent issues are:
August 1987: Duncan & Gibbs - Acquisition of Syntax in Panjabi and English
December 1987: Gibbon and Hardcastle - Articulatory Description and Treatment of 'lateral /S/ using Electropalatography: A Case Study
April 1988: Perry - Surgical Voice Restoration following Laryngectomy: The Tracheo-oesophageal fistula technique (Singer-Blom)
August 1988: Bryan - Assessment of Language Disorders after Right Hemisphere Damage; Lebrun - Language and Epilepsy: A Review

The journal is owned by the College of Speech Therapists, and the Editor is Elspeth McCartney of Glasgow University and Jordanhill College. Issues are published three times a year and annual volumes are of up to 500 pages.

ISSN: 0007 098X

THE BRITISH JOURNAL OF EXPERIMENTAL AND CLINICAL HYPNOSIS

This is the Journal of the British Society of Experimental and Clinical Hypnosis, a learned society which brings together appropriately qualified medical professionals who have a legitimate reason for using hypnosis in their work and who share a scientific interest in the research and practical application of hypnosis. The journal provides a forum for the critical discussion of ideas, theories, findings, procedures and social policies associated with the topic of hypnosis. It also disseminates information on all aspects of theory, research and practice. A book review section is included.

ISSN:0265 1033

Please send for the Cole & Whurr catalogue.

Cole & Whurr Ltd
19b Compton Terrace, London N1 2UN
01-359 5979